PRACTITIONER'S GUIDE TO EMPIRICALLY BASED MEASURES OF DEPRESSION

AABT CLINICAL ASSESSMENT SERIES

Series Editor

Sharon L. Foster
California School of Professional Psychology, San Diego, California

PRACTITIONER'S GUIDE TO EMPIRICALLY BASED MEASURES OF DEPRESSION
Edited by Arthur M. Nezu, George F. Ronan, Elizabeth A. Meadows, and Kelly S. McClure

A Continuation Order Plan is available for this series. A continuation order will bring delivery of each new volume immediately upon publication. Volumes are billed only upon actual shipment. For further information please contact the publisher.

PRACTITIONER'S GUIDE TO EMPIRICALLY BASED MEASURES OF DEPRESSION

Edited by

Arthur M. Nezu

MCP Hahnemann University
Philadelphia, Pennsylvania

George F. Ronan
Elizabeth A. Meadows

Central Michigan University
Mount Pleasant, Michigan

and

Kelly S. McClure

MCP Hahnemann University
Philadelphia, Pennsylvania

Published under the auspices of the Association for Advancement of Behavior Therapy

Kluwer Academic / Plenum Publishers
New York   Boston   Dordrecht   London   Moscow

ISBN 0-306-46246-X

©2000 Kluwer Academic / Plenum Publishers
233 Spring Street, New York, N.Y. 10013

http://www.wkap.nl/

10 9 8 7 6 5 4 3 2 1

A C.I.P. record for this book is available from the Library of Congress.

Printed in the United States of America

Series Preface

"Where can I find a copy of ...?"

"I have a client coming in who's depressed—do you have any good measures?"

Several times a year I look up from my desk to answer questions like these from graduate students and colleagues. My answers invariably disappoint them: I recite a litany of not very fruitful alternatives for finding the measures they seek. "Well, you can check the original article, but that probably won't have a copy. Or you can call the originator of the instrument. If you can't find the person or if he or she doesn't return your call, you can try getting a copy from someone who's used the instrument. But be sure to ask if it's copyrighted. Then make sure you look up the literature on its reliability and validity ..."

Difficulties in locating assessment devices and finding evaluative information on their psychometric properties vex researchers and clinicians alike. Such difficulty is likely to contribute to failure to use assessment tools that could greatly enhance a clinician's practice, and may contribute to continuing complaints about the schism between research and practice. Indeed, although many mental health professionals receive training in the scientific foundations of clinical practice, numerous surveys question their application of this training in practice settings after graduate school ends (e.g., Morrow-Bradley & Elliott, 1986; Swan & MacDonald, 1978).

The need for scientifically sound, but practical clinical tools is relevant for clinical assessment, intervention, and research. Increasing demands from third-party payers for accountability information has produced increased needs for practical assessment tools that yield useful information about changes in clients' functioning over time. Yet many graduate training courses provide little instruction in assessment other than traditional personality and intellectual assessment approaches (Aiken, West, Sechrest, & Reno, 1990), leaving many mental health professionals with limited information about alternatives to these approaches. As mentioned, obtaining copies of assessment devices for particular problem areas is a challenge because many are not readily available. Finally, although occasional reviews of assessment devices appear in the literature, few sources exist that enable clinicians and researchers to appraise reliability and validity evidence for particular assessment tools and to compare different instruments. This kind of information is essential in deciding whether the psychometric properties of measurement instruments are sufficiently strong to warrant their use.

The AABT Clinical Assessment Series, developed by the Association for Advancement of Behavior Therapy, addresses these issues. Each volume examines a different clinical problem area and provides critical overviews of key assessment issues and available assessment tools for use in that area. Convenient summary tables compare and contrast different instruments in terms of their time requirements and suitability for different assessment purposes. Finally, and most importantly, each volume provides a summary of reliability and validity information about each instrument along with sample copies of the instruments, or, for commercially available instruments, samples of the instrument content and information about how to purchase the assessment device. These compendia of information should serve as valuable resources for practicing clinicians and for researchers who wish to develop state-of-the-science assessment strategies for clinical problems and to make informed choices about which devices best suit their purposes. This volume, the first in the series, addresses depression. Subsequent volumes currently being developed will examine anxiety disorders in adults and child behavior problems in school settings.

The AABT Clinical Assessment Series was the brainchild of a number of individuals at the Association for Advancement of Behavior Therapy with the imagination and initiative to bring this project into being. Lizette Peterson and Linda Sobell deserve special recognition for their vision and persistence in launching this project. David Teisler provided invaluable support and liaison work between the editors and the organization. Mariclaire Cloutier at Kluwer Academic/Plenum Publishers greatly assisted with the production of the volume and in supporting the efforts required to bring this project to fruition. And of course, the editors of this volume—Art Nezu, George Ronan, Elizabeth Meadows, and Kelly McClure—collected massive amounts of information, reintegrating it in ways that are both scientifically sound and practically relevant. Chris Nezu also added valuable insights in her contributions to Chapter 3.

WHO SHOULD USE THIS BOOK?

This book is written for practitioners who assess and treat depressed clients and who wish to make their assessment practices more systematic, want to have assessment devices readily available, and want to expand their assessment practices with the most up-to-date approaches. Although the volume is produced in conjunction with the Association for Advancement of Behavior Therapy, the volume is not for behaviorists only—any empirically minded clinician should find this compendium valuable. In addition, the volume should prove useful for researchers who wish to compare and contrast various measurement tools for assessing depression and related constructs. Finally, the volume will prove invaluable for professors like myself in helping students and colleagues find easy answers to questions like those posed at the beginning of this preface.

Sharon L. Foster
Sacramento, CA

Preface

The words "depression" and "ubiquity" are often found in the same sentence. According to the World Health Organization, depression ranks first among women's most disabling diseases, and fourth among people overall. In the United States, approximately 18 million individuals experience depression at any given time. The costs to society in decreased work productivity and the expense of treatment have been estimated to be in excess of $16 billion per year. As such, it is highly likely that a significantly large percentage of patients a professional sees in *any* clinical setting (e.g., general medical/primary care practice, private mental health practice, hospital, community clinic) will be experiencing depression in some form, whether it is the core disorder (e.g., major depressive disorder) or concomitant symptoms related to the experience of a chronic medical illness, such as cancer. More importantly, recent research has strongly underscored the need to reconceptualize depression as a recurrent disorder (A. M. Nezu, Nezu, Trunzo, & McClure, 1998). In this light, reliable and valid assessment of depressive symptoms, as well as depression-related psychosocial vulnerability factors, becomes especially crucial. It is for this purpose that this volume was constructed.

Contained in this book are over 90 reviews of measures of depression and depression-related constructs. Included are structured interviews, self-report inventories, measures for adults, children, adolescents, and older persons, as well as measures for special populations (e.g., individuals with dementia, schizophrenia, or mental retardation). Reviews contain descriptions of the measures in addition to valuable information addressing their psychometric properties. Quick-view guides have been developed to provide a rapid method of identifying and comparing potentially useful measures. Moreover, 24 such measures are reprinted in Appendix B. Further, a chapter has been included (Chapter 3) to help clinicians engage in an effective decision-making process when selecting measures. This first volume in the Clinical Assessment Handbook Series should prove to be a valuable resource for any clinician's and researcher's library.

I would like to take this opportunity to extend my sincere thanks to the three Associate Editors of this volume—George Ronan, Elizabeth Meadows, and Kelly McClure. Their tenacity in obtaining accurate and comprehensive information for this book was astounding. I know they missed out on a lot of social activities in order to complete this volume. I am very grateful for their invaluable aid. I also give much thanks to the staff at the headquarters of the Association for Advancement of Behavior Therapy, especially David Teisler, who provided continual support for this project. Much thanks goes to the staff at Kluwer Academic/Plenum Publishers, who made this book a reality, and to Sharon Foster, Series Editor, who made this venture worthwhile. Last, I always give thanks to my wife, Chris, without whom I cannot do anything, much less complete a book. Even though she was not a coeditor of this volume, her influence on this effort is evident throughout.

Art Nezu
Philadelphia, PA

Contents

Part I. Guide to Volume I: Depression

Chapter 1.
INTRODUCTION 3

Background 3
Selection of Included Measures 3
Structure of the Book 4
Format of Instrument Descriptions 4
Guide to Quick-View Measurement Guides 7

Chapter 2
OVERVIEW OF DEPRESSION 9

Depression as a Diagnosis 9
Methods of Assessment 11
Assessment of Depression-Related Constructs 12
Major Treatment Models for Depression 12

Chapter 3
A 10-STEP GUIDE TO SELECTING ASSESSMENT MEASURES IN CLINICAL
AND RESEARCH SETTINGS (by Christine Maguth Nezu,
Arthur M. Nezu, & Sharon L. Foster) 17

Where to Begin? 17
Concluding Remarks 24

Part II. Assessment Instruments

Chapter 4
MEASURES OF DEPRESSION, DEPRESSIVE SYMPTOMATOLOGY, AND
DEPRESSIVE MOOD 27

Introduction 27

Beck Depression Inventory™-Second Edition (BDI-II)™ 29
Brief Psychiatric Rating Scale (BPRS) 32
Brief Symptom Inventory (BSI) 34
Carroll Depression Scales-Revised (CDS-R) 37
Center for Epidemiological Studies Depression Scale (CES-D) 39
Depression Anxiety Stress Scales (DASS) 42
Depression Questionnaire (DQ) 45
Depression 30 Scale (D-30) 47
Diagnostic Interview Schedule (DIS-IV) 49
Diagnostic Inventory for Depression (DID) 52
Hamilton Depression Inventory (HDI) 55
Hamilton Rating Scale for Depression (HRSD) 58
Hopelessness Depression Symptom Questionnaire (HDSQ) 61
Hospital Anxiety and Depression Scale (HADS) 63
Inventory of Depressive Symptomatology (IDS) 66
IPAT Depression Scale 69
Manual for the Diagnosis of Major Depression (MDMD) 71
Minnesota Multiphasic Personality Inventory 2 (MMPI-2) Depression Scale 73
Montgomery–Asberg Depression Rating Scale (MADRS) 75
MOS 8-Item Depression Screener (Screener) 78
Multiple Affect Adjective Checklist-Revised (MAACL-R) 81
Multiscore Depression Inventory for Adolescents and Adults (MDI) 84
Newcastle Scales 87
Positive and Negative Affect Scales (PANAS) 89
Primary Care Evaluation of Mental Disorders (PRIME-MD) 92
Profile of Mood States (POMS) 94
Raskin Three-Area Severity of Depression Scale 96
Revised Hamilton Rating Scale for Depression (RHRSD): Clinician Rating Form . . 99
Revised Hamilton Rating Scale for Depression (RHRSD): Self-Report Problem
    Inventory 101
Reynolds Depression Screening Inventory (RDSI) 104
Rimon's Brief Depression Scale (RBDS) 106
Schedule for Affective Disorders and Schizophrenia (SADS) Research Diagnostic
    Criteria (RDC) 108
State Trait-Depression Adjective Check List (ST-DACL) 111
Structured Clinical Interview for DSM-IV Axis I Disorders (SCID) 114
Symptom Checklist-90-Revised (SCL-90-R) 117
Zung Self-Rating Depression Scale (Zung SDS) 120

Chapter 5
MEASURES OF DEPRESSION: SPECIAL POPULATIONS 123

Introduction 123
Calgary Depression Scale for Schizophrenia (CDSS) 124
Children's Depression Inventory (CDI) 127
Children's Depression Rating Scale-Revised (CDRS-R) 129
Cornell Scale for Depression in Dementia (Cornell Scale) 133

Depression Rating Scale (DRS) 135
Geriatric Depression Scale (GDS) 137
Kiddie-Schedule for Affective Disorders and Schizophrenia for School-Age
Children-Present and Lifetime Version (K-SADS-PL) 140
Medical-Based Emotional Distress Scale (MEDS) 143
Multiscore Depression Inventory for Children (MDI-C) 145
Postpartum Depression Interview Schedule (PDIS) 147
Psychopathology Inventory for Mentally Retarded Adults (PIMRA) 150
Reynolds Adolescent Depression Scale (RADS) 152
Reynolds Child Depression Scale (RCDS) 154
Visual Analog Mood Scales (VAMS) 157
Youth Depression Adjective Checklist (Y-DACL) 159

Chapter 6
MEASURES OF DEPRESSION-RELATED CONSTRUCTS 163

Introduction 163
Actigraphy (Model 7164) 165
Anticipatory Cognitions Questionnaire (ACQ) 167
Attributional Style Questionnaire (ASQ) 169
Automatic Thoughts Questionnaire-Revised (ATQ-R) 172
Beck Hopelessness Scale™ (BHS)™ 175
Beck Scale for Suicide Ideation™ (BSS™) 177
Children's Attributional Style Questionnaire-Revised (CASQ-R) 179
Cognitive Bias Questionnaire (CBQ) 182
Cognitive Error Questionnaire (CEQ) (General and Lower Back Pain Versions) ... 185
Cognitive Events Schedule (CES) 187
Cognitive Triad Inventory (CTI) 189
Coping Inventory for Stressful Situations (CISS) 192
Coping Resources Inventory (CRI) 194
Coping Responses Inventory (CRI) 196
Depression Beliefs Questionnaire-Version I (DBQ-I) 199
Depression Check Questionnaire (DCQ) 202
Depression Proneness Rating Scale (DPRS) 204
Depressive Personality Disorder Inventory (DPDI) 207
Divorce Dysfunctional Attitudes Scale (DDAS) 209
Dysfunctional Attitude Scale (DAS) 212
Frequency of Self-Reinforcement Questionnaire (FSRQ) 214
Goal Orientation Inventory (GOI) 216
Interpersonal Events Schedule (IES) 219
Life Attitudes Schedule (LAS) 221
Pleasant Events Schedule (PES) 223
Pleasant Events Schedule-AD (PES-AD) 226
Positive Automatic Thoughts Questionnaire (ATQ-P) 228
Problem-Solving Inventory (PSI) 230
Reasons for Living Inventory (RFL) 233
Revised Grief Experience Inventory (RGEI) 235

Self-Control Questionnaire for Depression 238
Self-Control Schedule 240
Self-Esteem Worksheet 243
Social Adjustment Scale (SAS) 245
Social Problem-Solving Inventory-Revised (SPSI-R) 248
Social Resourcefulness Scale (SRS) 250
Sociotropy Autonomy Scale (SAS) 252
Suicide Ideation Questionnaire (SIQ) 255
Suicide Probability Scale (SPS) 258
Unpleasant Events Schedule (UES) 260
Ways of Coping Scale (WOC) 262
Ways of Responding (WOR) 265

Appendix A
QUICK-VIEW GUIDES 269

Table I. Assessment of Depression and Depressive Symptoms Among Adults
    (Chapter 4) 270
Table II. Measures of Depression: Special Populations (Chapter 5) 272
Table III. Measures of Depression-Related Constructs (Chapter 6) 273

Appendix B
REPRINTED MEASURES 277

Automatic Thoughts Questionnaire-Revised 277
Center for Epidemiological Studies Depression Scale 279
Cognitive Triad Inventory 280
Cornell Scale for Depression in Dementia 282
Depression Anxiety Stress Scales 284
Depression Check Questionnaire 286
Depression Proneness Rating Scale 288
Depression Rating Scale 290
Divorce Dysfunctional Attitudes Scale 292
Frequency of Self-Reinforcement Questionnaire 294
Geriatric Depression Scale 295
Hamilton Rating Scale for Depression 296
Hopelessness Depression Symptom Questionnaire 299
Inventory of Depressive Symptomatology (Self-Report) 303
Medically-Based Emotional Distress Scale 308
Pleasant Events Schedule 311
Positive and Negative Affect Scales 316
Raskin Three-Area Severity of Depression Scale 317
Revised Grief Experience Inventory 318
Rimon's Brief Depression Scale 320
Self-Control Schedule 321
Social Resourcefulness Scale 323

Sociotropy Autonomy Scale 325
Unpleasant Events Schedule 328

GLOSSARY (by Sharon L. Foster & Arthur M. Nezu) 335

REFERENCES 337

AUTHOR INDEX 349

Part I
Guide to Volume I: Depression

Chapter 1
Introduction

BACKGROUND

Depression continues to be considered the "common cold" of psychiatric disorders and represents one of the most significant mental health problems facing our nation. Despite its ubiquity, depression has been difficult to define and often means different things to different people (A. M. Nezu, Nezu, Trunzo, & McClure, 1998). However, during the past several decades, multiple models explaining the etiopathogenesis of depression have emerged, many of which have also engendered effective treatment approaches. In this context, a variety of efficacious psychosocial interventions have become available (Beckham & Leber, 1995; Gotlib & Hammen, 1992). Although a larger armamentarium of effective choices is obviously advantageous clinically, the average therapist may experience difficulty in keeping pace with these advances in research and technology. This first volume of the AABT Clinical Assessment Series was developed to serve as a rich resource for clinicians and researchers with specific regard to assessment issues of depression.

This volume is not a textbook for explaining the intricacies of measurement theory or how to best conduct a clinical interview. Rather, to facilitate breadth, it represents a comprehensive compendium of depression-related measures to help guide cognitive-behavior therapists in identifying appropriate assessment procedures in either a clinical or research setting. A cognitive-behavioral orientation underscores the close relationship between effective assessment and successful treatment (A. M. Nezu & Nezu, 1989a). This volume can serve as an invaluable resource helping to guide successful treatment by describing a variety of psychometrically sound and clinically useful assessment tools in a user-friendly manner.

SELECTION OF INCLUDED MEASURES

A major attempt was made to identify all relevant instruments for possible inclusion in this volume. This entailed multiple "calls" in professional journals, comprehensive literature reviews, and multiple computer searches. Despite these efforts, we may have missed an important instrument. If so, we take full responsibility and apologize in advance for any significant omissions. Final selection by the editorial staff was based on the following criteria:

- The measure must be available in English.
- The instrument must assess one of the following directly: depression, depressive symptoms, depressive mood, or a hypothesized mediator of depression (e.g., depression-vulnerability factor).
- The measure must have some relevance for the field of cognitive-behavior therapy broadly defined.
- The measure must be characterized by some known psychometric properties.

Some limits needed to be set for measures that are in the category of "depression-related constructs." Many of these instruments address variables that have been hypothesized and supported to be either etiologically related to depression or a significant mediator of depression. Examples include measures of cognitive distortions, coping skills, and pleasant events. We restricted such measures to those that have been actually shown to be related to depression in empirical studies. We do not include every measure of coping, for example. To do so would have far exceeded the goals of this book, as well as our page allotments.

STRUCTURE OF THE BOOK

The next chapter provides a brief overview of depression and various issues related to its assessment. In Chapter 3, Christine Maguth Nezu, Arthur M. Nezu, and Sharon L. Foster provide a general guide for selecting measures. Chapters 4–6 in Section II contain descriptions of over 90 depression-related measures. Specifically, Chapter 4 addresses instruments that measure depression and depressive symptomatology in adults. Included are structured interview procedures, clinician rating protocols, and a multitude of self-report inventories. Chapter 5 contains measures of depression geared for special populations, such as children, adolescents, persons with mental retardation, and schizophrenic patients. In Chapter 6, a wide variety of measures of depression-related constructs are reviewed, including coping skills, suicide, social support, and cognitive-behavior mediators. Appendix A contains the various quick-view guides, which provide for a user-friendly means of obtaining an overall summary of each measure reviewed in this volume. We also provide a Glossary of technical terms, and, in Appendix B, reprints of 24 measures.

Because many of the measures described in this volume are commercially published, we were unable to reprint them in their entirety. However, where possible, we provide sample items in order to provide the reader with a general sense of each instrument. Within this context, users are reminded to follow carefully copyright laws and to secure the appropriate permission, if necessary, prior to using a given measure. Different measures may require varying degrees of professional qualifications and knowledge of ethical guidelines. We strongly urge users of these test materials to follow the guidelines as specified by the *Standards for Educational and Psychological Testing* (American Psychological Association, 1985).

FORMAT OF INSTRUMENT DESCRIPTIONS

In each of these three measurement chapters, a standard outline, as noted below, is used to describe each instrument. Our intent is to provide relevant information in a user-friendly format that offers sufficient information to allow the reader to make informed and effective choices. To increase the breadth of our review, this information is somewhat truncated. For example, although specifics are provided about the psychometric properties of each measure, overwhelming details are not. However, relevant sources are provided if additional information is required.

Title

This is the title of the instrument.

Reference

This refers to the most direct literature citation for the measure. This can represent the manual if commercially published or a journal article that describes the instrument's initial development.

Purpose

This section describes the purpose of the instrument (e.g., to measure depressive symptom severity in geriatric samples, to assess problem-solving ability in adults).

Population

This is a brief description of the specific population for which the test was developed (e.g., adolescents aged 13 to 18 years, individuals with mild or moderate mental retardation).

Description

This section represents a brief overview of the structure and items of the instrument (e.g., 21-item, self-report measure), as well as the response format (e.g., 4-point Likert-type scale). If appropriate, various subscales are described.

Background

In this section, a brief overview of the rationale for developing the instrument is provided (e.g., to be consistent with DSM-IV criteria), as well as any important historical notes (e.g., previous versions of the instrument). For measures of depression-related variables, a brief description of its relationship to depression is given (e.g., relation of measure to a given model of depression).

Administration

This refers to the approximate time to complete measure or interview. If not formally noted in the source material, this estimate is based on the experience of the editors. Important administration concerns are also noted (e.g., need for adequate training in conducting a semistructured interview).

Scoring

This is a brief overview of the scoring procedure.

Interpretation

This section contains guidelines for interpreting test results (e.g., use of a cutoff score to designate level of depression). Often, the existence of norms will be noted indicating, for example, if such norms allow for the conversion of raw scores into standardized scores.

Psychometric Properties

Norms. This provides for a brief description of available norms.

Reliability. This section briefly describes relevant findings regarding internal stability and test–retest reliability.

Validity. This provides for a description of various validity estimates if available (e.g., content, concurrent, predictive, discriminant, construct, factorial, convergent).

Clinical Utility

Provides for a rating of "High" versus "Limited." "High" ratings indicate that a given instrument has been frequently used in clinical settings. "Limited" ratings suggest that such instruments have not been typically used in clinical settings or that clinicians might find the time or cost associated with these measures to be somewhat prohibitive. Note that these ratings are the opinions of the editors.

Research Applicability

Provides for a rating of "High" versus "Limited." "High" ratings suggest that the instrument has been used in research studies and found to be meaningful. "Limited" ratings indicate the absence of empirical studies that have used this measure. Note that these ratings are the opinions of the editors.

Source

This refers to the actual source of the measure (e.g., address and phone number of commercial publisher, address of agency or researcher).

Cost

This notes the current cost of the measure as of the date of publication of this volume.

Alternative Forms

This notes the availability of alternate forms (e.g., short versions, Spanish versions).

GUIDE TO QUICK-VIEW MEASUREMENT GUIDES

In order to provide for a quick means of identifying and evaluating a measure, we developed the quick-view guides located in Appendix A, which contain the following important information:

- Name of instrument (actual name of measure)
- Target population (age range, specific sample focus)
- Type of measure (e.g., self-report)
- Purpose (goal of measure; e.g., to assess depressive symptom severity)
- Time to complete (amount of time necessary to complete measure)
- Norms available? (whether normative data are available to compare with a particular client's score)
- Fee involved? (whether there is a cost involved in obtaining the measure)
- Availability of alternate forms (whether there are alternative forms available, e.g., foreign language versions, short-form versions)

Chapter 2
Overview of Depression

Feeling sad is virtually a universal phenomenon. Most people experience mild to moderate depressive symptoms from time to time. Depressed feelings may also occur normally in reaction to negative life events such as the death of a loved one or loss of a job. These symptoms may last from only a few days to several weeks. Depressive symptoms can range from mild negative emotion with a brief duration that passes quickly, to severe, chronic depressive symptoms. When depressive symptoms begin to become severe or last more than a few days or weeks, these symptoms may be considered a disease state or syndrome.

DEPRESSION AS A DIAGNOSIS

Currently, two major diagnostic systems, the *Diagnostic and Statistical Manual of Mental Disorders*, 4th ed. (DSM-IV; American Psychiatric Association [APA], 1994), and *The ICD-10 International Classification of Mental and Behavioural Disorders* (World Health Organization, 1992), are available and frequently used to diagnose depressive disorders. These nosological systems provide diagnostic guidelines based on clusters of symptoms rather than etiological conceptualizations.

In the first DSM (APA, 1952), the term "affective reactions" was used to include involutional melancholia as well as manic-depressive illness. The influence of psychodynamic theory, emphasizing theoretical notions of causality, led to the relabeling of depressive reactions to "depressive neuroses" in DSM-II (APA, 1968).

Due to dissatisfaction with the lack of standardized criteria, Feighner and his colleagues (Feighner et al., 1972) developed a classification system that grouped diagnostic categories together if they shared important clinical features, without making assumptions about etiology. The Feighner system, also known as Research Diagnostic Criteria (RDC), served as the basis for DSM-III (APA, 1980). In this version of the manual, all depressive disorders, regardless of severity, chronicity, or apparent association with precipitating stress, were grouped together. A distinction was made between affect (i.e., an immediately observed emotion, such as sadness) and mood (i.e., a more pervasive and sustained emotion). Three further distinctions were made regarding mood disorders: first, whether they were episodic or chronic; second, whether the affective episodes were limited exclusively to depressive periods (i.e., unipolar) or included at least one manic phase (i.e., bipolar); and third, whether the disorder was limited to a single index episode or involved recurring episodes.

In the subsequent revision of DSM-III, DSM-III-R, (APA, 1987), affective disorders were called "mood disorders" and were subdivided into bipolar and depressive disorders. DSM-IV (APA, 1994), the most recent version of the manual, continues with this distinction between nonbipolar and bipolar disorders.

According to DSM-IV, a "major depressive episode" involves the experience of five or more of the following symptoms over the course of a 2-week period representing a change from previous functioning:

- Depressed mood
- Markedly diminished interest or pleasure
- Significant weight change
- Sleep difficulties
- Psychomotor agitation or retardation
- Feelings of worthlessness or excessive guilt
- Concentration difficulties or indecisiveness
- Recurrent suicidal ideation or thoughts of death.

In addition, at least one of these five symptoms needs to be either depressed mood or loss of pleasure. Further, these symptoms must also cause clinically significant distress or impaired functioning.

Depressive "disorders," in DSM-IV, include Major Depressive Disorder (MDD)-Single Episode, MDD-Recurrent, Dysthymic Disorder, and Depressive Disorder-Not Otherwise Specified (NOS). A diagnosis of MDD can be made if an individual meets criteria for experiencing a major depressive episode. MDD becomes recurrent, according to DSM-IV, when a person experiences two separate depressive episodes, whereby an interval of at least two consecutive months occurs in which criteria for MDD cannot be met.

Dysthymic disorder is characterized by greater chronicity, but lesser severity, of similar symptoms to those involved in MDD. The core feature of dysthymic disorder is the chronic depressed mood occurring for most of the day, for most days, over a 2-year period. To meet diagnostic criteria, in addition to the chronic depressed mood, individuals with dysthymic disorder present with at least two of the following symptoms: poor appetite or overeating, insomnia or hypersomnia, low energy or fatigue, low self-esteem, poor concentration or difficulty making decisions, and feelings of hopelessness.

Depressive Disorder-NOS is the label given to disorders which have depressive features, but whose symptoms do not fully meet criteria for other depressive disorders such as MDD or Dysthymic Disorder. Unlike the other depressive disorders, Mood Disorder Due to a General Medical Condition and Mood Disorder Due to a Substance are diagnosed according to their presumed etiologies (i.e., the direct physiological effects of general medical condition and substances, respectively). The subtypes "With Depressive Features" and "With Major Depressive-Like Episode" are specified for Mood Disorder Due to a General Medical Condition.

Although it is not specified as a disorder in the DSM-IV, the category of "double depression," defined as the cooccurrence of MDD and Dysthymic Disorder, has been described by Keller and Shapiro (1982). This disorder is conceptualized as an acute phase of MDD that is superimposed over the more chronic Dysthymic Disorder. This differentiation is significant because researchers have found that rates of recovery and relapse differ widely between individuals with double depression and MDD when receiving the same treatment.

The ICD-10, which is used more widely in international research, contains categories and definitions of depressive disorders that are compatible with the DSM-IV. Both are nosological systems which classify depressive syndromes according to the presence and severity of clinical symptoms and functional impairment. In addition, with the exception of depression due to a medical condition or substance, both are based upon clusters of symptoms rather than etiological explanations. No clear delineations between categories are readily apparent in either system. Rather, differences between categories of depression were determined by teams of experts in the area of depression.

Whereas the classification systems described above provide operational definitions for typical patterns of depressive symptoms, they do not advise professionals on how to go about gathering the information necessary to make these diagnoses. A great deal more is considered when attempting to measure depression. Depending upon its purpose, the assessment may require consideration of the presence or absence of depressive symptoms, the severity of symptoms, the presence or absence of a full-blown depressive syndrome, the presence or severity of depression-related constructs, or any combination of these. The professional must consider the short-term and long-term goals when developing and conducting an assessment. Decision-making guidelines are provided in the next chapter.

METHODS OF ASSESSMENT

A large percentage of the measures described in this volume address depression and depressive symptoms. In general, they can be classified as either self-report inventories or clinician-rating procedures.

Self-Report Questionnaire

The self-report measure is a method of assessment whereby the participant answers specific questions in the form of a questionnaire or inventory. Typically, this method of assessment is conducted using a paper-and-pencil format. However, the questionnaire may also be completed via computer. Depending upon the questionnaire, this method can be relatively brief (taking as few as 10 minutes) and the client may complete the questionnaire outside of session. In fact, some empirically validated treatments include periodic self-monitoring with self-report questionnaires (e.g., J. S. Beck, 1995).

The self-report method for assessing depression has its limitations. In keeping with the decision-making guidelines provided in Chapter 3, it is important to understand the purpose for which self-report questionnaires are to be used. Although many are commonly used for idiographic assessments in clinical settings, they may not have been validated for that purpose. For example, self-report questionnaires may not be sufficient as the sole approach to measure suicidal ideation. Further, it may be very tempting to use a cutoff score on a self-report inventory as the single means of deriving a diagnosis, a practice that should be avoided.

Structured Interviews and Clinician-Rated Measures

Clinician ratings may include questions similar to those included in a self-report questionnaire. However, as indicated by its name, it is completed by the clinician, usually following a structured clinical interview. This method of assessment has numerous benefits. First, it provides a standardized format for the clinician to follow. This can improve the reliability of longitudinal assessment, as well as provide a method by which to compare information gathered by a clinical interview to normative data. A clinician-rated questionnaire can also facilitate a complete assessment which includes all biopsychosocial aspects of depression. The clinician-rated questionnaire can be conducted periodically to review patient symptoms and evaluate which have remitted and which are still present. This type of format also allows the clinician to inquire further about responses that may be inconsistent or provide an incomplete picture.

A clinician-rated questionnaire may also be a preferred method of assessment when other, cooccurring disorders interfere with patients' abilities to complete self-report questionnaires. For example, Addington, Addington, and Maticka-Tyndale (1993) found that although assessments using the Beck Depression Inventory (BDI; A. T. Beck, Ward, Mendelson, Mock, & Erbaugh, 1961) and the Calgary Depression Scale (Addington, Addington, & Schissel, 1990; Addington, Addington, Maticka-Tyndale, & Joyce, 1992) produced comparable results among a group of people with schizophrenia, more than one third of the psychiatric inpatients who participated had difficulty completing the BDI and 6% of the sample did not complete it at all.

ASSESSMENT OF DEPRESSION-RELATED CONSTRUCTS

Professionals may also be interested in measuring depression-related constructs. Assessing in this way can help identify potential mediators of depressive symptoms or other depression-related phenomena (e.g., suicide ideation). These data can be helpful for case conceptualization, formulating intermediate goals for therapy, understanding factors that contribute to the onset or maintenance of depressive symptoms or syndromes, or identifying problems that increase the risk of relapse or recurrence. This is especially relevant to depression since it is more and more considered a long-term, recurrent, chronic disorder (see A. M. Nezu, Nezu, Trunzo, & McClure, 1998, for a review of depression relapse and maintenance issues). Many depression-related constructs have been identified in the literature (A. M. Nezu & Nezu, 1989b). However, the costs of assessing every mediator of depression for every patient would greatly outweigh the benefits. Rather, the clinician is advised to use the guidelines described in Chapter 3 and other decision-making models to select which depression-related constructs are most applicable to each individual patient (see also A. M. Nezu & Nezu, 1989b, 1993). As a resource, the next section provides a brief overview of several psychosocial models of the treatment of depression.

MAJOR TREATMENT MODELS FOR DEPRESSION

Lewinsohn's Behavioral Model

Lewinsohn (1974) and his colleagues conceptualized depression within the framework of learning theory and extended earlier behavioral formulations (Ferster, 1973; Skinner, 1953) that emphasized the reduced frequency of overall activity as the primary defining characteristic of depression. The guiding theoretical assertions of Lewinsohn's work are (a) that depression is a function of the degree to which an individual's activity level is maintained by positive reinforcement, and (b) that deficits in various social skills play an influential role in determining the rate of such reinforcement for one's behavior. Research indicates, for example, that depressed persons exhibit fewer interpersonal behaviors than nondepressed persons and elicit minimal social reinforcement from others (Gotlib & Robinson, 1982; Libet & Lewinsohn, 1973).

Based on such a formulation, Lewinsohn and his colleagues developed a brief (12 session), structured, behaviorally oriented program geared to change the quality and quantity of depressed patients' interactions with their environment. Patients are taught relaxation skills, cognitive self-management, stress management skills, and provided feedback as a means of reducing the intensity and frequency of aversive events and to increase their rate of engaging in pleasant activities. A more recent revision of this behavioral approach, entitled the Coping with Depression course (Lewinsohn, Antonuccio, Breckenridge, & Teri, 1987), broadened its skills training to include four general domains: relaxation training, increasing pleasant activities, cognitive restructuring, and improving social interactions. Controlled outcome studies provide support for this program's effectiveness in reducing depression (Brown & Lewinsohn, 1984; Hoberman, Lewinsohn, & Tilson, 1988; Steinmetz, Lewinshon, & Antonuccio, 1983).

Social Skills Training

Similar to Lewinsohn's focus on interpersonal skills, Becker and his colleagues (e.g., Becker & Heimberg, 1985; Becker, Heimberg, & Bellack, 1987) and Bellack, Hersen and their colleagues (e.g., Bellack, Hersen, & Himmelhoch, 1981, 1983; Hersen, Bellack, Himmelhoch, & Thase, 1984), developed treatment programs geared to improve the social skills of depressed individuals in order to decrease their emotional distress. In these treatment programs, the hypothesized mechanism of action centered around a person's ability to engage in those activities that would facilitate the quantity and quality of social interactions in order ultimately to increase the amount of response-contingent positive reinforcement (e.g., Becker & Heimberg, 1985). Several outcome studies conducted by these investigators demonstrate the efficacy of this overall approach for the treatment of depression (see above citations).

McLean (1979) also viewed depression as resulting from ineffective coping and social skills and developed a 10-week program that included training in these domains (i.e., communication, behavioral productivity, social interaction, assertiveness, decision making, problem solving, cognitive self-control) as a means of developing prosocial behaviors and prevention against relapse. An evaluation of this approach conducted by McLean and Hakstian (1979) provide strong support for its efficacy as a treatment approach for depression.

Rehm's Self-Control Therapy

Rehm's (1977) conceptualization of depression was originally based on Kanfer's (1971) general self-control model that placed major significance on an individual's ability to achieve goals through three sequential processes, namely, self-monitoring, self-evaluation, and self-reinforcement. Rehm posited that depressed individuals demonstrate deficits in each of these self-control processes. For example, Roth and Rehm (1980) compared self-monitoring in depressed and nondepressed psychiatric patients. They found that when allowed to choose the type of performance feedback (e.g., correct versus incorrect responses), depressed patients more frequently selected negative feedback, whereas nondepressed patients more frequently chose positive feedback. Further, a comparison of depressed and nondepressed psychiatric patients showed that although the two groups had equivalent performances on a memory task, depressed individuals punished themselves more, and rewarded themselves less, than did nondepressed patients (Rozensky, Rehm, Pry, & Roth, 1977).

Self-control therapy, similar to other behaviorally oriented protocols, is structured and time-limited. In addition, it focuses on training in the three major deficit areas described above. For example, patients are taught to (a) maintain a daily record of positive experiences and their associated mood, (b) develop specific, overt, and reachable goals concerning positive activities, and (c) identify reinforcers and to administer these rewards to themselves upon successfully achieving a goal. Studies conducted by Rehm and others based on this model of treatment demonstrate the efficacy of self-control therapy for depression (e.g., Fuchs & Rehm, 1977; Rehm, Fuchs, Roth, Kornblith, & Romano, 1979; Roth, Bielski, Jones, Parker, & Osborn, 1982).

Nezu's Problem-Solving Therapy

A problem-solving model of depression focuses on the depressogenic vulnerability caused by deficits in one's overall problem-solving ability to cope with both major and minor stressful events. Borrowing from a transactional problem-solving model of stress (A. M. Nezu & D'Zurilla, 1989), A. M. Nezu and his colleagues conceptualize the etiopathogenesis of depression to lie within the reciprocal relations among daily problems, major stressful life events, immediate emotional states, and problem-solving coping (A. M. Nezu & Perri, 1989). For example, if the outcome of these interactions within this framework is negative, primarily as a function of ineffective problem-solving ability (i.e., unsuccessful problem resolution or poor coping with stressful events), then depression is likely to occur (A. M. Nezu, 1987). Deficits or dysfunctions in problem solving can exist in any of the major skill domains: problem orientation (i.e., set of generalized orienting responses regarding problems in living and one's ability to cope with such problems), problem definition and formulation (i.e., ability to understand the nature of a problem, identify obstacles to goals, delineate realistic objectives, perceive cause–effect relationships), generation of alternatives (i.e., ability to brainstorm multiple solution ideas), decision making (i.e., ability to identify potential consequences, predict the likelihood of such consequences, and conduct a cost–benefit analysis of desirability of these outcomes), and solution implementation and verification (i.e., ability to optimally carry out a solution, monitor its effects, troubleshoot if solution is not effective, and self-reinforce if outcome is satisfactory). Ample research exists supporting this model. For example, problem-solving skills have been found to be negatively correlated with depressive symptoms (D. J. Dobson & Dobson, 1981; Gotlib & Asarnow, 1979; Heppner & Anderson, 1985; A. M. Nezu, 1986a), as well as serving as an important moderator of the stress–depression relationship (e.g., A. M. Nezu, Nezu, Saraydarian, Kalmar, & Ronan, 1986; A. M. Nezu & Ronan, 1985, 1988).

The associated model of treatment, Problem-Solving Therapy (PST), has four specific goals: (a) to help depressed individuals identify previous and current life situations that are antecedents of a depressive episode, (b) to minimize the extent to which their depressive symptoms impact negatively on current and future attempts at coping, (c) to increase the effectiveness of their problem-solving attempts at coping with current problems, and (d) to teach general skills that will enable them to deal more effectively with future problems in order to prevent future depressive episodes (A. M. Nezu, Nezu, & Perri, 1989). Treatment involves training in each of the above problem-solving component processes and skills (A. M. Nezu, Nezu, & Perri, 1990).

Studies conducted to investigate the efficacy of PST for depression demonstrate its effectiveness with clinically depressed adults (A. M. Nezu, 1986b; A. M. Nezu & Perri, 1989), geriatric patients (Arean et al., 1993; Hussian & Lawrence, 1981), and primary care patients (Mynors-Wallis, Gath, Lloyd-Thomas, & Thomlinson, 1995). In both the A. M. Nezu (1986b) and A. M. Nezu and Perri (1989) studies, follow-up assessments revealed treatment gains to be maintained 6-months posttreatment.

Behavioral Marital Therapy for Depression

Research has recently pointed to the strong relationship between depression and marital distress. For example, Weissman (1987) found that the 6-month prevalence rate of major depression in a community sample of women who reported marital distress was 45.5%. Hoover and Fitzgerald (1981) reported that both unipolar and bipolar patients reported greater conflict in their marriages than did nondepressed controls. A study by Gotlib and Whiffen (1989) revealed that among a sample of couples wherein the wife met diagnostic criteria for clinical depression, both husbands and wives reported greater marital dissatisfaction as compared to a group of nondepressed control couples.

Based on these findings, several research teams have evaluated the efficacy of Behavioral Marital Therapy (BMT) as a treatment for depression. For example, O'Leary and Beach (1990) demonstrated that BMT was as effective as individual cognitive therapy in reducing depression, as assessed at posttreatment and a 1-year follow-up; however, only BMT significantly impacted on marital adjustment. Similar results were obtained in a study by Jacobson, Dobson, Fruzetti, Schmaling, and Salusky (1991). In a study that compared individual Interpersonal Psychotherapy (IPT; see below) with a couples version of IPT, both treatment approaches were found to produce significant and comparable reductions in depressive symptoms (Foley, Rounsaville, Weissman, Sholomskas, & Chevron, 1989).

Beck's Cognitive Therapy

The most prevalent cognitive model of depression is that posited by A. T. Beck (1976; A. T. Beck, Rush, Shaw, & Emery, 1979) and is composed of three key elements: (a) negative cognitive triad, (b) negative schemas, and (c) cognitive distortions. The cognitive triad consists of three patterns of negative ideas and attitudes that characterize depressed individuals and includes negative views of the self, the world, and the future.

Schemas are stable, long-standing thought patterns representing a person's generalizations about past experiences. They serve to organize from past experiences information relevant to a current situation and serve to determine the manner in which information is perceived, remembered, and later recalled. Depression-prone individuals tend to respond to their environment in a fixed, negative manner involving specific distortions responsible for the way the depression-prone individual perceives and interprets new experiences in a logically inaccurate manner. Cognitive errors include arbitrary inference, selective abstraction, overgeneralization, magnification/minimization, personalization, and dichotomous thinking.

Cognitive Therapy (CT) is perhaps the most recognizable and popular form of psychosocial treatment for depression. Large numbers of controlled outcome studies have been conducted during the past two decades supporting the efficacy of CT. Results from two recent meta-analyses (K. Dobson, 1989; Robinson, Berman, & Neimeyer, 1990), as well as numerous reviews (e.g., Hollon, Shelton, & Loosen, 1991), underscore its relative efficacy, its comparability to psychopharmacological approaches, and occasional superiority to other psychosocial therapies with regard to depression.

Interpersonal Model

The IPT was originally developed by Klerman and his colleagues (Klerman, Weissman, Rounsaville, & Chevron, 1984) based on more psychodynamically oriented formulations emphasizing the primacy of interpersonal relationships (e.g., Sullivan, 1953). Similar to all of the above treatment models, IPT is a time-limited, manualized intervention for depression. However, unlike the above models, IPT places less emphasis on the etiological directionality of interpersonal functioning and depression. Rather, depression is conceptualized as occurring within an interpersonal context and often impairing interpersonal functioning; impaired interpersonal functioning is not necessarily viewed as the *cause* of a depressive episode. In contrast, CT, PST, and the other models described above give a strong causal role to the mechanism of action identified as treatment targets. IPT, on the other hand, "avoids etiological statements about whether untoward psychosocial events cause depression or vice versa; indeed, for clinical purposes, causality may not matter" (Markowitz & Weissman, 1995; p. 376).

For IPT, the mechanism of action is interpersonal functioning, especially within the context of four specific problem areas: grief, role dispute, role transition, and interpersonal deficits. The IPT therapist identifies which particular problem area is salient for a given patient and attempts to help depressed patients by (a) facilitating the mourning process, (b) encouraging the patient to explore potential options to change a relationship associated with interpersonal disputes, (c) facilitating the patient's adjustment to new interpersonal situations, and/or (d) reducing the patient's social isolation and encouraging experimentation with new social relationships. Significant evidence exists in support of IPT's efficacy as a treatment for depression (Markowitz & Weissmann, 1995).

Chapter 3
A 10-Step Guide to Selecting Assessment Measures in Clinical and Research Settings

Christine Maguth Nezu, Arthur M. Nezu, and Sharon L. Foster

> There are no such things as applied sciences, only applications of science
> —Louis Pasteur

WHERE TO BEGIN?

This volume provides many of the best assessment resources that clinical science has to offer for assessing depression and depression-related constructs. However, as one approaches assessment of a clinical problem or contemplates the optimal assessment strategy for a research design, the need for effective decision making clearly emerges. More selections and choices regarding assessment strategies and tools are available now than ever before. Where does one begin when faced with the range of possible alternatives?

A series of decision-making guidelines can be gleaned from the behavioral assessment and treatment literature that begin with the awareness of potential clinical judgment biases and end with a systematic way of "solving the problem" of assessment strategy selection (A. M. Nezu & Nezu, 1989a; 1993). Detailed presentations and discussion can be found in other sources concerning the deleterious effects of human judgmental errors and decision-making bias when the selection of assessment tools is not carefully planned (Arkes, 1981; Dawes, 1986; Kahnemann & Tversky, 1973; A. M. Nezu & Nezu, 1989a). One important maxim that can be drawn from this literature is that, although excellent assessment tools exist for many different clinical problems, the tools are only as good as the skill of the craftsperson who uses them.

17

This chapter is designed to outline a decision-making process for the selection of assessment measures for a given patient. Because so many assessment approaches exist, and because each patient's difficulties are unique, no definitive cookbook or strategy exists that applies to all problem areas. Nonetheless, a few guidelines are generally applicable across clients and problem areas regarding the selection of assessment tools. To facilitate the effectiveness of this decision-making process, we present a 10-step set of heuristics.

Step 1: Determine the Goal of Assessment

There are many different possible contexts, reasons, or goals for assessment (Cone, 1998a; Evans, 1985; C. M. Nezu & Nezu, 1995). These are listed and described below:

- Screening
- Diagnosis and classification
- Description of problem areas and symptoms
- Case formulation and clinical hypothesis testing
- Treatment planning
- Prediction of behavior
- Outcomes evaluation

Screening helps to provide a quick indication of whether further assessment is warranted. To be useful, scores from screening instruments should correlate highly with scores produced by lengthier assessment devices which provide more comprehensive assessments of the presence or absence of the disorder being assessed. This ordinarily involves assessment of the criterion-related validity of the screening instrument. Cutoff scores are often required to use screening instruments, along with information about the types of errors made when using those cutoffs. Errors are typically expressed in terms of the percentages of false-positive and false-negative results that emerge when comparing the results of the screening device with a more in-depth assessment. For example, the number of clients designated as "depressed" using particular cutoff scores on a screening device could be compared with the number who turned out actually to be depressed after further comprehensive assessment. When the screening measure leads to errors in classification, it is generally more important that it make errors of inclusion (e.g., screening in some clients who will later be excluded) than errors of exclusion (e.g., keeping needy clients from receiving services).

Diagnosis and classification are frequent goals in both clinical and research settings. Diagnostic grouping provides a common clinical language and a topic area by which to search the scientific literature for accurate, reliable, and valid evaluation and treatment procedures. Regarding research, such classifications provide important delineations among clinical samples and improve the validity and replicability of findings. Many assessment tools address particular diagnostic areas and focus on descriptions of specific symptoms of a particular group, providing measurement of symptom range, severity, or frequency. These tools often provide specific idiographic information for persons within a specific diagnostic group. Such measures can be particularly useful for evaluating changes in diagnostic symptoms or assessing intervention outcomes. Instruments that are designed specifically for formulating diagnoses warrant particular scrutiny for their content validity; a diagnostic instrument should contain content that clearly corresponds to the criteria required for diagnosis by the DSM or other classification system. The content should exclude extraneous material and weight symptoms as required by the classification system. In addition, the diagnosis that the instrument leads to should be reliable over time, and when clinician judgment is involved, should demonstrate good interclinician agreement when the system is implemented by independent clinicians evaluating the same client.

In order to develop an accurate *case formulation*, it is important to understand the etiology, function, and maintaining factors of an individual's complaints. As such, in this context, assessment focuses on hypothesized mechanisms of action. These may involve cognitive, emotional, behavioral, or biomedical factors that are theoretically or empirically linked to the symptoms or complaints for which an individual is seeking treatment. Rosen and Proctor (1981) referred to these as instrumental outcomes. These factors serve as instruments to effect change in the chief problem areas or the major reasons for seeking treatment. These later variables (or dependent variables) are referred to by Rosen and Proctor as ultimate outcomes. Within this framework, changes in instrumental outcomes (e.g., coping skills) potentially lead to changes in ultimate outcomes (e.g., psychological distress).

Assessment of instrumental variables helps the clinician to *formulate a treatment plan* (A. M. Nezu & Nezu, 1989a). A relevant example involves evaluating cognitive distortions in an individual who complains of depression. In such a case, the assessor is not only measuring depression (i.e., the referral complaints or ultimate reason for seeking treatment), but also a cognitive mediational style that is hypothesized to serve as an important causal factor of depression (an instrumental outcome). As such, the clinician would be able to determine if a cognitive model of depression may be applicable to a specific patient. If so, then a cognitive therapy approach may be recommended. If not, such an intervention might be inappropriate, and, thus, potentially ineffective. Therefore, measures of instrumental outcomes can be useful for evaluating the idiographic importance of various mechanisms of action that are nomothetically linked to the clinical phenomena of interest. Measurements of both types of variables also underscore the importance of outcomes assessment in both clinical and research settings (A. M. Nezu, 1996). To be especially useful for predicting which treatments are likely to work and which will not, a measure should ideally provide some evidence that its use leads to more effective or efficient treatment than would occur in its absence.

Assessment is also used for behavioral *prediction* in academic, research, and clinical settings. Particularly relevant to clinical situations is the prediction of behavior that carries a high risk of danger to self or others. Examples include assessment of the likelihood of suicide or violence. Other examples include evaluating the likelihood that an individual will benefit from an educational or therapeutic experience. Here previous studies of predictive validity are important, so the clinician can gauge how well the assessment tool actually predicts the outcome for which it was intended, and the nature and range of errors of prediction that occur.

Assessment devices also help to monitor client progress and *evaluate treatment outcome*. This requires, first, that the content of the measure address the behaviors targeted by the treatment plan. Second, the measure should be stable in the absence of conditions that produce change (i.e., show good test–retest reliability in the absence of treatment or changes in the client's circumstances). Third, the measure should be sufficiently sensitive to detect change. This is ordinarily shown by studies that demonstrate that scores on the measure change significantly during treatment, but not in the absence of treatment. Studies of whether changes in scores on the measure following treatment correlate highly with changes in scores on other measures of the same construct also provide some evidence of treatment sensitivity, as well as convergent validity.

Finally, there may be multiple goals of assessment. An example involves a situation when both diagnosis and treatment recommendations are desired. This would require assessment tools that classify, as well as tools that might increase the therapist's understanding of patient problem areas. As such, a crucial first step toward effective selection of assessment instruments rests in the accurate determination of assessment goals.

Step 2: Adopt a Systems Approach

With regard to selecting assessment strategies and identifying potential patient target problems, we advocate a multimethod, systems-oriented approach as an overall plan (A. M. Nezu, Nezu, Friedman, & Haynes, 1997). As indicated above, in most clinical situations, there are multiple goals of assessment, including accurate diagnosis, prediction, explanation, and monitoring of symptoms. Regarding any one of these goals, several additional subareas will almost inevitably warrant assessment. Many pathways can connect a particular set of experiences or circumstances with the ultimate clinical manifestation a given individual presents. Therefore, clinicians generally need to assess a variety of factors, including emotional experiences, thought patterns, behavioral sequences, impact of the social or physical environment, physiological correlates, important developmental experiences, and ethnocultural information. These variables may serve to act and interact as causal or maintaining factors concerning the client's presenting complaints. Moreover, a systems-based approach can be improved by incorporating a constructional philosophy (Evans, 1985). This philosophy emphasizes the value in building upon or adding areas of strength or adaptive behavioral repertoires, rather than focusing assessment solely on deficits or pathology. This approach adds more complexity to the assessment enterprise by encouraging the clinician to assess strengths and competencies, as well as pathology.

Finally, for each assessment purpose and for each focal problem area, the use of multiple assessment methods can increase the reliability, validity, and utility of the information obtained. Thus, it makes sense to adopt a strategic approach in which the clinician uses a range of strategies and assessment procedures. Different assessment procedures include role plays, observational methods, interviews, self-report inventories, and ratings of physical or medical functioning.

Step 3: Individualize Assessment and Identify Obstacles

Each patient presents unique obstacles to assessment. Examples of obstacles include motivational variance, language difficulties, specific emotional, cognitive, or intellectual impairments, coexisting physical problems, or unresponsiveness. In addition, clinicians also present unique obstacles. Limited time or lack of resources may limit access to psychophysiological equipment, expensive inventories or questionnaires, or laboratory tests. Limited experience may reduce a therapist's familiarity with specific problems or disorders. For example, a therapist who specializes in depression may be less familiar with substance abuse or compulsive behavior; yet such disorders coexist with some frequency in clinical settings. Individualizing assessment necessarily involves identifying the idiographic problems present in each assessment situation, as well as formulating an assessment plan to work around or overcome those obstacles.

Step 4: Adapt Assessment to Overcome Obstacles

The first step in overcoming obstacles to effective assessment is to identify any areas of difficulty involved in conducting each type of assessment the clinician requires. We view this as an important problem to solve—failure to do so can lead to clinicians who, over time, become tolerant and uncritical of poor-quality information and are therefore likely to make less effective decisions. Resolution of potential assessment problems involves closely approx-imating the needed information that is required, while accepting the limitations imposed by either patient or therapist factors. For example, when assessing panic disorder or sexual arousal disorders, physiological arousal is generally an important factor to assess. The clini-cian who lacks optimal instrumentation for this assessment may not be able to capture the "purest" measure of arousal, but is able to obtain a viable approximation to this needed infor-mation, for example, by asking the client to define his or her bodily sensations when anxious, and then devising a plan for the client to track those sensations using a self-monitoring procedure. As another example, if the ethnocultural background of the provider and patient is discrepant or unfamiliar, it is important to select tools using a culturally informed assessment process (Tanaka-Matsumi, Seiden, & Lam, 1996). This might involve adapting one's tools or questioning, translating instruments into another language, or carefully discussing assessment with the client and listening carefully for any reservations the client might voice about the procedures.

Whether or not major impediments to systematic assessment are present, selection of an assessment strategy requires answers to the question, "Which assessment procedures should I incorporate to maximize the chances of obtaining valid, reliable, and comprehensive informa-tion about this client for my particular assessment goal?" This challenging task can be approached through the following steps. When the practitioner identifies difficulties that are likely to interfere with assessment, he or she should state goals that explicitly incorporate these impediments. For example, even when a specific goal is clear (e.g., treatment planning), the question should be stated as, "How can I obtain valid, reliable and comprehensive data relevant to treatment planning about this client who is poorly motivated ... or has a disability ... or in a way that is culturally sensitive?" Different strategies and instruments will have greater and lesser utility for different situations. When instruments have not been developed or evaluated for their utility in the identified circumstances, a search for information on how best to apply or to adapt the available tools may need to be pursued. Examples involve using the culturally informed assessment procedure developed by Tanaka-Matsumi et al. (1996) or adapting assessment tools originally developed for other populations to a population with developmental disabilities (C. M. Nezu, Nezu, & Gill-Weiss, 1992).

Step 5: For Each Clinical Focal Area, Generate a Variety of Assessment Strategies

Different ways of accessing information about the focal problem areas (i.e., referral symptoms and instrumental outcomes) should be considered in producing a list of possible ways of assessing areas of concern. For example, if one focal area for the client involves interpersonal problems, potential assessment methods might include self-report inventories, interview procedures with the client, interview procedures with relevant collaterals, behav-ioral observation, and structured role plays.

Step 6: For Each Strategy, Generate Multiple Ideas

Each strategy will likely have many different "tactics" or instruments available from which to choose. For example, possible alternatives for the previously mentioned strategy of collateral interviews might include in-session or telephone interviews or surveys with family members, friends, or coworkers. To increase possibilities, one can combine various tactics across strategies to produce novel approaches (e.g., family members complete self-report inventories assessing various problem areas related to treatment goals). This volume specifically provides a compendium of instruments that can be used to assess depression, and can be a valuable resource in expanding clinicians' knowledge of the range of "tactics" available to them.

Step 7: Conduct a Cost-Benefit Analysis

For each assessment subgoal and range of measurement alternatives, evaluate the potential effects of using each, based on the answers to the following criteria-related questions.

Likelihood of Effects:
1. What is the likelihood that the measure will provide needed information and produce reliable, valid, and comprehensive information about this area/focal problem? This evaluation will be based upon data provided by the empirical literature (e.g., data concerning reported reliability and validity of a particular self-report measure).
2. What is the likelihood that the therapist and patient will carry out this procedure optimally in order to obtain the needed information? If not, what help, adaptations, or modifications are required in order to increase the chance that this assessment can be carried out?

Value of Outcome:
1. What is the extent of time and effort involved for the patient, and does the benefit of the information yielded by the assessment outweigh the amount of time and effort required to complete this assessment?
2. What is the extent of time and effort that will necessarily be expended by the therapist? Is additional training required in order to administer the desired assessment instrument optimally or ethically? For example, if psychophysiological assessment is required, does the information provided add sufficient value to the assessment to warrant the additional cost and time?
3. Is the procedure consistent with the morals, values, and ethics of both the therapist and patient?
4. What is the emotional impact (i.e., cost versus gain) on both the therapist and the patient?
5. Could the assessment result in any physical danger or predictable untoward side effects to the patient?
6. What are the effects, if any, of the assessment on other people involved (e.g., family members, friends, individuals in the community)?
7. What are the short-term effects and long-term effects of the selected assessment strategy and tactics? For example, does participating in the assessment have therapeutic benefit for the patient (e.g., by helping the person become more aware of the connection between symptoms and the circumstances that elicit them; by helping the client see the gradual, incremental gains he or she is making)?
8. How much unique information does this measure offer? If it offers redundant information, will that information help to assess the validity of information gathered via a different method?

Step 8: Based on a Comparison of these Criteria Ratings, Choose the One(s) with the Highest "Utility"

Several authors have suggested that the "best" assessment measures to employ for a clinical problem are the ones with the highest functional utility in a given situation (Cone, 1998b; A. M. Nezu & Nezu, 1989a). By evaluating assessment tactics according to the above criteria, the clinician can determine those with the highest ratings. These will predictably be the ones with the highest utility:cost ratio. Choices are likely to include those with the highest criteria ratings or several measures that collectively yield the highest ratings as a group.

Step 9: Implement Assessment Procedures

As mentioned above, specific situational contexts may require adaptation of a particular measure. This may reduce the user's confidence regarding applicability of the psychometric information about the instrument to the adapted version or raise issues concerning the external validity of the information the tactic produces. Although clearly devices should be used as designed whenever possible, specific clinical situations may require adaptation to solve implementation problems illuminated when the clinician considers obstacles to assessment. In these circumstances, the clinician should interpret the information from the instrument in light of the nature and extensiveness of the adaptions that he or she made to the instrument. In addition, collecting information about the same issue using a different source or method can help the clinician appraise informally the convergent validity of the information produced by the adapted instrument.

Step 10: Monitor the Effects

Essential to monitoring the effects is to observe whether the assessment procedure generated useful, valid, and reliable information about a focal problem area. This involves comparing the predicted outcome of the assessment plan with actual results achieved. If the match is satisfactory, that is, the goals of this particular assessment is achieved with a level of confidence that is both required and comfortable, then the therapist can "exit" from the decision-making process for the present time.

It is important to underscore that different reasons for assessment often reemerge during the course of therapy. Therefore, in a sense, "assessment" is a continuous process *throughout the course of treatment*. For example, new symptoms may emerge, or new reasons for assessment may occur. One such case may include the individual who came to treatment for reduced anxiety and stress management, but later reveals problems that involve potential risk of injury that require assessment specifically focused on risk prediction.

If the predicted assessment outcome is unsatisfactory, it is important to assess the reason for this discrepancy. For example, were the goals of assessment not clear? Was there suboptimal implementation of assessment procedures? Did the clinician fail to recognize or identify incipient problems at the start of assessment, such as low client motivation which impeded completion of various inventories? These obstacles require correction through either reformulation of the assessment, improved implementation of assessment procedures, selection of other measures that can be better implemented, or improved client motivation for assessment.

This troubleshooting involves recycling through the problem-solving processes until the goals are achieved.

CONCLUDING REMARKS

This 10-step approach may leave readers initially somewhat exhausted as they anticipate the complexities involved in every selection of assessment instruments. However, with the daunting range of possible assessment tools from which to choose, we believe that such a guided metacognitive task can ultimately save valuable professional time and increase the efficacy of assessment for both research and clinical settings. After all, much of therapy involves assessment; the therapist continuously collects information and bases various treatment decisions on that information. The question is not whether to assess; rather it is *how* to assess—how to select and use assessment tactics in systematic ways that improve treatment decisions, and how to evaluate the quality of the information that those tactics produce.

Part II
Assessment Instruments

Chapter 4
Measures of Depression, Depressive Symptomatology, and Depressive Mood

INTRODUCTION

In this chapter, a variety of measures are described that assess depression and depressive symptoms for adults and adolescents. Included are structured interview protocols, clinician ratings, and self-report measures. Several specifically address the construct of depression and depressive symptoms, whereas others focus on more generalized mood or psychiatric symptomatology. Although this latter group involves measures that are broader in scope, each does include a scale or subscale focused on depression or depressive mood. The following is a listing of these measures by category. However, note that the assessment tools are listed in this chapter by alphabetical order.

Structured Interview Procedures

- Diagnostic Interview Schedule
- Schedule for Affective Disorders and Schizophrenia Research Diagnostic Criteria
- Structured Clinical Interview for DSM-IV Axis I Disorders

Clinician-Rated Protocols

- Brief Psychiatric Rating Scale
- Hamilton Rating Scale for Depression
- Manual for the Diagnosis of Major Depression
- Montgomery–Asberg Depression Rating Scale
- Newcastle Scales
- Primary Care Evaluation of Mental Disorders
- Raskin Three-Area Scale
- Revised Hamilton Rating Scale for Depression: Clinician Rating Form
- Rimon's Brief Depression Scale

Self-Report Inventories

- Beck Depression Inventory-Second Edition
- Carroll Depression Scales-Revised
- Center for Epidemiological Studies Depression Scale
- Depression Questionnaire
- Depression 30 Scale
- Diagnostic Inventory for Depression
- Hamilton Depression Inventory
- Hopelessness Depression Symptom Questionnaire
- Inventory of Depressive Symptomatology
- IPAT Depression Scale
- Minnesota Multiphasic Personality Inventory 2 Depression Scale
- MOS 8-Item Depression Screener
- Multiscore Depression Inventory for Adolescents and Adults
- Positive and Negative Affect Scales
- Revised Hamilton Rating Scale for Depression: Self-Report Problem Inventory
- Reynolds Depression Screening Inventory
- State Trait-Depression Adjective Check Lists
- Zung Depression Self-Rating Depression Scale

Measures of General Mood or Psychiatric Symptomatology

- Brief Symptom Inventory
- Depression Anxiety Stress Scales
- Hospital Anxiety and Depression Scale
- Multiple Affect Adjective Checklist-Revised
- Profile of Mood Scales
- Symptom Checklist-90-R

BECK DEPRESSION INVENTORY™-SECOND EDITION (BDI-II)™*

Original Citation

Beck, A. T., Steer, R. A., & Brown, G. K. (1996). *Manual for the BDI-II*. San Antonio, TX: The Psychological Corporation.

Purpose

To assess the severity of depressive symptoms.

Population

Adults and adolescents aged 13 years and older.

Description

The BDI-II is a 21-item self-report measure of depressive symptoms that was developed in concert with criteria for diagnosing depressive disorders contained in the DSM-IV. Each item represents a symptom characteristic of depression, such as sadness, guilt, suicidal thoughts, and loss of interest. Nineteen items include a 4-point scale ranging from 0 to 3, representing ascending levels of severity, from the absence of a given symptom (e.g., "I do not feel sad") to an intense level (e.g., "I am so sad or unhappy that I can't stand it"). The remaining two items (i.e., changes in sleeping patterns, changes in appetite) allow the respondent to indicate increases *or* decreases in these behaviors. Respondents are requested to read each statement and to chose the *one* statement that best describes themselves during the past two weeks.

Two sample items are reprinted below with permission of the publisher.

14. Worthlessness
    0   I do not feel I am worthless.
    1   I don't consider myself as worthwhile and useful as I used to.
    2   I feel more worthless as compared to other people.
    3   I feel utterly worthless.
21. Loss of Interest in Sex
    0   I have not noticed any recent change in my interest in sex.
    1   I am less interested in sex than I used to be.
    2   I am much less interested in sex now.
    3   I have lost interest in sex completely.

Background

This version represents the third generation of the Beck Depression Inventory, the original having been developed by A. T. Beck, Ward, Mendelson, Mock, and Erbaugh (1961). During the past three decades, the BDI has become the most widely used self-report instrument for measuring depressive symptom severity in both research and clinical settings (see A. T. Beck, Steer, and Garbin, 1988, for a review of the applications and psychometric properties of the original BDI).

In 1979, a modified version of the BDI (BDI-IA) was published (A. T. Beck, Rush, Shaw, & Emery, 1979; technical manual published in 1987 by A. T. Beck and Steer) to eliminate alternative wordings for the same symptoms and to avoid the use of double negatives. Unlike the BDI-IA, the BDI-II represents a significant modification over the BDI, based on changes in diagnostic criteria, as exemplified in DSM-III to DSM IV. The BDI-II was developed to replace these earlier versions.

Administration

In general, the BDI-II requires 5–10 minutes to complete.

Scoring

The BDI-II is scored by summing the ratings for the 21 items. The maximum score is 63. Higher scores indicate higher levels of depressive symptoms.

Interpretation

According to A. T. Beck et al. (1996), the following cutoff scores can serve as guidelines for understanding BDI-II scores: minimal depression (0–13), mild depression (14–19), moderate depression (20–28), and severe depression (29–63). Caution, however, is underscored by the test developers to not use such scores as the sole source of information for diagnostic purposes.

Psychometric Properties

In the manual, norms and psychometric properties are based on two samples: a group of 500 patients (317 men; 183 women) from four psychiatric outpatient facilities and a group of 120 college students (67 men; 53 women). Additional information beyond the material contained in the manual about the psychometric properties of the BDI-II can be found in Dozois, Dobson, and Ahnberg (1998).

Norms.   Means and standard deviations for the BDI-II are provided in the manual for both above samples and by diagnostic group (i.e., mood disorders, anxiety disorders, adjustment disorders, and other disorders). The mood disorders category is further broken down into major depression-single episode, major depression-recurrent episode, dysthymia, bipolar, and depression not otherwise specified.

Reliability. With regard to internal consistency, coefficient alpha estimates were found to be .92 and .93 for the psychiatric outpatient sample, and .93 for the college students. Test–retest reliability was estimated based on 26 outpatients who completed the BDI-II twice, 1 week apart. This stability correlation was .93.

Validity. One estimate of the construct validity of the BDI-II concerns its significant correlation (i.e., .93) with an earlier version of this inventory, the BDI-IA. With regard to concurrent validity, the BDI-II was found to correlate .71 with the Hamilton Rating Scale for Depression (p. 58). As an indication of its construct validity, the BDI-II correlates .68 with a measure of hopelessness (Beck Hopelessness Scale, p. 175) and .37 with a measure of suicide ideation (Beck Scale for Suicide Ideation; p. 177), both constructs generally viewed to be conceptually related to depression. Intercorrelations among the 21 items provided in the manual offer evidence of the BDI-II's factorial validity.

Based on a series of iterated principal factor analyses, two major factors appear to underlie this inventory's structure. For the psychiatric outpatient sample, the two factors can best be described as a somatic-affective dimension and a cognitive dimension. For the student sample, the two factors can be labeled as cognitive-affective and somatic dimensions.

Clinical Utility

High. This new version of the BDI has improved clinical sensitivity and has been developed specifically to be consistent with DSM-IV criteria.

Research Applicability

High. The original BDI is probably the widest used self-report measure to assess severity of depressive symptoms in major research studies.

Source

The Psychological Corporation, 555 Academic Court, San Antonio, TX 78204-2498. Phone: 800-211-8378.

Cost

$53.00 for manual and 25 record forms.

Alternative Forms

Spanish record forms are available.

BRIEF PSYCHIATRIC RATING SCALES (BPRS)

Original Citations

Lukoff, D., Liberman, R. P., & Nuechterlein, K. H. (1986). Symptom monitoring in the rehabilitation of schizophrenic patients. *Schizophrenia Bulletin*, *12*, 578–602.

Overall, J. E. & Gorham, D. R. (1962). The Brief Psychiatric Rating Scale. *Psychological Reports*, *10*, 799–812.

Purpose

To assess psychiatric symptoms and severe psychopathology.

Population

Adults with severe psychiatric disorders.

Description

The BPRS was developed to measure patient change. The expanded version contains 24 items that are grouped into five syndromes (thought disorder, withdrawal, anxiety-depression, hostility-suspicion, and activity). Each item represents a discrete symptom (e.g., depression). Sophisticated clinical interviewers, using both patient reports of symptoms experienced over the preceding 2 weeks and behavioral observations made during a semistructured interview, complete the ratings. The manual for the expanded BPRS (reprinted in Lukoff et al., 1986) contains an interview schedule, symptom definitions, and specific anchor points for rating symptoms. Interviewers rate symptom severity on a 7-point scale from 1 (absent) to 7 (extremely severe). Each scale point is associated with a specific description.

Background

The original BPRS (Overall & Gorham, 1962) is described as a symptom-construct rating scale intended for use by clinically sophisticated interviewers. It contains 16 items and yields four syndrome subscales: thinking disturbance, hostile-suspicious, withdrawal-retardation, and anxious-depression. Operational definitions for each of the 16 symptoms are provided, as well as guidelines for standardized administration.

Two items (disorientation and excitement) were added to the scale in 1966. The expanded BPRS (Lukoff et al., 1986) includes new items for schizophrenia (bizarre behavior, self-neglect, and suicidality) and mania (elevated mood, distractibility, and motor hyperactivity).

The BPRS remains a popular measure of patient change in psychopharmacology research. It has also been used to develop clinical prediction models for treatment response expectations and to describe, measure, and empirically classify psychiatric patients. It is also frequently used as a clinical tool to examine and evaluate psychiatric diagnosis.

Administration

Administration of the interview and rating of symptoms takes 10–40 minutes depending on the interviewer's familiarity with the patient, the number of symptoms present, and other patient characteristics.

Scoring

Item ratings are summed to compute a total pathology score. In addition, summing items within each of the five subscales produces syndrome scores.

Interpretation

The total score provides a global index of psychopathology, but tracking changes across only one or two syndrome scales is appropriate for some diagnoses. Additionally, changes in ratings on individual items over time can be interpreted as changes in symptom status.

Psychometric Properties

Norms. None.

Reliability. A comprehensive review (Hedlund & Vieweg, 1980) suggests adequate interrater reliability. Interrater reliability estimates for the items range from .67 to .88. Interrater reliabilities ranging from .85 to .94 have been reported for the total pathology and syndrome subscale scores.

Validity. Hedlund and Vieweg's (1980) comprehensive review also addresses the validity of the BPRS. They note a variety of treatment studies which report the BPRS to consistently track changes in psychiatric symptoms that are corroborated and supported by other clinical ratings. They also note a number of studies which have found moderate to high correlations between the BPRS and other clinical scales (e.g., Minnesota Multiphasic Personality Inventory, MMPI; p. 73, item composites; and the Multiple Affective Adjective Checklist; p. 81). They conclude that these studies provide evidence of concurrent and construct validity for the instrument. Evidence of predictive and construct validity also comes from studies that have successfully employed the BPRS when developing and testing diagnostic classifications and treatment response typologies. Finally, the large number of factor analytic studies that support the five-syndrome subscale structure establishes the internal or structural validity of the BPRS.

Clinical Utility

High. The BPRS is one of the most widely used instruments for evaluating symptom levels in schizophrenia and major mood disorders. Research with the instrument over the past 30 years suggests that this measure provides an accurate assessment of important symptom constructs and is sensitive to changes in symptom severity.

Research Applicability

High. The BPRS has been used in clinical research in psychopathology for over 30 years. However, it is best suited for the assessment and description of severe psychopathology. It is designed to be administered by trained professional interviewers.

Source

Printed in Overall and Gorham (1962) and Lukoff et al. (1986).

Cost

Information regarding the use of the BPRS should be obtained from the Department of Health and Human Services, Public Health Service, National Institute of Mental Health, Center for Studies on Schizophrenia, Rockville, MD 20857.

Alternative Forms

The BPRS has been translated into a number of European languages including German, Czech, French, and Spanish.

BRIEF SYMPTOM INVENTORY (BSI)

Original Citation

Derogatis, L. R. (1993). *Brief Symptom Inventory (BSI) administration, scoring, and procedures manual* (3rd ed.). Minneapolis, MN: National Computer Systems.

Purpose

To measure psychological symptoms reported by psychiatric patients, medical patients, and nonpatients.

Populations

Adolescents and adults.

Description

The BSI is a 53-item self-report inventory. Each of the symptoms contained is rated on a 5-point scale of distress ranging from 0 ("not at all") to 4 ("extremely"). In addition to three global distress indices (general severity index, positive symptom distress index, and positive symptom total), the BSI provides information on nine primary symptom dimensions. The primary symptom dimensions include anxiety, depression, hostility, interpersonal sensitivity, obsessive-compulsive, paranoid ideation, phobic anxiety, psychoticism, and somatization. The Depression scale of the BSI contains six items reflecting a range of indicators of clinical depression (e.g., feelings of sadness, feelings of worthlessness).

Background

The BSI was derived from the Symptom Checklist 90-R (SCL 90-R; p. 117). The correlation between the primary symptom dimensions associated with the BSI and the same primary symptom dimensions associated with the SCL 90-R ranges from .92 to .99. Of particular interest to the current review is the .95 correlation between the primary symptom dimension of depression on the BSI and the SCL 90-R.

Administration

The BSI takes approximately 10 minutes to complete.

Scoring

Computer and hand scoring of the BSI are available. Hand scoring is completed using plastic scoring templates. A work sheet is also available for recording raw scores on the nine symptom dimensions and the three global indices. Raw scores are plotted on a profile sheet and *T*-score conversion allows for an analysis across scores. Profile sheets are available for patient and nonpatient samples.

Interpretation

High scores indicate severer symptoms. The manual suggests first evaluating the global indices to gain an understanding of the overall level of distress. The second step involves looking at the primary symptom dimensions. The manual suggests that such an analysis can provide information regarding specific concerns. Finally, the manual also suggests perusing the discrete items to identify specific symptoms that need to be addressed.

Psychometric Properties

Norms.   Data are available for psychiatric inpatients ($N = 310$), psychiatric outpatients ($N = 1002$), and nonpatient respondents ($N = 719$).

Reliability.   A sample of 1,002 psychiatric outpatients was used to estimate coefficient alpha for the nine primary symptom dimensions. Estimates range from .71 to .85; the estimate for the primary symptom dimension of depression was .85. Sixty nonpatients were tested at a 2-week interval to obtain stability estimates. Test–retest reliability estimates for the three global indices ranged from .80 to .90. Similar estimates for the primary symptom dimensions ranged from .68 to .91, with a value of .84 for the primary symptom dimension of depression.

     Validity.   Several of the BSI scales have been found to correlate with related constructs measured using the MMPI (p. 73). Nevertheless, the same lack of specificity noted for the primary symptom dimensions associated with the SCL 90-R (p. 117) is likely to be found for the BSI (e.g., Hayes, 1997). For instance, the BSI depression scale was significantly related to the Wiggins Depression Content Scale ($r = .72$) and the Tyron Depression Cluster Scale ($r = .67$), as well as a variety of scales not conceptually related to depression (MMPI Scale 8, $r = .52$; MMPI Scale 7, $r = .46$; and Tyron Autism Cluster Scores, $r = .43$). Similar to the SCL 90-R, the BSI is probably best thought of as a general screening device that measures global levels of psychopathology.

Clinical Utility

     Limited. As a general measure of psychopathology, the measure has high clinical utility. For instance, the measure possesses enough sensitivity that it can be used repeatedly to assess changes in psychiatric symptoms as a result of treatment. Unfortunately, the primary symptom dimension of depression has not been well validated and 87% of the items are conceptualized as not specific to depression.

Research Applicability

     Limited. As a general measure of psychopathology the measure has considerable utility. For instance, the measure could clearly be used to equate samples for overall levels of psychopathology. Unfortunately, the primary symptom dimension of depression lacks the specificity and sensitivity that is often required by researchers evaluating levels of depression.

Source

     National Computer Systems, Assessment Sales Dept., 5605 Green Circle Drive, Minnetonka, MN 55343. Phone: 800-627-7271. Website: www.ncs.com.

Cost

     A variety of options are available (e.g., Starter Kit, Preview Kit, Computer Generated Interpretative Reports, Audiocassette Version, Large Print Version, Hand Scoring Keys, etc.). The Hand Scoring Starter Kit costs $104. Contact National Computer Systems for additional prices.

Alternative Forms

     Alternate forms are available in Spanish and 13 other languages.

CARROLL DEPRESSION SCALES-REVISED (CDS-R)

Original Citation

Carroll, B. (1998). *Carroll Depression Scales-Revised (CDS-R): Technical manual.* Toronto: Multi-Health Systems, Inc.

Purpose

To assess the severity of depressive symptoms.

Population

Adults age 18 years and over.

Description

The CDS-R is a 61-item self-report inventory geared to assess one's depressive symptomatology over the past few days. Respondents are requested to read each statement and indicate YES or NO. Statements address the following areas: depression, guilt, suicide, initial insomnia, middle insomnia, late insomnia, work and interests, retardation, agitation, psychological anxiety, somatic anxiety, gastrointestinal, general somatic, libido, hypochondriasis, loss of insight, and loss of weight. Sample items (reprinted with the permission of the publisher © 1998, Multi-Health Systems, Inc.) are noted below:

2.	I have dropped many of my interests and activities.	YES	NO
5.	I am miserable or often feel like crying.	YES	NO
7.	I feel worthless and ashamed about myself.	YES	NO
9.	I feel in good spirits.	YES	NO
11.	I get hardly anything done lately.	YES	NO
12.	I am exhausted much of the time.	YES	NO

Background

The CDS-R is the newly revised version of the Carroll Rating Scale for Depression (CRS; Carroll, Feinberg, Smouse, Rawson, & Greden, 1981). The CRS was designed following an empirical investigation of self-report versus clinician-completed depression rating scales. Results of these studies indicated variable concordance rates, leading Carroll et al. (1973) to suggest that neither self-report nor clinician-administered depression scales should be used in making a diagnosis by themselves. Because the Hamilton Rating Scale for Depression (HRSD; p. 58) is a widely used observer scale, the CRS was developed to match the items and purpose of the HRSD in a self-report format. The CDS-R was developed to build upon the original CRS and to make it compatible with the DSM-IV.

Administration

When self-administered, the CDS-R takes under 20 minutes to complete.

Scoring

Items are scored either 0 or 1, yielding a total score range of 0–61. Forty statements, when answered Yes, are indicative for depression; in the remaining 21 statements No is indicative of depression. Higher scores indicate higher levels of depression.

Interpretation

Carroll et al. (1981) suggest a cutoff score of 10 as a screen for depression.

Psychometric Properties

Psychometric properties for the CDS were established in several samples. These are briefly described within each section for which they were used. It is noted in the manual that although the data reviewed were drawn from CDS ratings, they are directly applicable to the CDS-R as well.

Norms.   In a sample of 559 depressed patients, the mean CDS score was 27.0 (SD = 8.9). In a nonpsychiatric sample of 119 employees of the University of Michigan Medical Center (ages 18–64 years), the mean score was 4.6 (SD = .40) and the median score was 3.

Reliability.   Split-half reliability was calculated using 3,725 CDS scores at the University of Michigan, with the correlation between halves at .87. In addition, scores on the half-sets had a strong correlation with scores on the whole set (rs = .97 and .96). Internal consistency was examined in a sample of 559 depressed patients and 129 community controls; alphas for both the CDS and the Brief CDS were high, .95 and .90, respectively. Item-total correlations from a sample of 278 University of Michigan respondents were moderate, ranging from .02 to .83 with a mean correlation of .56. Finally, test–retest reliability was examined in a sample of 16 patients who provided a total of 42 pairs of ratings, with intervals ranging from 5 hours to 4 weeks between testings. Results indicated excellent stability over time (r = .97). However, it should be noted that this correlation may be misleadingly high: Only patients whose concurrent HDRS ratings did not vary by more than two points across the two testing sessions were included in this analysis due to the CDS being a state, rather than trait measure, and thus being expected to change due to changes in clinical state over time.

Validity.   The CDS was validated against a number of clinician- and self-rated measures of depression. In a sample of 279 ratings from depressed inpatients who completed the CDS, HRSD, and BDI on the same day, the CDS demonstrated good convergent validity (BDI, r = .86; HRSD, r = .71). Slightly higher correlations with the HRSD were found in separate samples of 97 patients diagnosed with major depression (r = .80) and 198 patients with a variety of diagnoses (r =.75). When compared with clinician ratings from the Montgomery–Asberg Depression Rating Scale (MADRS; p. 75) in a sample of 559 depressed patients, both the CDS and Brief CDS showed significant correlations ($rs =$. 71 and .67, respectively). A similar correlation was found between the CDS and clinician-rated global depression ratings ($r = .63$) in a sample of 2,331 paired ratings and between the CDS and the Center for Epidemiological Studies Depression Scale (CES-D; p. 39), $r = .67$.

Discriminant validity was established by examining a sample of 30 patients diagnosed with depression or anxiety who completed both the CDS and the State-Trait Anxiety Inventory (STAI; Spielberger, Gorsuch, & Lushene, 1970). The correlation between the CDS and STAI was not statistically significant ($r = .26$).

Clinical Utility

High. The CDS-R can be used as a brief screening measure that closely corresponds to a recognized clinician-rated measure.

Research Applicability

High. The HRSD is one of the most widely used clinician-rated measures of depression and has been included in many clinical research studies. The CDS-R provides a similar measure of depression in a self-report format.

Source

Multi-Health Systems, Inc., 908 Niagara Falls Blvd., North Tonawanda, NY 14120-2060. Phone: 800-456-3003.

Cost

A CDS kit, including the manual and 25 CDS-R forms, is available for $70. Packages of 25 or 100 CDS-R forms are $30 and $100, respectively.

Alternative Forms

A 12-item version, the Brief CDS, is also available; both the CDS-R and the Brief CDS are available in a version for French-Canadian subjects. A German translation has also been studied and found to have adequate psychometric properties (Merten & Siebert, 1997).

CENTER FOR EPIDEMIOLOGICAL STUDIES DEPRESSION SCALE (CES-D)

Original Citation

Radloff, L. S. (1977). The CES-D Scale: A self-report depression scale for research in the general population. *Applied Psychological Measurement*, *1*, 385–401.

Purpose

To measure the current level of symptoms which accompany depression in a general population.

Population

Adults.

Description

The CES-D is a 20-item self-report measure of depressive symptoms. Each item provides a statement representing a symptom characteristic of depression (e.g., "I had crying spells"), followed by a 4-point Likert-type response scale ranging from "rarely or none of the time" (less than 1 day) to "most all of the time" (5–7 days). Respondents are instructed to circle the number of each statement which best describes how often they felt or behaved this way during the past week. Sixteen of these scales range from 0 to 3 representing ascending frequency. The remaining four scales range from 3 to 0, representing descending levels of frequency.

Based on a principal components factor analysis of data from the general population samples, four major factors underlie this inventory's structure. These factors have been described as depressed affect, positive affect, somatic and retarded activity, and an interpersonal factor. The factor structure was similar across subgroups and with the general population (a requirement for any instrument intended for epidemiological studies, and therefore to be generalized across subgroups).

Background

The CES-D was developed to be used in epidemiological studies of depression in the general population. Therefore, it was designed to measure the current level of depressive symptomatology, and not to diagnose depression or measure symptom severity. Items of the CES-D were selected from a pool of items included in other valid measures of depression at the time.

Administration

This instrument was designed to be brief and usable by lay interviewers. It takes less than 10 minutes to complete.

Scoring

The CES-D is scored by summing the ratings of the 20 items. Scores range from 0 to 60.

Interpretation

Higher scores indicate higher frequency of depressive symptoms experienced during the past week. The authors of the CES-D caution that individual scores should not be interpreted, as it was not developed as a diagnostic tool. Investigators have designated a cutoff score of 16 as a suitable indicator to differentiate depressed from nondepressed patients (Comstock & Helsing, 1976). However, no indicators have been designated to discriminate depressive subtypes or to distinguish primary from secondary depression.

Psychometric Properties

Norms and psychometric properties based on three community samples and two psychiatric patient samples have been described by Radloff (1977). The groups were comprised of 2,514 White nonpatient adults, 1,060 White nonpatient adults, 1,422 White nonpatient adults, and 70 White adult psychiatric patients.

Norms.   Means and standard deviations for the CES-D are provided by Weissman, Sholomskas, Pottenger, Prusoff, and Locke (1977) for males and females in a variety of populations.

Reliability.   With regard to internal consistency, coefficient alpha estimates were found to be .85 for the general population and .90 for the patient sample. Test–retest correlations were examined on 419 participants who completed the CES-D 2, 4, 6, or 8 weeks after their original interviews. Correlations ranged from .51 to .67. Another group of 1,552 respondents were reinterviewed 3, 6, or 12 months after their first interview. Stability correlations for this group ranged between .32 and .54.

Validity.   One test of the validity of the CES-D concerns its ability to discriminate between psychiatric inpatient groups and the general population. CES-D scores were significantly and substantially different between these groups. Further examination of the concurrent validity involved comparing mean scores on the CES-D to scores on other empirically validated ratings of depressive severity. Correlation with the HRSD (p. 58) was .44 and correlation with the Raskin Three-Area Scale (p. 96) was .54. These correlations increased to .69 and .75, respectively, after 4 weeks of treatment. The discriminant validity of the CES-D was also supported by its negative correlation with the Bradburn Positive Affect Scale (Bradburn, 1969) and its low correlation with nondepression variables such as medications, disability days, social functioning, and aggression.

Consistent with research demonstrating the relationship between mental illness and significant life events (Dohrenwend & Dohrenwend, 1974), higher depression scores were found among participants who experienced negative life events. The relationship between the CES-D and life events also supports the instrument's sensitivity to mood state.

Weissman et al. (1975, as cited in Radloff, 1977) also demonstrated that CES-D scores decreased after treatment.

Clinical Utility

Limited. Although this instrument has good specificity as well as sensitivity, it is intended for research purposes only.

Research Applicability

High. This is a useful tool for epidemiological studies of depression. Although research on other uses is not as well supported, it has been used to measure change in depressive symptomatology over time and as a screening tool for inclusion in treatment studies.

Source

The CES-D is reprinted in the Appendix. For more information, contact Epidemiology and Psychopathology Research Branch, Room 10C-05, National Institute of Mental Health, 5600 Fishers Lane, Rockville, MD 20857.

Cost

None.

Alternative Forms

The CES-D has been used in many countries in addition to the United States. It has also been used in computer-assisted and telephone interviews. These alternative versions have been adapted by the investigators of each study, but the NIMH does not keep a comprehensive list of alternative forms.

DEPRESSION ANXIETY STRESS SCALES (DASS)

Original Citation

Lovibond, S. H., & Lovibond, P. F. (1995). *Manual for the Depression Anxiety Stress Scales.* Sydney: The Psychology Foundation of Australia. Reprinted with permission from Peter Lovibond.

Purpose

To assess aspects of depression, anxiety, and stress using a dimensional approach.

Population

Adolescents and adults.

Description

The DASS is a 42-item self-report measure. Items fall into three scales: Depression (D), Anxiety (A), and Stress (S), with 14 items per scale. Scales are further divided into subscales of two to five similar items each. Each item is scored from 0 ("did not apply to me at all") to 3 ("applied to me very much, or most of the time") in terms of how much the item applied within the past week.

Background

The DASS was initially developed to assess anxiety and depression while removing the overlap between the two constructs. Specifically, the authors developed the DASS to include all core symptoms of anxiety and depression, while maintaining maximum discrimination between these two scales. The Stress scale was added as factor analyses early on indicated the presence of this factor. The first version of the measure was called the Self-Analysis Questionnaire (SAQ; Lovibond, 1982), which included the same three scales, but with varying numbers of items per scale. The measure was developed using what the authors termed simultaneous multiscale dimensioning, in which item analyses are conducted repeatedly to refine the measure; thus, the measure was revised as data continued to be collected with additional samples, leading to the current DASS.

Administration

Administration time is not specified in the manual, but should range from about 10 to 20 minutes on average. A briefer version, the DASS21, should take approximately half the administration time as the full measure. Both measures may be administered either individually or in groups.

Scoring

Scoring consists of summing the scores for the 14 items within each scale. If using the DASS21, scores may be converted to equivalent DASS scores by multiplying by 2. Scoring templates are included with the manual, as are tables for conversion to Z-scores.

Interpretation

The manual lists cutoff scores for each scale in terms of raw scores, Z-scores, and percentiles. For the Depression Scale, scores 0–9 are considered Normal, 10–13 Mild, 14–20 Moderate, 21–27 Severe, and above 28, Extremely Severe.

Psychometric Properties

Psychometric properties for the DASS were determined based on six samples of nonclinical subjects, for a total of 1,044 men and 1,870 women ranging in age from 17 to 69 years. Several more recent studies (Antony, Bieling, Cox, Enns, & Swinson, 1998; Brown, Korotitsch, Chorpita, & Barlow, 1997) have examined the psychometric properties of the DASS in clinical samples as well.

Norms.   Overall the means and (standard deviations) for the three scales are Depression 6.34 (6.97), Anxiety 4.70 (4.91), Stress 10.11 (7.91). Norms broken down by age and gender are detailed in the manual.

Reliability.   Test–retest data were not described in the manual, but are available for the clinical samples, with the DASS showing good temporal stability (correlations ranging from .71 to .81 with a 2-week interval). Internal consistencies for both normal and clinical samples were high. For the normal sample, alphas were 0.91 for Depression, 0.84 for Anxiety, and 0.90 for Stress, with somewhat lower alphas for the DASS21 scales.

Validity.   The DASS was validated against several standardized measures of the constructs each scale purports to measure. Comparisons with the BDI (BDI; p. 29) and the Beck Anxiety Inventory (BAI; A. T. Beck & Steer, 1990) indicated that the DASS scales differentially correlated with the Beck measures as follows, indicating good convergent and discriminant validity of these two scales: DASS-D and BDI, .74; DASS-D and BAI, .54; DASS-A and BDI, .58; DASS-A and BAI, .58. Comparisons of DASS scales across clinical anxiety and mood disorder diagnostic groups, conducted in the clinical studies referred to above, also supported the validity of the scales.

Clinical Utility

High. The DASS is fairly quick to administer and score, and provides useful information regarding not only depression, but related problems with anxiety and stress, in a way that allows for discriminating among them.

Research Applicability

High. Emotion researchers have noted frequently the degree to which aspects of negative affect such as anxiety and depression overlap, despite the distinction generally drawn between them. The DASS allows for a dimensional assessment of three forms of negative affect, with relatively minimal overlap among these forms. In addition, the DASS has already been used in a number of studies in large research groups.

Alternate Forms

The DASS-21, consisting of half the items of the full DASS, is also available. A Cantonese translation of the DASS is available through Dr. Calais Chan at Prince of Wales Hospital in Hong Kong; e-mail: calaischan@cuhk.edu.hk.

Source

The DASS is reprinted in Appendix B. For additional information, contact The Psychology Foundation, Room 1017A, Level 10 Mathews Building, University of New South Wales, Sydney NSW 2052, Australia. Website: http://www.psy.unsw.edu.au/dass.

Cost

The DASS can be downloaded directly from the website listed above, at no charge. The manual is available at the above address for $25 in Australian or U.S. dollars, or UK£15.00.

DEPRESSION QUESTIONNAIRE (DQ)

Original Citations

Bertolotti, G., Zotti, A. M., Michielin, P., Vidotto, G., & Sanavio, E. (1990). A computerized approach to cognitive behavioural assessment: An introduction to CBA-2.0 Primary Scales. *Journal of Behavior Therapy and Experimental Psychiatry, 21,* 21–27.

Sanavio, E., Bertolotti, G., Michielin, P., Vidotto, G., & Zotti, A. M. (1988). *CBA-2.0 Cognitive behavioral assessment: Scale Primarie. Manuale.* Florence: Organizzazioni Speciali.

Purpose

To measure clinically significant depression, subclinical depressive symptoms, and depression associated with other disturbances.

Population

Adults.

Description

The DQ is a 24-item self-report measure of depressive symptoms developed in Italy. Each item provides a statement (e.g., "I often feel like crying"), and respondents are requested to indicate in a yes/no format whether the statement correctly describes the way they feel "right now." Twenty-two of the items represent the presence of a specific depressive symptom. The remaining 2 items are structured to allow the respondent to deny the presence of a depressive symptom, so that the answer "no" represents higher symptomatology.

Background

Sanavio et al. (1986) developed an instrument entitled the Cognitive Behavioral Assessment-2.0 (CBA-2.0) to evaluate a wide range of behavioral and psychological characteristics, which include anxiety, personality traits, psychophysiological disorders, depressive symptoms, and obsessions and compulsions. Believing that other depression instruments were inadequate for their purposes, the CBA team designed the DQ to assess depressive characteristics to be part of the CBA-2.0. Other depression measures considered by the CBA team were perceived as being too lengthy, had only modest clinical utility and discriminant validity, had not been adequately validated for Italian-speaking participants, had limited utility with subclinically depressed populations, and provided poor translations or limited use in Italy. The DQ was designed to assess depression while overcoming the limitations of these instruments.

Administration

Paper-and-pencil, as well as computerized, versions of the DQ are available. The instrument was designed to be brief and takes approximately 20 minutes to complete.

Scoring

"Yes" responses are scored as 1 point and "no" responses are scored as 0, with two exceptions. For the items which deny a manifestation of depression, "no" responses are scored as 1 point and "yes" responses as 0. The total score is obtained by summing the scores of the individual items. Scores range from 0 to 24. Computer scoring is available for this instrument.

Interpretation

High scores indicate greater depressive symptomatology. A score of 15 has been identified as an appropriate cutoff score to differentiate depressed from nondepressed patients.

Psychometric Properties

Norms.   Bertolotti et al. (1990) provide means and standard deviations for a variety of groups which are subdivided by age and gender. These norms are based on samples of 337 normal adults, 86 adult medical inpatients awaiting endocavitary or retroperitoneal surgery, and 50 adults with chronic pain. All participants were in Italy.

Reliability.   An estimate of the internal consistency of the DQ yielded a Cronbach's alpha estimate of .86. Test–retest correlations were .88 with a 7-day lapse between administrations, and .72 with a 30-day lapse between administrations.

Validity.   Scores on the DQ were compared to scores on the Italian translation of the BDI (p. 29) among 46 depressed psychiatric patients in order to assess the instrument's construct validity. Correlation between the instruments was .56, which was strong enough for the developers to consider the construct valid, and low enough for them to conclude that the DQ measures some things that the BDI does not. Examination of the discriminant validity of the DQ found only one false positive and three false negatives using a cutoff score of 15.

A monofactorial structure was found upon a factor analysis of the DQ using Varimax rotation. A second interpretation of the factor analysis identifies five factors consisting of performance of habitual activities, relationship with others/wish to cry or be dead, oral disturbance, strain, and thoughts of suicide.

Clinical Utility

High. This instrument can be used to discriminate depressed from nondepressed patients, especially in medical settings, or when medical and psychiatric diagnoses cooccur.

Research Applicability

High. This instrument provides a systematic decision-making guideline that increases diagnostic validity and reliability in research settings.

Source

Giorgio Bertolotti, Fondazione Salvatore Maugeri, Clinica del Lavoro e Della Riabilitazione, D.P.R. n. 991 del 15.06.65, Istituto di Ricovero e Cura a Carattere Scientifico, Centro Medico di Tradate, Servizio di Psicologia, Via Roncaccio, 16, I-21049 Tradate, Varese, Italy. Phone: 0331.829630/829631.

Cost

None.

Alternate Forms

Italian, English, and computer-administered forms are available.

DEPRESSION 30 SCALE (D-30)

Original Citation

Dempsey, P. (1964). A unidimensional depression scale for the MMPI. *Journal of Consulting Psychology*, 28, 364–370.

Purpose

To measure depressive symptoms.

Population

Adults.

Description

The D-30 contains 30 MMPI items that are endorsed in a true–false format ("I cry easily," "I brood a great deal"). High scores are associated with an increase in depressive symptoms.

Background

The D-30 was developed from the 60 items originally associated with the Minnesota Multiphasic Personality Inventory-Depression Scale (MMPI-D; p. 73). The MMPI-D Scale was developed to identify depressed people, as well as personality features associated with depression that separate depressed from nondepressed individuals. The D-30 was developed to provide a unidimensional measure of depressive symptoms.

Administration

The D-30 can be administered in an individual or a group format. The entire test requires approximately 10 minutes to complete.

Scoring

A score is derived from summing the items responded to in the keyed direction. The original article contains a table for converting raw scores to T-scores.

Interpretation

The typical interpretive strategy for the D-30 entails determining whether there is a significant T-score elevation. A T-score elevation greater than 70 is considered clinically significant. Perusing the items endorsed in the keyed direction can also be helpful.

Psychometric Properties

Norms.   The normative sample was composed of 280 normal subjects and 144 hospitalized psychiatric patients. The original article contains information for converting raw scores to T-scores.

Reliability.   Split-half reliability estimates using four different samples ranged from .84 to .95. Test-retest reliability for male college students was .92; a similar estimate for female college students was .88.

Validity.   The original article uses a sample of 280 nonpsychiatric patients and a sample of 144 hospitalized psychiatric patients to explore the usefulness of adopting a cutoff score of 70. More recent research (e.g., Fullerton, Wenzel, Lohrenz, & Fahs, 1968; Russo, 1994; Wierzbicki & Bartlett, 1987) presents additional data on the validity of this measure.

Clinical Utility

Limited. This measure is likely to provide a reasonable qualification of depressive symptoms. Unfortunately, the copyrights for the items rest with the University of Minnesota and it may prove difficult to get permission for routine clinical use. In addition, National Computer Systems does not support the stand-alone use of MMPI item parcels.

Research Applicability

High. The D-30 is likely to prove a useful measure of depressive symptoms in research studies.

Source

Items are contained in Dempsey (1964).

Cost

Although the items appear in a variety of published manuscripts (Dempsey, 1964; Russo, 1994), the University of Minnesota retains copyright over the Minnesota Multiphasic Personality Inventory items and permission should be sought prior to duplication. The phone number is (612) 617-1963. Note that the licensed distributor, National Computer Systems, does not provide support for the administration of item parcels.

Alternative Forms

Alternate forms are available in Spanish and other languages.

DIAGNOSTIC INTERVIEW SCHEDULE (DIS-IV)

Original Citation

Robins, L. N., Helzer, J. E., Croughan, J. L., & Ratcliff, K. S. (1981). National Institute of Mental Health Diagnostic Interview Schedule: Its history, characteristics, and validity. *Archives of General Psychiatry*, *38*, 381–389.

Purpose

To diagnose DSM-IV disorders.

Population

Adults.

Description

The DIS-IV is a highly structured interview designed to allow laypersons to determine DSM diagnoses. It consists of 22 individual modules, most of which focus on specific diagnoses (e.g., generalized anxiety disorder) or groups of diagnoses (e.g., specific phobia/social phobia/agoraphobia/panic). Several modules focus on other areas such as demographics and a summary of the interview. Questions are structured so that the interviewer can exit the module at various points as it becomes determined that the disorder in question is not present. All answers are coded according to explicitly stated guidelines, with the coded answers entered into a computer to yield specific diagnoses. Module F assesses depression/dysthymia.

Sample questions, reprinted with the permission of the author, are as follows:

F1.	In your lifetime, have you ever had at least two weeks when nearly every day you felt sad, depressed, or empty most of the time?
F2.	Have you ever had a period of at least two weeks when you lost interest in most things or got no pleasure from things which would usually have made you happy?
F4.	(While) you (were feeling sad, empty or depressed/had lost interest in most things) have you ever had a period of at least two weeks in a row when there was a change in things like your sleeping, your appetite, your energy, or your ability to concentrate and remember?
F25.	Since you first (were depressed/lost interest) for two weeks or longer, have you ever had 2 or more months in a row when you felt OK?
	A. Once you felt OK for two months or longer after an episode, did you ever have another period of (feeling depressed/lost interest) for two weeks or longer?
	B. How many episodes have you had altogether that had at least 2 months of your feeling OK between them?
F30.	When did (your last/the) episode end, when you had (been feeling depressed/lost interest) and had some of these problems nearly every day for at least two weeks?
F32.	Was there any time in the last 12 months when you wanted to talk to a doctor or other health professional about feeling depressed or uninterested in things?

Background

The DIS-IV is the sixth version of the Diagnostic Interview Schedule, which was initially developed in 1978 for use in the National Institute of Mental Health's (NIMH) Epidemiological Catchment Area (ECA) Program. The goal of the ECA Program was to determine the prevalence and incidence rates of various psychiatric disorders in the United States. Given the incredibly large number of diagnostic interviews that needed to be conducted to meet this goal, the need arose for an interview that could be conducted by trained laypeople; this was the impetus for the development of the DIS, which allowed for the assessment of specific diagnostic categories within the DSM-III (the then-current DSM version).

The DIS has been revised during the past several years to meet the needs of a changing system. The major revision is to keep the DIS compatible with the current DSM; thus, the DIS-IV is compatible with the DSM-IV. Other changes have been made as well. For example, categories not included in earlier DIS versions, such as diagnoses arising in childhood (e.g., separation anxiety disorder), are included in the DIS-IV. Also, additional questions have been added to allow for more specificity regarding the course of a disorder, treatment seeking, and links with physical causes, among other areas. Other changes removed aspects of the previous DIS, such as questions related to non-DSM diagnostic systems (e.g., the Feighner system), so as to limit the length of the interview.

Administration

The DIS requires between 90 and 120 minutes for completion, although the authors list several ways in which the interview may be shortened without compromising its validity (e.g., dropping modules not of interest). Note that extensive training of lay interviewers is required.

Scoring

Individual responses are scored according to explicitly stated guidelines, each symptom scored as either Yes or No, without decision-making on the part of the interviewer. These responses are then keyed into a computer, which yields DSM-IV diagnoses based on the patterns of responses provided.

Interpretation

The DIS-IV does not include specific interpretation guidelines. It yields DSM-IV diagnoses, as well as additional information regarding related areas (e.g., treatment utilization and health behaviors).

Psychometric Properties

Norms.   Not applicable.

Reliability.   Test-retest reliability was calculated for the depression module of the DIS-IV in a sample of 140 persons each interviewed twice about depression. Of this sample, 35% were positive for a major depressive episode, and the test–retest kappa was found to be .63 (range .49–.77). The sample was 56% African-American, and 44% female, with a mean age of 36 years.

Validity.   Comparing the DIS to other measures has been difficult since there are few measures that cover the full range of DSM diagnoses. Alternatively, investigators have compared results of the DIS obtained by lay interviewers to results obtained by trained psychiatrists and found that, in general, the scores are comparable (Robins, Helzer, Croughan, & Ratcliff, 1981). The DIS also showed high sensitivity and specificity for lifetime diagnoses of depression with values of 80% and 84%, respectively (Robins, Helzer, Croughan, & Ratcliff, 1981).

Clinical Utility

Limited. The DIS is a lengthy interview, designed for use by highly trained laypersons. Thus, it is unlikely to be useful to professional clinicians whose training allows them access to interviews with better psychometric properties should they wish to use structured diagnostic interviews.

Research Applicability

High. Although a number of questions regarding the validity of the DIS have been raised over the years, it is the most widely used interview for laypersons and is likely to continue to be important in epidemiological research.

Source

DIS Orders, % Lee N. Robins, Ph.D., Department of Psychiatry, Campus Box 8134, Washington University School of Medicine, 4940 Children's Place, St. Louis, MO 63110.

Cost

$50 for DIS-IV interview. Mock interviews for training purposes are available for $25, and two scoring software programs are available as well ($75 for the scoring only, $200 for a program including data entry, cleaning, and scoring).

Alternate Forms

The DIS is available in a number of other languages. A Diagnostic Interview Schedule for Children is also available.

DIAGNOSTIC INVENTORY FOR DEPRESSION (DID)

Original Citation

The DID is currently being developed by Mark Zimmerman, M.D., and his colleagues. Therefore, a primary reference is not available at this time. Expect more information to appear in the literature in the future.

Purpose

To diagnose DSM-IV Major Depressive Disorder, as well as depression-related symptom severity, psychosocial impairment, and life satisfaction.

Population

The original validation studies of the DID were conducted with psychiatric outpatients. Since this instrument is currently being developed, its applicability to other populations has not been examined.

Description

The DID is a 38-item self-report questionnaire that is comprised of three subscales: symptom items, psychosocial functioning, and quality of life. Respondents are requested to answer each question according to how they have been feeling during the past week. Each symptom item addresses a specific DSM-IV (APA, 1994) major depressive symptom. These items include 5-point response scales, ranging from 0 to 4 representing ascending levels of severity. The psychosocial functioning and quality of life scales ask respondents to indicate how much difficulty they have had and how satisfied they have been with specific areas of their lives (e.g., "relationships with your friends"). Responses are indicated according to a 5-point scale ranging from 0 (no difficulty) to 4 (extreme difficulty). A sample item from the symptom scale, with the permission of the author, is reprinted below:

1. During the past week, have you been feeling sad or depressed?
   - 0 No, not at all.
   - 1 Yes, a little bit.
   - 2 Yes, I have felt sad or depressed most of the time.
   - 3 Yes, I have been very sad or depressed nearly all the time.
   - 4 Yes, I have been extremely depressed nearly all the time.

Background

The DID was specifically designed to identify cases of major depression as defined by DSM-IV (APA, 1994) criteria. The authors believe that it improves upon other depression instruments by providing *a priori*-determined cutoffs, as well as an algorithmic approach to diagnosis, that reflects the DSM-IV diagnostic procedure. In this way, the DID minimizes variability between studies that occur when investigators use different cutoff scores. In addition, it reflects clinical diagnostic procedures. The DID is the only self-report instrument for major depression that assesses symptom severity and duration, as well as psychosocial impairment, due to depression and quality of life.

Administration

The DID takes approximately 25 minutes to complete.

Scoring

This instrument uses an algorithmic scoring approach similar to that used in the DSM-IV (APA, 1994).

Interpretation

Results are described according to the following categories: nondepressed, borderline, mild, moderate, and severe.

Psychometric Properties

Norms.   Since the DID is a newly developed instrument, norms are not available at this time.

Reliability.   Internal consistency reliability was measured in a sample of 400 psychiatric outpatients for the 19 symptom items, as well as for the psychosocial functioning and quality of life subscales. Estimates were .91, .90, and .91, respectively. Test–retest reliability coefficients were .93 for the depression subscale, .81 for the psychosocial functioning subscale, and .82 for the quality of life subscale. This test was conducted with a subsample of 74 patients who completed a second DID within 1 week after completing the first.

Validity.   The validity of the DID was examined in a number of ways. First, the DID symptoms scale was compared to the Beck Depression Inventory (p. 29) and showed a correlation of .83. A correlation of .73 was also found between the DID and an extracted Hamilton Rating Scale for Depression (p. 58) score derived from the Schedule for Affective Disorders and Schizophrenia (p. 108). In addition, a correlation of $-.44$ was found between the psychosocial functioning subscale of the DID and the Global Assessment of Functioning Scale DSM-IV (APA, 1994) . Other tests of the validity of the DID showed significant differences between the severity ratings produced by the DID and demonstrated good sensitivity (88.3%) as well as specificity (71.3%).

Clinical Utility

Limited. The DID has not been widely used. However, its close ties to the DSM-IV, its ability to differentiate between levels of symptom severity, and its measurement of psychosocial functioning and quality of life make the DID a promising new measure.

Research Applicability

Limited. Again, the DID is newly developed. The authors hope that this instrument will decrease the diagnostic variability often found between research studies.

Source

Mark Zimmerman, M.D., Rhode Island Hospital, Outpatient Psychiatry, Bayside 5, 235 Plain Street, Providence, RI 02905.

Cost

Information about the cost of the DID is not available at this time. Interested investigators can contact Dr. Zimmerman for more details.

Alternative Forms

None.

HAMILTON DEPRESSION INVENTORY (HDI)

Original Citation

Reynolds, W. M., & Kobak, K. A. (1995). *Hamilton Depression Inventory (HDI): Professional manual.* Odessa, FL: Psychological Assessment Resources.

Purpose

To assess an individual's current level of depressive symptomatology.

Population

Adults aged 18–89 years.

Description

The HDI is a self-report measure of depressive symptoms that was based on the original Hamilton Rating Scale for Depression (p. 58). Although the HDI technically contains 23 items, respondents are requested to answer 38 questions, as certain items contain several parts. For example, one item contains 4 questions concerning the frequency of experiencing four different types of physical symptoms (i.e., heart pounding, sweating, gastrointestinal problems, headaches). Respondents are asked to use the past 2 weeks as the frame of reference. Sample items, reprinted with the permission of the publisher, include the following*:

*Reproduced by special permission of the Publisher, Psychological Assessment Resources, Inc. © 1995 by PAR, Inc.

    1d. How often do you cry or feel like crying?
        0) Rarely.
        1) Slightly more than usual for me.
        2) Quite a bit more than usual for me.
        3) Nearly all the time.
    10a. How often have you felt anxious or nervous over the past 2 weeks?
        0) Not at all or rarely (if 0, skip to Question 11).
        1) Occasionally.
        2) Often (about half the time).
        3) Very often.
        4) Almost all of the time.
    10b. On average, how bad was the feeling of anxiety or nervousness over the past 2 weeks?
        1) Mild.
        2) Moderate.
        3) Severe.
        4) Very severe.
    19. Do you feel helpless or incapable of getting everyday tasks done?
        0) Not at all.
        1) Occasionally.
        2) Often.
        3) Almost constantly.
    23. Over the past 2 weeks, how often did you have difficulty making decisions?
        0) Not at all or rarely.
        1) Occasionally.
        2) Often (about half of the time).
        3) Very often.
        4) Almost all of the time.

In addition to the basic 23-item HDI, a 17-item version can be derived (HDI-17) that parallels the content and scoring of the original, standard 17-item clinician-administered HRSD. Further, a 9-item short-form version is available that can be used as a brief screening device in either clinical or research settings. Last, an HDI melancholia subscale exists to provide information specifically concerning the presence and severity of melancholic features associated with depressive disorders as delineated in DSM-IV.

Background

The HDI was developed to provide for a self-report version of the HRSD, as well as to be more consistent with DSM-IV criteria. In addition, the authors indicate that unlike other self-report measures of depression, the HDI contains questions that are geared to assess both the frequency and severity of a given symptom in order to provide for greater precision. The HDI evolved from earlier work these authors engaged in concerning a computer-administered version of the HRSD.

Administration

The full-scale HDI requires approximately 10–15 minutes to complete.

Scoring

Instructions are provided on how to derive the various raw scores (e.g., full-scale HDI; 17-item HDI; melancholia subscale). Some norms are also provided in the manual to allow for the conversion of raw scores into percentile ranks and T-scores. The range of the total HDI score is 0–73. The higher the score, the more severe the depressive symptoms.

Interpretation

For the full-scale HDI, a raw score of 19, which represents a T-score of 71, can be used as the cutoff to designate individuals as candidates for treatment referral.

Psychometric Properties

Norms. Normative data were gathered from 506 adults (235 men, 271 women) living in a variety of community settings from the midwestern and western parts of the country. The ages ranged from 18 to 89 years.

Reliability. Internal consistency estimates range from .90 for the HDI-17 version to .93 for the full-scale HDI. With regard to test–retest reliability, the correlation was found to be .95 over a period of about 1 week.

Validity. Based on a sample of 403 interviews with adults, the HDI was found to correlate .94 with scores using the clinician-rated HRSD. It is also highly correlated with other self-report measures of depression (e.g., BDI; p. 29) and depression-related constructs (e.g., suicide questionnaire, hopelessness).

Clinical Utility

High. Research contained in the manual points to the substantial degree of clinical efficacy and utility regarding the HDI when it is used to discriminate between depressed and nondepressed adults based on the single cutoff score.

Research Applicability

Unknown at present, although it would seem to be high given that the HDI appears to possess strong psychometric properties and has significant clinical utility.

Source

Psychological Assessment Resources, Inc., P. O. Box 998, Odessa, FL 33556. Phone: 800-331-TEST.

Cost

$79 for manual, five test booklets, 25 summary sheets, 25 answer sheets, and five short-form booklets.

Alternative Forms

A nine-item short form exists.

HAMILTON RATING SCALE FOR DEPRESSION (HRSD)

Original Citations

Hamilton, M. (1960). A rating scale for depression. *Journal of Neurology, Neurosurgery and Psychiatry, 23,* 56–62.

Hamilton, M. (1967). Development of a rating scale for primary depressive illness. *British Journal of Social and Clinical Psychology, 6,* 278–296.

Purpose

To assess the severity of depressive symptoms as well as to measure changes in a patient's condition over time.

Population

Adults who have been diagnosed with a depressive disorder.

Description

The HRSD is a 21-item clinician-rated instrument that is completed following a thorough clinical interview. Each item presents a symptom of depression (e.g., depressed mood, guilt, insomnia) and is rated according to its severity as experienced by the patient *during the past few days or week.* Of the 17 items whose scores are considered, 9 items include 5-point scales ranging from 0 to 4 which represent ascending levels of severity. The remaining 8 items include 3-point scales ranging from 0 to 2, also representing ascending levels of symptom severity.

Hamilton (1967) recommended that clinicians interview other informants whenever the accuracy of patient reports is in doubt. He also recommended that clinicians keep direct questions to a minimum, and that they ask questions in a variety of manners (e.g., ask "How badly do you sleep?" as well as "How well do you sleep?"). The HRSD does not provide specific probes.

Background

The original HRSD was developed by Hamilton to quantify the information obtained after interviewing patients who had already been diagnosed with depression. Results of a more detailed factor analysis supporting its validity were published seven years later (Hamilton, 1967). Since then, researchers have produced numerous variations of the HRSD which may alter, add, or delete items. For example, the NIMH Early Clinical Drug Evaluation Program produced a version of the HRSD which included anchor points describing different levels of each item. Another modified version was used in the NIMH Treatment of Depression Collaborative Research Program, which added items to assess hypersomnia, weight gain, and increased appetite. Other versions can be located on various websites such as www.glaxowellcome.com. Two forms of the Revised Hamilton Rating Scale for Depression are described on pp. 99 and 101 in this book.

Administration

Hamilton (1967) suggests that clinicians take at least 30 minutes to conduct a clinical interview in order to obtain adequate information for completing the HRSD. Once the information has been solicited, the questionnaire takes approximately 10 minutes to complete.

Scoring

Approaches to scoring vary among the different versions of the HRSD. The original 21-item version of the HRSD is scored by summing the ratings for each item to produce total scores ranging from 0 to 50. Hamilton (1960) recommended that two interviewers conduct a joint interview, then complete separate rating scales and add their scores to produce a total score ranging from 0 to 100. It is important to note the method employed for scoring when reporting results of studies using the HRSD.

Interpretation

Higher scores indicate greater severity of depressive symptoms. Some factor analyses have identified two relatively stable factors in the HRSD representing a general factor of depressive illness and a bipolar factor representing varying degrees of psychomotor symptoms ranging between agitation and retardation. A comprehensive review of factor analysis of the HRSD is provided by Hedlund and Vieweg (1979).

Psychometric Properties

Numerous investigations of the psychometric properties of the HRSD have been conducted. However, attempts to compare these studies have met with difficulty since there are so many variations of the HRSD and the changes have not always been reported. The psychometric properties reported here are based on a comprehensive review provided by Hedlung and Vieweg (1979) of the psychometric properties of the original 21-item version.

Norms.   Not applicable.

Reliability.   Most interrater reliability coefficients have been ≥ .84. One study of the internal consistency of the HRSD reported correlations between individual items and the total score ranging from .45 to .78 (Schwab, Bialon, & Holzer, 1967).

Validity.   The validity of this instrument has been established by comparing HRSD scores to scores on numerous self-report and clinician rated measures for depression. Comparisons with the BDI (p. 29) yielded correlations ranging from .21 to .82 with a median of .58, and comparisons with the Zung Self-Rating Depression Scale (p. 120) ranged from .38 to .62 with a median of .45. Comparisons were made among samples of depressed patients prior to treatment, and these relationships generally increased after treatment. See Hedlund and Vieweg's (1979) extensive review of the validity data for the HRSD for further details.

Clinical Utility

High. The HRSD is one of the most widely used instruments to quantify data gathered from clinical interviews.

Research Applicability

High. The HRSD has been used extensively to measure the treatment effects of various psychotherapies as well as pharmacological interventions for depression. Researchers are urged to note which version of the HRSD was used when reporting research results.

Source

The HRSD is in the public domain, and variations of the instrument can be found in a number of sources. The original HRSD is printed in Hamilton's (1967) article, and an adapted version is published in Hedlund and Vieweg's (1979) article. The instrument can be found in other depression and assessment guides, and on websites on the internet such as www.glaxo-wellcome.com. It is also reprinted in Appendix B.

Cost

None.

Alternative Forms

Many variations of the HRSD are available, and professionals should note which version is being employed when selecting the instrument or reporting results.

HOPELESSNESS DEPRESSION SYMPTOM QUESTIONNAIRE (HDSQ)

Original Citation

Metalsky, G. I ., & Joiner, T. E. (1997). The Hopelessness Depression Symptom Questionnaire. *Cognitive Therapy and Research, 21,* 359–384.

Purpose

To measure symptoms related to the hopelessness subtype of depression.

Population

Adults.

Description

The Hopelessness Depression Symptom Questionnaire (HDSQ) is a 32-item self-report measure of "hopelessness depression." Each item consists of four statements regarding a particular component of hopelessness depression. Respondents are requested to read each group of statements and to choose the statement that best describes themselves during the past 2 weeks. The 32 items form eight subscales: motivational deficit, interpersonal dependency, psychomotor retardation, anergia, apathy/anhedonia, insomnia, difficulty in concentration/brooding, and suicidality.

Background

Hopelessness depression has been proposed as a specific subtype of depression that is characterized by a specific etiology, course, and treatment (Abramson, Metalsky, & Alloy, 1989). The HDSQ was developed so that the symptoms thought to be associated with hopelessness depression, rather than with depression per se, could be adequately assessed. The authors note that existing measures of depression are not sufficient to measure hopelessness depression due to their omission of some relevant symptoms and/or inclusion of nonrelevant ones. They further note that sadness was not included in the original HDSQ due to the large number of measures already including that symptom, but that a sadness subscale as well as a "mood-exacerbated negative cognitions" subscale are currently being added to the measure.

Administration

When self-administered, the HDSQ can be completed in under 10 minutes. It can be administered either individually or in group formats.

Scoring

Scores are obtained by summing the rating for each item, both within the eight subscales and for total scores. Scores for each subscale range from 0 to 12, and total scores from 0 to 96, with higher scores reflecting greater levels of hopelessness depression.

Interpretation

Cutoff scores are not provided, although scores may be compared with norms compiled on undergraduate samples, as listed below.

Psychometric Properties

Psychometric properties are based on 435 undergraduate students (248 female, 187 male). Of these, 174 students completed the HDSQ a second time, 10 weeks following their first administration.

Norms.   The mean score was 11.38 (SD = 9.67), with scores ranging from 0 to 58. Mean scores for the subscales, each comprised of four items, ranged from .40 (SD = 1.25) for suicidality to 2.36 (SD = 1.71) for dependency.

Reliability.   Internal consistency was high, with an alpha value of .93 for the full HDSQ. Alphas for the subscales ranged from .70 (motivational deficit) to .86 (both anergia and suicidality). Test–retest reliability over a period of several weeks was moderate (r = .58; T. Joiner, personal communication, February 19, 1999).

Validity.   Factor analyses yielded eight factors that matched the eight subscales of the HDSQ, supporting the first-order structure of the measure. The second-order model, positing the 8 subscales as all part of the higher order factor of hopelessness depression, was then tested using a LISREL approach in which the one latent variable (hopelessness depression) was measured by eight observed variables. This model fit the data well, with a goodness of fit index of .98 and adjusted goodness of fit index of .97, as well as a χ^2 (df = 18) of 27.63.

Clinical Utility

High. The HDSQ is relatively quick to complete, and provides information on a specific type of depression not well measured by other available instruments.

Research Applicability

High. For researchers examining the hopelessness theory of depression especially, the HDSQ should prove useful. It is the only measure including symptoms specifically thought to be related to this subtype of depression.

Source

The HDSQ is reprinted in Appendix B. For additional information, contact Gerald I. Metalsky, Ph.D., Department of Psychology, Lawrence University, P.O. Box 599, Appleton, WI 54912-0599, or Thomas Joiner, Ph.D., Department of Psychology, Florida State University, Tallahassee, FL 32306-1270.

Cost

None.

Alternative Forms

None.

HOSPITAL ANXIETY AND DEPRESSION SCALE (HADS)

Original Citation

Zigmond, A. S., & Snaith, R. P. (1983). The Hospital Anxiety and Depression Scale. *Acta Psychiatrica Scandinavica, 67*, 361–370.

Purpose

To screen for mood disorders among nonpsychiatric hospital patients.

Population

Medical (nonpsychiatric) outpatients between the ages of 16 and 65.

Description

The HADS is a 14-item self-report instrument that measures symptoms of depression and anxiety. Items which reflect symptoms of both emotional disorder and physical disorder (e.g., dizziness) were purposely excluded from the HADS in order to reduce the probability of false-positive diagnoses. Seven of the items reflect symptoms of depression and the other 7 reflect symptoms of anxiety. Each item presents a statement and is followed by a 4-point Likert-type response scale representing increasing or decreasing levels of frequency. Respondents are requested to read each item and underline the reply which comes closest to how they have been feeling during the past week. Responses to the items alternate so that the first response indicates maximum severity in one item, and the last response indicates maximum severity in the next item. Sample items are reprinted below with the permission of the publisher, NFER-NELSON.

I still enjoy the things I used to enjoy:
 Definitely as much
 Not quite so much
 Only a little
 Hardly at all
I can laugh and see the funny side of things:
 As much as I always could
 Not quite so much now
 Definitely not so much now
 Not at all
I can enjoy a good book or radio or TV programme:
 Often
 Sometimes
 Not often
 Very seldom

Background

This instrument was developed in response to the perceived need for clinicians to be able to quickly screen for emotional disorders in nonpsychiatric hospital clinics. Standard depression instruments produced biased results because they were unable to discriminate between the physiological symptoms of psychiatric illness versus medical illness. One goal of the HADS is to allow patients to quickly complete it while waiting for their medical appointments. In order to keep the questionnaire brief, the authors decided to assess only for depression and anxiety since these are the most prevalent emotional disorders seen in hospital practice.

Another aim of the authors was to provide an instrument that could distinguish between symptoms of depression and symptoms of anxiety.

Administration

The scale takes about 10 minutes to complete and instructions for the patient are included on the form.

Scoring

The anxiety and depression subscales are scored separately for this instrument simply by adding the scores of each item for each subscale. Scores range from 0 to 21 for both the anxiety and depression subscales.

Interpretation

Higher scores indicate greater depression or anxiety. Zigmond and Snaith (1983) found that cutoff scores of ≤ 7 for noncases, 8–10 for doubtful cases, and ≥ 11 for definite cases produced the best diagnostic sensitivity and specificity for both the anxiety and depression scales.

Psychometric Properties

Norms. Moorey et al. (1991) examined HADS scores of 573 people with cancer at the time of their initial diagnosis or first recurrence. Mean depression scores among this population were 5.44 (SD = 4.07, range 0–19). Less than 9% of this group scored above the cutoff.

Reliability. The psychometric properties of the HADS were tested on 100 general medical outpatients. The internal consistency, which was measured by calculating Spearman correlations between each item and the total score of the remaining items for each of the first 50 participants, yielded a range of .60–.30 for the depression subscale. Another test of the internal consistency of the HADS yielded a Cronbach's alpha of .90 for the depression scale in a sample of 568 cancer patients (Moorey et al., 1991).

Validity. The concurrent validity was tested by comparing scores on the HADS to 5-point psychiatric ratings of the 100 general medical patients described above (Zigmond and Snaith, 1983). Using the cutoff scores of ≤ 7 for normal, 8–10 for borderline, and ≥ 11 for affected cases, these comparisons yielded a 1% false-negative rate and a 1% false-positive rate for the HADS. The psychiatric interview and HADS correlated .79 for the depression subscale.

A factor analysis by Moorey et al. (1991) showed that the total HADS measures two factors among a population of cancer patients. This study supports the author's assertion that the anxiety and depression scales measure separate constructs.

Clinical Utility

High. The low rates of false positives and false negatives make the HADS a useful screening tool and the cutoff scores help identify probable clinical levels of depression. Its brief administration is also preferable for medical settings.

Research Applicability

Limited. Initial psychometric data on the HADS look promising. More research is needed to support the utility of the HADS among various medical populations in addition to general medical outpatients and cancer patients.

Source

Zigmond and Snaith (1983). Test materials, which include scoring templates, are also available from NFER-Nelson Publishing Company, Ltd., Darville House, 2 Oxford Road East, Windsor, Berkshire, SL4 1DF, U.K. Phone: 011 44 1753 858 961.

Cost

None if obtained through Zigmond and Snaith (1983). Prices vary depending upon the amount of forms requested through NFER-Nelson.

Alternative Forms

Arabic, Dutch, French, German, Hebrew, Swedish, Italian, and Spanish versions of the HADS are available at no charge from R. P. Snaith. Norwegian, Danish, and Cantonese versions have also been reported in the literature.

INVENTORY OF DEPRESSIVE SYMPTOMATOLOGY (IDS)

Original Citation

Rush, A. J., Gullion, C. M., Basco, M. R., Jarrett, R. B., & Trivedi, M. H. (1996). The Inventory of Depressive Symptomatology (IDS): Psychometric properties. *Psychological Medicine, 26,* 477–486.

Purpose

To measure overall depressive symptom severity, discriminate between depressed and euthymic states, and provide a sensitive measure of symptom change during treatment.

Population

Adult inpatients and outpatients with Major Depressive Disorder (MDD).

Description

The IDS is available in both self-report (IDS-SR) and clinician-rated (IDS-C) forms. Both forms contain 30 items which measure ascending levels of frequency, duration, and intensity/severity of symptoms along a 4-point response scale ranging from 0 to 3. The response scales are identical for both forms, and the items are accounted for by three factors: (a) a cognitive/mood factor, (b) an anxiety/arousal factor, and (c) sleep regulation for both forms, but also appetite regulation and leaden paralysis for the IDS-SR.

Clinicians administering the IDS-C ask respondents scripted questions about how they have been feeling during the past 7 days (e.g., "How have you been sleeping in the past week?"). Then they choose the answer that best represents the respondent's reply, considering the frequency, duration, and intensity/severity of the symptom. Each item of the IDS-SR presents a specific depressive symptom (e.g., "Feeling Sad") and asks respondents to choose the answer that best describes them during the past 7 days (e.g., "I feel sad more than half the time.")

Background

Believing that the Hamilton Rating Scale for Depression (Hamilton, 1960; p. 58) inadequately covered the symptoms of depression and did not produce clear categories of depressive symptoms upon factor analysis, Rush et al. (1986) developed a 28-item version of the IDS-C. Their aim was to cover a more complete range of criterion symptoms, reduce the amount of confounded items (items which measured more than one symptom at once), exclude items that are infrequently observed in depression (e.g., obsessions and compulsions), and measure only one factor or several clearly defined factors of depression. The IDS-SR was developed in order to provide a comparable self-report version that could be directly compared to the IDS-C, while also improving upon the content-related limitations of the Carroll Rating Scale for Depression (Carroll et al., 1981; p. 63), the most commonly used self-report comparison to the HRS-D.

Two additional items were later added to the 28-item versions of the IDS-C and IDS-SR in order to assess atypical symptom features as defined in the DSM-IV. Although the 28-item version of the IDS is still available, the developers recommend the 30-item version because it is more complete.

Administration

The IDS-C and the IDS-SR each takes approximately 30–45 minutes to complete.

Scoring

Because the IDS-C and the IDS-SR contain identical items, they are scored in the same manner. Although the instruments contain 30 items, respondents reply to only 1 of 2 items assessing both appetite and weight change (either for increase or decrease). Therefore, only 28 of the 30 items are scored, and the scores of these items are summed to provide a total score. The maximum score is 90. Higher scores indicate higher severity of symptoms.

Interpretation

The authors provide the following cutoff scores to describe symptom severity for the 30-item version of the IDS-C: ≤ 13, normal; 14–22, mild; 23–30, moderate; 31–38, moderate to severe; 39+, severe. The following cutoff scores are provided for the 30-item version of the IDS-SR: ≤ 15, normal; 16–24, mild; 25–32, moderate; 33–40, moderate to severe; 41+, severe. However, the authors note that these cutoff scores are solely based on clinical judgment, and not empirical data. Results of an analysis suggest that the optimal cutoff point to distinguish between symptomatic and euthymic subjects is ≥ 13 for the IDS-C and ≥ 18 for the IDS-SR (Rush et al., 1996).

Psychometric Properties

The psychometric properties of the IDS-C and the IDS-SR 30-item versions are based on 337 adult outpatients with current MDD and 118 adult euthymic subjects.

Norms.   Means and standard deviations are reported for the 28-item versions of the IDS-C and IDS-SR in Rush et al. (1996). Other norms can be obtained from the author.

Reliability. Cronbach's alpha was used to measure internal consistency of 30-item versions of the IDS-C and the IDS-SR. Estimates were found to be .94 for both forms when all subjects were included in the analysis. However, estimates were .67 and .77, respectively, when only the subjects with current MDD were included. Other estimates of the internal consistency were .77 for the IDS-C and .81 for the IDS-SR among patients with MDD. Interrater reliability for the IDS-C, using intraclass correlations, was found to be .96.

Validity. In one study estimating both instruments' concurrent validity, the IDS-C and the IDS-SR, along with the HRSD (p. 58) and the BDI (p. 29), were compared to subjects' clinical severity as described by the DSM-III-R fifth digit. The IDS-C and the IDS-SR (30-item versions) correlated with the DSM-III-R fifth digit .62 and .54, respectively. These relationships were comparable to those found for the HRSD (.48) and the BDI (.62). The discriminant validity of the IDS-C and IDS-SR was also demonstrated by their ability to significantly differentiate groups of depressed and euthymic individuals ($p < .0001$). Specificity was found to be .95 for the IDS-C and .94 for the IDS-SR. Sensitivity was found to be .997 for both versions.

Clinical Utility

High. The IDS-C and IDS-SR rate symptom severity based on time experienced rather than intensity, making them compatible with DSM-III-R and DSM-IV diagnostic criteria, the most widely accepted clinical approaches for diagnosing depression.

Research Applicability

High. Research shows that the IDS-C and the IDS-SR are sensitive to treatment effects.

Source

The IDS is reprinted in Appendix B. For more information, contact Dr. A. John Rush, Department of Psychiatry at St. Paul, POB 1, Suite 600, 5969 Harry Hines Boulevard, Dallas, TX 75235-9101.

Cost

None.

Alternative Forms

An Italian record form of the IDS is available. Results of one study using this form can be found in Tondo, Burrai, Scamonatti, Weissenburger, and Rush (1988).

IPAT DEPRESSION SCALE

Original Citation

Krug, S. E., & Laughlin, J. E. (1976). *Handbook for the IPAT Depression Scale*. Champaign, IL: Institute for Personality and Ability Testing.

Purpose

To measure depressive symptoms.

Population

Males and females age 16 years and older.

Description

The IPAT Depression Scale contains 36 items that assess thoughts and feelings related to depression (e.g., "My zest for work is high," "I feel my health is run down and I should see a doctor soon"). Respondents are asked to check one of three options for each item. Four additional items are used to moderate the relationship between the IPAT Depression Scale and measures of anxiety. Subjects respond to each item using a 3-point scale of agreement.

Background

Krug and Lauglin (1976) developed the IPAT Depression Scale based on seven depression factors including such traits as somatic complaints, feelings of guilt, and excessive self-criticism. Because the scale was significantly correlated with anxiety, four additional items were added. These items relate to anxiety and are used to suppress the relationship between the scale and measures of depression.

Administration

The IPAT Depression Scale requires 10–20 minutes to complete and can be administered in an individual or a group setting.

Scoring

The scorer should first check to make sure there are no patterns to the answers that might suggest deliberate distortion. A scoring key is then placed over the answer sheet and the 36 depression items are scored and added together. Finally, the 4 suppressor items are scored, added together, and subtracted from the total for the 36-item depression score.

Interpretation

The IPAT Depression Scale generates a score that reflects the overall level of depression. High scores indicate the endorsement of more depression-related symptoms.

Psychometric Properties

Norms.   Norms were developed from over 1,000 individually diagnosed psychiatric cases and several thousand normal controls who were randomly selected from more than 60 testing sites. Norms are provided for converting raw scores to Sten scores and/or percentiles. Data are available on a variety of clinical groups.

Reliability.   Reliability was examined on a number of different groups, including depressives ($N = 67$), clinical samples (excluding depressives) ($N = 728$), prisoners ($N = 211$), alcoholics ($N = 195$), narcotic addicts ($N = 69$), college students ($N = 458$), and adult controls ($N = 632$). Coefficient alpha estimates ranged between .88 and .93. Comparisons were also conducted on reliabilities between uncorrected and corrected scores within male convicts ($N = 59$), college undergraduates ($N = 79$), and college females ($N = 109$). Coefficient alpha estimates ranged from .85 to .94.

Validity.   Validity of the test was examined through an evaluation of its underlying factor structure, ability to discriminate among different groups, and theoretical consistency with other constructs. Results found the IPAT Depression Scale to be quite satisfactory within each of the areas mentioned. With regard to how well the test score correlates with depression, an obtained correlation of .88 between the scale and a "pure depression factor" was observed using 1,904 normal and clinical cases.

Clinical Utility

High. The IPAT Depression Scale is a useful self-report measure of depression. To minimize concerns that could arise when asking clients to complete a measure of depression, the booklet refers to the scale as a "Personal Assessment Inventory." The questionnaire is easily administered and can serve as a screen for depression-related symptoms. Norms are available for a variety of samples.

Research Utility

High. The IPAT Depression Scale can be easily administered in an individual or group format. Hand scoring keys simplify the scoring process and the high degree of internal consistency makes it a valuable measure of depressive symptoms. The availability of a correction factor that controls for the covariation of anxiety-related symptoms would also prove useful in depression-related studies.

Source

Institute for Personality and Ability Testing, P. O. Box 1188, Champaign, IL 61824. Phone: 800-225-IPAT.

Cost

A variety of options are available (e.g., manual, scoring key, test booklets, testing kit, etc.). For up-to-date information, contact IPAT.

Alternative Forms

None.

MANUAL FOR THE DIAGNOSIS OF MAJOR DEPRESSION (MDMD)

Original Citation

Huyser, J., De Jonghe, F., Jonkers, F., & Schalken, H. F. A. (1996). The manual for the Diagnosis of Major Depression (MDMD): Description and reliability. *International Journal of Methods in Psychiatric Research*, 6, 1–4.

Purpose

To diagnose major depression and its subtypes (except "with psychotic features") as defined by DSM-III-R.

Population

Adults.

Description

The MDMD is a clinician-rated instrument that includes a guideline for conducting a diagnostic interview, a glossary, and a scoring form. Clinicians rate the severity of depressive symptoms as experienced "during the worst period of the current episode" (pp. 2–3).

Background

The MDMD was developed for use in psychiatric outpatient clinics. It was designed to obtain the same amount of information as a fully structured interview while being less rigid and allowing clinicians to stay within the time restraints of an outpatient appointment. It is intended for use when a diagnosis of major depression is suspected and provides clinicians with guidelines for confirming or ruling out this diagnosis.

Administration

The MDMD takes approximately 20–30 minutes to complete. Assuming that the clinician already has sufficient training in DSM-III-R diagnosis and clinical interviewing, 2–4 hours of training on administering the MDMD is adequate. When conducting the MDMD, it is assumed that organic mental disorders, psychotic disorders (including psychotic depression), and bipolar disorder have already been ruled out.

Scoring

The MDMD provides categorical results indicating inclusion in or exclusion from the diagnosis of major depression and its subcategories.

Interpretation

Results of the MDMD allow clinicians to diagnose or rule out major depression. When a diagnosis of major depression is present, results are further divided into the subcategories of "single type," "recurrent type," and "chronic type."

Psychometric Properties

Norms.   Not applicable.

Reliability.   Test-retest reliability was tested on a sample of 50 psychiatric outpatients in an academic medical center in Amsterdam. The lapse between administration ranged from 4 to 95 days, and the raters were different for each administration. The test–retest reliability coefficient was .82 for the overall diagnosis of major depression, .46 for melancholic type, .72 for single type, .78 for recurrent type, and .70 for chronic type.

Validity.   Not available.

Clinical Utility

Limited. However, results look promising and Huyser et al. (1996) report that clinicians are satisfied with its utility. However, more research is needed on its reliability and validity in order to support the meaning of the MDMD results.

Research Applicability

Limited. Although applicable to research settings, more research is needed to support the meaning of the MDMD results.

Source

Frans de Jonghe, M.D., Ph.D., van Breestraat 41, 1071 ZG Amsterdam, The Netherlands.

Cost

None.

Alternate Forms

None.

MINNESOTA MULTIPHASIC PERSONALITY INVENTORY 2 (MMPI-2) DEPRESSION SCALE

Original Citation

Butcher, J. N., Dahlstrom, W. G., Graham, J. R., Tellegren, A., & Kaemmer, B. (1989). *Minnesota Multiphasic Personality Inventory-2 (MMPI-2): Manual for administration and scoring*. Minneapolis, MN: University of Minnesota Press.

Purpose

To assess levels of psychiatric symptoms and personality patterns in adults. The D-Scale was designed to measure level of depressive symptoms, as well as several personality features associated with depression.

Population

Adults.

Description

The MMPI-2 contains 567 items that are endorsed in a true-false format. Items are organized into three basic validity scales and 10 basic clinical scales. *T*-score conversions are used so that across-scale comparisons can be made. The Depression Scale (D-Scale) is one of the 10 basic scales and contains 57 true-false items (e.g., "My sleep is fitful and disturbed," "I brood a great deal"). High scores indicate greater levels of depression. The D-Scale is not unidimensional.

Background

The MMPI was first published in 1942 (Hathaway & McKinley, 1942) and was designed to help mental health workers assess a variety of psychiatric disorders. Butcher et al. (1989) revised the original version, which resulted in the publication of the MMPI-2. Surveys of test usage in the United States have consistently found the MMPI-2 rated as the most frequently employed objective personality measure (e.g., Lubin, Larsen, & Matarazzo, 1984). The D-Scale in the original version contained 60 items. Three of these items were dropped due to objectionable content; thus, the MMPI-2 D Scale contains 57 items.

Administration

The entire test requires approximately 90 minutes to complete. The D-Scale requires approximately 12 minutes to complete.

Scoring

A raw score is derived from summing the D-Scale items responded to in the keyed direction. This raw score can then be converted to a T-score.

Interpretation

The typical interpretive strategy for the D-Scale entails first looking at whether this scale has a significant T-score elevation. The manual suggests that T-score elevations greater than 65 are significant. If the T-score is significant, then a more thorough review using the Harris–Lingoes Depression Subscales is warranted. Finally, a perusal of the items endorsed may also prove beneficial.

Psychometric Properties

Norms.   The restandardization sample consisted of 1,138 males and 1,562 females. The sample approximated national norms regarding age, geographic distribution, income, marital status, and race. The manual contains information for converting raw scores to T-scores.

Reliability.   Coefficient alpha estimates for the 10 clinical scales range from .34 to .87. Estimates for the D-scale range from .59 for males ($N = 1,095$) to .64 for females ($N = 1,374$). Test–retest reliability estimates for the 10 clinical scales range from .72 to .92. One-week test–retest reliability for the D-Scale is estimated at .75.

Validity. Literally thousands of published studies have used the MMPI and reviews have consistently appeared in the *Mental Measurement Yearbook* (e.g., Archer, 1992; Nicholas, 1992). Recent research on the D-Scale suggests problems with sensitivity and positive predictive power (e.g., Elwood, 1993). A particular concern relates to the fact that it is not unidimensional. A fairly sophisticated analysis of the D-Scale found the 57 items could be organized into two different groupings (Chang, 1996). Chang described these parcels as reflecting either mental or physical depression.

Clinical Utility

Limited. Because the MMPI-2 contains 567 items, the time required to administer and score the inventory would seem greater than the potential benefit. Although the items contained in the D-Scale are readily available in a variety of places (e.g., Graham, 1993; Chang, 1996) and raw score to *T*-score conversions are also available, National Computer Systems does not provide support for single-scale administration.

Research Utility

Limited. Although considerable research exists on both the MMPI-2 and the D-Scale, some of the research on the D-Scale has not been positive (e.g., Elwood, 1993). Indeed, D-Scale elevations are not easily interpretable given that the scale does not reflect a unidimensional construct (e.g., Chang, 1996).

Source

National Computer Systems, Assessment Sales Dept., 5605 Green Circle Drive, Minnetonka, MN. Phone: 800-627-7271. Website: www.ncs.com.

Cost

Contact NCS for current prices, as multiple options are available.

Alternative Forms

Alternate forms are available in Spanish and other languages.

MONTGOMERY–ASBERG DEPRESSION RATING SCALE (MADRS)

Original Citation

Montgomery, S. A., & Asberg, M. (1979). A new depression scale designed to be sensitive to change. *British Journal of Psychiatry, 134*, 382–389.

Purpose

To assess depression symptoms, focusing on effects of antidepressant treatment.

Population

Adults receiving antidepressant medication treatment.

Description

The MADRS is a clinician-rated measure of depressive symptoms. The measure consists of 10 items, each representing depressive symptoms that are sensitive to change, such as sadness, sleep, and inner tension. Items are rated on a 7-point scale with descriptive anchors at even-numbered ratings (e.g., "No sadness," "Looks dispirited, but does brighten up without difficulty"). The authors note that ratings are based on a clinical interview, but that information from other sources should be used to fill in missing information when necessary.

Two sample items are printed below, with permission of the publisher and authors:

> Item #1: Apparent Sadness
> Representing despondency, gloom and despair (more than just ordinary transient low spirits), reflected in speech, facial expression, and posture. Rate by depth and inability to brighten up.
> 0—No Sadness.
> 1
> 2—Looks dispirited but does brighten up without difficulty.
> 3
> 4—Appears sad and unhappy most of the time.
> 5
> 6—Looks miserable all the time. Extremely despondent.
>
> Item #5: Reduced Appetite
> Representing the feeling of a loss of appetite compared with when well. Rate by loss of desire for food or the need to force oneself to eat.
> 0—Normal or increased appetite.
> 1
> 2—Slightly reduced appetite.
> 3
> 4—No appetite. Food is tasteless.
> 5
> 6—Needs persuasion to eat at all.

Background

The MADRS was developed to detect changes in depressive symptoms following antidepressant medication treatment. The authors noted that existing depression scales often fail to detect differences between active drugs, or between drug versus placebo, and that this may be because the scales were not developed to be sensitive specifically to these effects.

Item selection for the MADRS was based on ratings from 106 depressed patients on the

Comprehensive Psychopathological Rating Scale (CPRS; Asberg, Montgomery, Perris, Schalling, & Sevall, 1978) both prior to and following a 4-week treatment period.

Administration

The measure is rated simultaneously with the administration of a clinical interview, and requires approximately 5 minutes to complete. The measure does not require specialized training in its administration.

Scoring

Scoring may include both individual item ratings and summed scores, both of which can be included as change scores to assess medication outcome.

Interpretation

The MADRS has been used primarily in examining change scores on either individual items or summed scores.

Psychometric Properties

Norms. The MADRS was developed using a sample of 106 patients with primary depressive illness that was otherwise heterogeneous in nature, including both outpatients and inpatients, with endogenous or reactive, psychotic or nonpsychotic, and bipolar or unipolar depression. Patients were drawn from two countries (England and Sweden) to reduce cultural bias in the selection of items. Their ages ranged from 18 to 69 years.

Reliability. Interrater reliability was assessed, using the sample described above, between two English raters ($r = .90$), two Swedish raters ($r = .95$), and one English and one Swedish rater ($r = .97$), as well as between psychiatrist and general practitioner ($r = .97$) and psychiatrist and nurse ($r = .93$), demonstrating adequate interrater reliability among a variety of professionals. No information was provided on test-retest reliability. Correlations between change scores on individual items and total change scores ranged from 0.34 (agitation) to 0.84 (apparent sadness).

Validity. The MADRS was compared with the Hamilton Rating Scale for Depression (p. 58) in terms of differentiating responder status based on clinical global judgment. Both scales correlated significantly with each other and with the clinician judgments.

Clinical Utility

High. The MADRS is simple to administer for both trained and untrained raters, takes little time to administer, and has few items to score.

Research Applicability

Limited. In the one study referred to above, the MADRS did better differentiate between medication responders and nonresponders than did the HRDS. However, more research is required before definitive statements can be made.

Source

Marie Åsberg, Professor, M.D., Psychiatric Clinic, Karolinska Hospital R500, SE-171 76, Stockholm, Sweden (measure is reprinted in referenced article).

Cost

None.

Alternative Forms

A self-assessment version is currently undergoing evaluation in Sweden.

MOS 8-ITEM DEPRESSION SCREENER (SCREENER)

Original Citation

Burnam, M. A., Wells, K. B., Leake, B., & Landsverk, J. (1988). Development of a brief screening instrument for detecting depressive disorders. *Medical Care, 26,* 775–789.

Purpose

To provide a quick screen for the presence of major depression and dysthymia.

Population

Adults.

Description

The Screener is an eight-item self-report measure. The first six items focus on symptoms, asking how often in the past week the symptom has been experienced; these have possible values of 0 ("rarely or none; less than 1 day") to 3 ("most or all; 5–7 days"). The last two items focus on duration, and have only two possible answers: yes (scored 1) or no (scored 0).

Background

The Screener was initially developed for use in the National Study of Medical Care Outcomes (MOS). This study required a very brief screen that could be included, along with several other instruments, in a 10-minute self-report measure. The requirements for the screener were (a) that it would be very sensitive to depressive disorders, and (b) that it would have a fairly high positive predictive value, to reduce the number of clinical interviews that would need to be conducted to identify depression cases.

To develop the Screener, the authors reviewed a number of existing measures, choosing the Center for Epidemiological Studies Depression Scale (CES-D, p. 39) as the basis for their symptom items. Two items related to duration of symptoms (required for DSM diagnosis/caseness) were drawn from the Diagnostic Interview Schedule (DIS, p. 49).

Administration

When self-administered, the Screener takes less than 5 minutes to complete.

Scoring

Each of the first six items is scored 0–3 as noted above; 1 item ("I enjoyed life") is reverse-scored. The last two items are scored 0 (if no) or 1 (if yes). These scores are then weighted to form a prediction equation as follows:

$$P = e^{a+Bx}/(1 + e^{a+Bx})$$

where e is the base of natural logarithms, $a = -6.543$, and
$$Bx = (1.078 \times \text{Item 1}) + (0.185 \times \text{Item 2}) + (0.269 \times \text{Item 3}) + (0.329 \times \text{Item 4})$$
$$- (0.280 \times \text{Item 5}) + (0.288 \times \text{Item 6}) + (2.712 \times \text{Item 7}) + (2.182 \times \text{Item 8})$$

Interpretation

A variety of cutoffs of the above equation have been used. A cutoff of .006 sensitivity was adequate only for recent depression; sensitivity to episodes farther back in time was not acceptable. A cutoff of .009 demonstrated good sensitivity for both current and lifetime depression, although with lower specificity, especially decreasing positive predictive values for recent depression. Additional information on results with various cutoff points can be found in the primary reference.

Psychometric Properties

Two samples provided the data used in developing and evaluating the Screener (both included the measures from which the Screener items were drawn—the CES-D and DIS— rather than the Screener itself). These two samples were 3,132 adults in the Los Angeles sample of the Epidemiological Catchment Area (ECA) study, and 525 adults from the Psychiatric Screening Questionnaire for Primary Care Patients (PSP) study.

Norms. As the Screener is a measure of caseness rather than of severity, no norms are available.

Reliability. Both the CES-D and the DIS, from which the Screener items are drawn, have acceptable test–retest reliabilities. One study (Wells, Burnam, Leake, & Robins, 1988) comparing in-person and telephone administration of DIS items found acceptable test–retest reliability, both in terms of percentage agreement and kappas, which the authors suggest supports the test–retest reliability of the DIS items administered in various ways as in the Screener.

Validity. Both sensitivity and specificity of the Screener as a screening instrument, validated against the full DIS, were acceptable for major depression and dysthymia at several time frames. Although these can be adjusted by changing the cutoff score, cutoffs were identified that allow for both adequate sensitivity and specificity. Positive predictive value was also adequate, although this also can be adjusted by varying the cutoff score used. In general, the false-negative rate was considerably higher for individuals with disorders other than depression.

Clinical Utility

Limited. The Screener is unlikely to be of use to mental health practitioners, due to the complicated predictive equation that is recommended for scoring the inventory.

Research Applicability

High. It has already been used in a large-scale national study (MOS).

Source

M. Audrey Burnam, Ph.D., The RAND Corporation, 1700 Main St., Santa Monica, CA 90406-2138 (scale is within primary reference).

Cost

None

Alternate Forms

None.

MULTIPLE AFFECT ADJECTIVE CHECKLIST-REVISED (MAACL-R)

Original Citation

Zuckerman, M., & Lubin, B. (1985). *Manual for the MAACL-R: The Multiple Affect Adjective Checklist-Revised.* San Diego, CA: EdITS.

Purpose

To assess state and trait anxiety, depression, hostility, positive affect, and sensation-seeking.

Population

Adolescents and adults.

Description

The MAACL-R is a 132-item checklist of individual adjectives related to anxiety (A), depression (D), hostility (H), positive affect (PA), and sensation-seeking (SS). There are two forms available, one assessing *state affect* with the instructions to check words describing how one feels "now—today," and one assessing *trait affect* with the instructions to check words describing how one "generally feel(s)." The two checklists themselves are identical, with each listing the 132 words that respondents check by marking a box beside each applicable item.

Background

The MAACL was initially published in 1965 (Zuckerman & Lubin, 1965) and consisted of only three scales: anxiety, depression, and hostility. It has been used in hundreds of published studies since that time, and was revised in 1985 to address psychometric difficulties of the original scale. These included high intercorrelations among the subscales and the need to minimize the influence of an acquiescence response set on subscale scoring. Further, the MAACL initially used a bipolar affect scale, whereas empirical evidence now supports the use of independent positive and negative affect scales. These have been incorporated into the MAACL-R. Finally, factor analyses conducted with the new scale suggested 2 new subscales based on combinations of the existing ones, and thus the MAACL-R also includes subscales of Dysphoria (Dys; combining Anxiety, Depression, and Hostility), and Positive Affect-Sensation Seeking (PASS; combining those two individual scales). Sample items are reprinted below, with permission of the publisher:

    1. active
  19. calm
  36. discontented
  37. discouraged
123. unsociable

Administration

The MAACL-R can be administered either individually or in groups; in both methods instructions are to be read aloud by the administrator. Answers are marked by checking a box beside each word to be endorsed. Administration time is not specified in the manual, but should range from about 5 to 10 minutes on average. Training is not required for administration.

Scoring

Scoring consists of summing the number of items checked within each of the five primary scales, with one exception: For the SS scale, four of the items within that scale are counted if they are *not* checked. The additional scales (Dys and PASS) are obtained by summing the raw scores of the individual scales comprising them, as noted above. Both hand scoring and computer scoring are available.

The MAACL-R is considered invalid if no items are checked, or if more than 92 (trait form) or 93 (state form) items are checked.

The manual includes tables with which to obtain standardized T-scores; although not strictly necessary, these scores reduce the impact of response sets.

Interpretation

If using T-scores, these scores may be compared with those of the sample population; scores may also be compared, either in raw or standard form, within subjects over time. No cutoff scores are provided.

Psychometric Properties

Psychometric properties for the state form of the MAACL-R were established with a sample of 536 undergraduate students who completed the measure twice, with a maximum 5-day interval between administrations. The trait form was administered to 1,543 subjects by a commercial polling company using a national stratified sample, with retests at between 2 and 8 weeks. Both forms were also administered to a sample of 746 adolescents.

Norms.   Norms broken down by a number of variables, such as gender, race, age, and education, among others, are provided in the manual. To provide one example, in the trait form sample, women endorsed significantly more items (on average, 31.2 versus 28.7 items) than did men overall. Women scored higher than men on the subscales of Anxiety (1.53 versus .93), Positive Affect (10.92 versus 10.06), and Dysphoria (.85 versus .53); whereas men scored higher than women on Sensation Seeking (5.83 versus 5.50).

Reliability. Test–retest reliabilities were calculated for both the state and trait versions, although a state measure would be expected to have a lower test–retest reliability than a trait measure. Test–retest reliabilities for the state scale were low, with most correlations not meeting statistical significance. The trait form demonstrated higher test-retest reliabilities, ranging from .10 to .92, with most correlations above .45 and reaching statistical significance. Internal consistencies for both state and trait were also satisfactory, with the exception of trait SS.

Validity. MAACL-R responses were compared with self-ratings, peer ratings, and observer ratings of affect to assess convergent and discriminant validity. Self-rating comparisons indicated good convergent validity for all scales but H and SS, with less satisfactory discriminant validity (adequate only for A and D scales). Peer ratings supported all the subscales on the trait form, but only the D and H scales of the state form. Observer ratings also significantly correlated with MAACL-R scores, but to a lesser degree. The MAACL-R was also compared with other, more standardized measures such as the Profile of Mood States (POMS; p. 94), and the Minnesota Multiphasic Personality Inventory (MMPI; p. 73), and also with psychiatric diagnoses, with mixed results. It should be noted that the highest correlations between the MAACL-R and MMPI were seen on the MMPI Depression scale, which was positively correlated with the MAACL-R Dys scale and negatively correlated with the MAACL-R PA scale.

Clinical Utility

Limited. It is unlikely that many clinicians will find the time required to administer and score the MAACL-R worthwhile, as the items included are also those likely to be evident during routine consultations. So far, the MAACL-R does not appear to have advantages over either general clinical interviews or more standardized complex measures of mood and affect, although studies are continuing and thus this may change.

Research Applicability

High. As noted previously, the MAACL has been used in hundreds of published studies, and thus considerable data are available that future researchers may wish to use as comparison data in their own studies.

Source

Educational and Industrial Testing Service, P. O. Box 7234, San Diego, CA 92167. Phone: 800-416-1666.

Cost

Specimen sets (manual plus one copy of all MAACL-R forms) are $28.50. Packages of hand-scoring and machine-scoring forms are available at $9.50 for 25 forms, with discounts for larger amounts. Scoring keys and other related products, including scoring itself, are also available for additional charges.

Alternate Forms

None.

MULTISCORE DEPRESSION INVENTORY FOR ADOLESCENTS AND ADULTS (MDI)

Original Citation

Berndt, D. J. (1986). *Multiscore Depression Inventory (MDI) manual.* Los Angeles: Western Psychological Services.

Purpose

To measure the severity of depression.

Population

The MDI has been used with groups ranging from bright junior high school students to the oriented elderly. Normative data are available for individuals as young as 13 years and range into late adulthood.

Description

The MDI is a 118-item self-report questionnaire. Each item presents a statement that describes a symptom or feature of depression. Respondents indicate in a true/false format whether each statement is representative of how they usually feel, think, or behave. The MDI provides for a full-scale score, as well as scores for the following 10 subscales: low energy level, cognitive difficulty, guilt, low self-esteem, social introversion, pessimism, irritability, sad mood, instrumental helplessness, and learned helplessness. Sample items, reprinted with the permission of the publisher, are noted below:

1. I often feel droopy and tired.
2. My thought processes are crisp and precise.
3. I often have a heavy conscience.
4. I generally feel inferior.

5. The fewer people around me, the better I feel.
6. My future seems to get better and better.
7. I flare up when someone crosses me.
8. I am a happy person.
9. People do not treat me fairly.

Background

The MDI was designed to be sensitive to the symptoms and features of mild levels of depression found in syndromes such as cyclothymic and dysthymic disorder. The developers believed that other instruments measuring severity of depressive symptoms exhibited a "floor effect," where low-grade depressive symptoms were undifferentiated from normal, or non-depressed, mood states. The authors also sought to provide more specific details about the experience of the depressive syndrome in addition to a global rating.

Administration

This instrument takes approximately 20–25 minutes to complete.

Scoring

Users can purchase a microcomputer diskette that can be used to administer and score the MDI. A mail-in service is also available for scoring and interpretation. In addition, a scoring key is available which provides transparent overlays to differentiate the subscales. The full scale score ranges from 0 to 118. Each subscale score ranges from 0 to 12, except the Guilt subscale, which ranges from 0 to 10. Higher scores indicate higher severity of depressive symptoms.

Interpretation

The manual cautions that MDI scores should not be used to diagnose depression; rather, they should be used as part of an overall assessment battery that includes an interview. The manual provides detailed conversion tables where raw scores can be translated into T-scores and percentiles. Users can develop visual representations of the subscale profiles for individuals, and the manual provides guidelines for interpreting these profiles. In addition, validity scores can be obtained to examine the probability of faking, sabotage, or atypical responses.

Psychometric Properties

Norms. The manual provides normative data for ages ranging from 13 years to late adulthood. In addition, normative data are provided for special populations of anorexic, bulimic, and weight-preoccupied respondents, college students, high school students, high-striving adolescents, and family practice outpatients.

Reliability.   The internal consistency of the MDI was measured in a variety of samples. Reliabilities of the full scale scores ranged from .96 to .97, whereas the subscale scores ranged from .70 to .91. Test–retest reliabilities were tested among two samples of college students. In the first sample ($N = 107$), the test–retest reliability was .82 after a 3-week interval, and reliabilities of the subscales ranged from .38 to .86. The second sample ($N = 71$) was retested immediately and 3 weeks after the first test. Results were $r = .94$ for immediate retest and .82 after a 3-week interval. Reliability correlations for subscale scores ranged from .81 to .93 upon immediate retest and from .65 to .86 after 3 weeks.

Validity.   The concurrent validity of the MDI was measured by comparing scores on this instrument to scores on the BDI (p. 29) and the trait version of the Depression Adjective Check List (p. 111) in a sample of 200 college students. Correlations were .69 and .77, respectively. Another study compared the MDI Full Scale score to the Hamilton Rating Scale for Depression (p. 58), where the correlation between these scores was .66. The item selection strategy, which included a point biserial item correlation and is detailed in the manual, also demonstrated the convergent and divergent validity of the individual items of the MDI. A role-play simulation strategy demonstrated its face validity.

A principal components factor analysis ($N = 263$) using Varimax rotation, which supports the construct validity of most of the MDI subscales, identified eight factors. These factors were identified as instrumental helplessness, cognitive difficulty, social introversion, irritability, pessimism, guilt, low energy level/sad mood, and learned helplessness/low self-esteem. A second factor analysis using hierarchical cluster analysis supported the construct validity of six of the subscales (Berndt, 1981).

Clinical Utility

High. The MDI provides a tool for understanding symptoms of milder manifestations of depressive symptoms and syndromes. Scores on the MDI can help clinicians generate hypotheses, identify strengths and problem areas for individual patients, and detect remission and relapse.

Research Applicability

High. The psychometric properties of the MDI have been supported by extensive data collected on several large samples. It is able to detect slight changes in depressive symptoms, even among the milder manifestations of depressive disorders.

Source

Western Psychological Services, 12031 Wilshire Boulevard, Los Angeles, CA 90025. Phone: 800-648-8857.

Cost

$112 for a kit which includes 50 hand-scored test/answer sheets, 50 profile forms, one set of hand-scoring keys, one manual, and two Western Psychological Services test report prepaid MDI mail-in answer sheets for computer scoring and interpretation.

Alternate Forms

A 47-item short form is available.

NEWCASTLE SCALES

Original Citation

Carney, M. W. P., Roth, M., & Garside, R. F. (1965). The diagnosis of depressive syndromes and prediction of ECT response. *British Journal of Psychiatry*, *111*, 659–674.

Purpose

To differentiate between endogenous and reactive depression.

Population

Adults diagnosed with major depressive disorder.

Description

The Newcastle Scale was developed to differentiate subtypes of major depression, specifically endogenous versus reactive depression. The scale contains 10 items (e.g., absence of psychological stressors), all of which represent clinical features of endogenous depression (i.e., weight loss, motor agitation/retardation). Carney et al. (1965) provide definitional guidelines to aid the identification of symptom features. Sophisticated clinical interviewers score these items based on information obtained during a semistructured interview. The Newcastle Scale is frequently administered with the Hamilton Rating Scale for Depression (p. 58). It should be noted that although the Newcastle Scale is a frequently used measure in Europe, the scale has received little attention in North America.

Background

The original Newcastle Scale was slightly modified by Carney and Sheffield (1972) with the redefinition of one item. A second version of the scale, the Newcastle II (described by Bech et al., 1983), is also composed of 10 items which represent features of melancholic, or endogenous, depression. Although there is some correspondence between the scales, there are differences in the content and the range of weights assigned to each item. Therefore, the Newcastle II is not considered an alternate or expanded version of the original. Three positively scored items are contraindicative of endogenous depression and the remaining items have various negative weights.

Administration

Administration of the interview and rating of symptoms takes 10–30 minutes, depending on the number of symptoms present and other patient characteristics. Each symptom is rated as either absent or present and multiplied by an assigned weighting.

Scoring

Each item is rated as either 0 (absent) or 1 (present) and each item score is multiplied by the weighting provided for that item. Some items are weighted positively and some items are weighted negatively. A single scale score is computed by summing both the positive and negative weighted-item scores.

Interpretation

According to Carney et al. (1965), a score of +6 or more is indicative of endogenous depression and a score of +5 or less indicates no endogenous depression. More recent validation studies (Zimmerman, Coryell, Pfohl, & Stangl, 1987; Zimmerman, Pfohl, Stangl, & Coryell, 1986) recommend using a cutoff score of +5 to identify those with endogenous depression.

The Newcastle II also identifies endogenous depression using cutoff scores. Scores of −20 or less are associated with endogenous depression, scores ranging from −12 to −19 make a diagnosis of endogenous depression doubtful, and scores of −11 or more suggest absence of endogenous depression (cited in Bech et al., 1983).

Psychometric Properties

Norms. None.

Reliability. The original authors report acceptable levels of interrater reliability (Carney & Sheffield, 1972) and a more recent study demonstrated acceptable agreement between independent raters. Bech et al. (1983) report 90% and 91% agreement in categorizing patients for the Newcastle and Newcastle II, respectively. Intraclass correlation, an index of reliability of all raters, was 0.81 for the Newcastle and 0.77 for the Newcastle II.

Validity. The majority of validity studies examined the relationship between phenomena associated with endogenous depression and the Newcastle Scale. This measure consistently discriminated on biological markers associated with endogenous depression (e.g., dexamethasone suppression test, Holden, 1983; electroconvulsive therapy response, Vlissides

& Jenner, 1982). Additional findings have extended to discriminating psychosocial factors. Zimmerman et al. (1987) report that patients categorized as endogenously depressed on the Newcastle Scale differ from other depressives on psychosocial variables associated with endogenous depression. As predicted, the endogenous group was older, more severely depressed, had better social support, fewer life events, less personality disorder, and a lower morbid risk of alcoholism.

The scale's construct validity is supported by its moderate to high correlations with the Newcastle II. In addition, both the Newcastle Scale and Newcastle II are significantly correlated with the Melancholia Scale (Bech et al., 1983).

Clinical Utility

Limited. The Newcastle Scales distinguish among subgroups of depressives, namely those with endogenous symptoms and those without. However, at this time, the distinction between those two subgroups has limited clinical application.

Research Applicability

High. The Newcastle Scale has been shown to have adequate reliability and validity. It continues to be used more frequently than the Newcastle II. Nonetheless, both are frequently used research assessment devices in Europe. Two recent validation studies by Zimmerman and colleagues (Zimmerman et al., 1986; Zimmerman et al., 1987) suggest that the Newcastle Scales can be used just as effectively in the United States.

Source

Printed in Carney et al. (1965).

Cost

None.

Alternative Forms

None.

POSITIVE AND NEGATIVE AFFECT SCALES (PANAS)

Original Citation

Watson, D., Clark, L. A., & Tellegen, A. (1988). Development and validation of brief measures of positive and negative affect: The PANAS scales. *Journal of Personality and Social Psychology, 54*, 1063–1070.

Purpose

To assess the two independent dimensions of positive and negative affect.

Population

Adults.

Description

The PANAS includes two 10-item scales, one assessing positive affect (PA) and the other negative affect (NA). Each item consists of a single adjective (i.e., "enthusiastic"), which is rated on a scale ranging from 1 ("very slightly or not at all") to 5 ("extremely"). Instructions can vary to allow for different time periods assessed. For example, the authors noted seven different time periods they have assessed, ranging from, "Indicate to what extent you feel this way right now, that is, at the present moment," to, "Indicate to what extent you generally feel this way, that is, how you feel on the average." Intermediate time frames can include "today," "the past few days," or "the past week."

Background

The PANAS was developed to assess independently the two dimensions of positive and negative affect in accordance with contemporary theories of emotion (e.g., Watson & Tellegen, 1985) that describe these dimensions as orthogonal, rather than as opposite poles of a single dimension. The authors and their colleagues initially developed measures including far more items to assess these moods, while developing and clarifying their theories, and then developed the PANAS so these dimensions could be assessed briefly.

Administration

When self-administered, the PANAS takes less than 5 minutes to complete, and can be administered both individually and in group format.

Scoring

The PANAS is scored by summing the responses within each scale, yielding separate scores for PA and NA that each range from 10 to 50.

Interpretation

Cutoff scores are not provided, although scores may be compared with norms compiled on undergraduate samples.

Psychometric Properties

Psychometric properties for the PANAS were established with samples of undergraduate students, university employees, and other adults. No differences were found among these samples and they were then combined to determine psychometric data. Data were collected using seven different time frames, with samples of 586–1,002 subjects largely, but not completely, independent. A smaller psychiatric inpatient sample ($N = 61$) was also assessed, but is not included in the general data listed below unless noted specifically.

Norms. Norms are listed for each of the seven time frames in the source article. Using the "today" time frame, the mean PA score was 29.1 ($SD = 8.3$) and the mean NA score was 16.3 ($SD = 6.4$). In general, PA scores are higher than NA scores on all time frames, and both PA and NA scores rise as the time frames expand.

Reliability. Test–retest reliabilities were calculated using a sample of 101 subjects who completed all seven time frames of the PANAS twice, with an 8-week interval between retests of the same time frame. Test–retest reliability ranged from .39 to .71, with greater stability exhibited for the longer time periods assessed. Internal consistencies for both PA and NA scales were high in all time frames for both clinical and nonclinical samples.

Validity. Factor analyses supported both the convergent and discriminant validity of the PA and NA scales. The PANAS was compared with other brief affect measures as well, with these analyses further supporting the convergent and discriminant validity of the scales. Specifically, for scales of positive affect, the PA scale was highly correlated and the NA scale correlations were quite low, with opposite results seen for scales of negative affect. The PANAS was also compared with three standardized measures of psychopathology: the Hopkins Symptom Checklist (HSCL; Derogatis, Lipman, Rickels, Uhlenhuth, & Covi, 1974); the Beck Depression Inventory (BDI; p. 29), and the State-Trait Anxiety Inventory, State Form (STAI-S; Spielberger et al., 1970). In these comparisons, the PA scale correlations ranged from $-.19$ to $-.36$ and the NA scale correlations ranged from .51 to .74, again supporting the validity of the PANAS scales. PANAS scores for the clinical sample were higher than for the normative sample, which the authors noted may further support the scales' validity, but should be interpreted with caution due to the small size of that sample.

Clinical Utility

High. The PANAS is quick to complete, and can be used as an easily repeated measure of mood.

Research Applicability

High. The PANAS has been used in a large number of studies already, and may be especially important for researchers needing independent assessments of positive versus negative affect.

Source

The PANAS is reprinted in Appendix B. For more information, contact David B. Watson , Ph.D., Department of Psychology, University of Iowa, 11 Seashore Hall E, Iowa City, IA 52242-1407.

Cost

None, when used for noncommercial purposes. A manual for the PANAS is available from the author for a nominal charge.

Alternate Forms

A German translation of the PANAS has been validated by Krohne, Egloff, Kohlmann, and Tausch (1996). Other languages in which the PANAS is available include French, Spanish, Russian, Polish, and Norwegian; a Swedish version will also be available shortly. An expanded version of the PANAS (PANAS-X) includes the original PANAS as well as 11 additional scales assessing specific types of affect such as joy and fear, for use by researchers needing a more comprehensive assessment of affect.

PRIMARY CARE EVALUATION OF MENTAL DISORDERS (PRIME-MD)

Original Citation

Spitzer, R. L., Williams, J. B. W., Kroenke, K., Linzer, M., deGruy III, F. V., Hahn, S. R., & Brody, D. (1993). *PRIME-MD: Clinician evaluation guide*. New York: Pfizer, Inc.

Purpose

To diagnose and identify five mental disorders and problems (mood, anxiety, somatoform, alcohol, eating disorders) commonly encountered in primary care settings.

Population

Adults.

Description

PRIME-MD contains two components: a one-page patient questionnaire (PQ) and a 12-page clinician evaluation guide (CEG). The PQ is completed by the patient prior to seeing the primary care physician (PCP) and consists of 26 yes/no questions inquiring about symptoms that were present during the past month. These questions are divided into the five diagnostic areas noted above. "Yes" responses to certain questions serve as triggers for the physician to follow up with certain modules contained in the CEG. These critical items were derived from the DSM-III-R. With regard to the mood module, a positive answer to one of two questions (i.e., sad mood, loss of pleasure) serves as a critical item.

The CEG is administered during the patient visit and consists of multiple questions divided into the five modules representing 18 different diagnostic categories, 9 of which correspond to specific DSM-III-R diagnoses. With regard to mood disorders, these include major depressive disorder (MDD), partial remission or recurrence of MDD, and dysthymia. The mood module contains 17 questions reflecting DSM-III-R criterion symptoms (e.g., poor appetite, trouble concentrating) that are embedded in a decision tree that facilitates accurate diagnosis. The diagnostic findings are recorded on a summary sheet.

Background

Research has shown that more patients are treated in the primary care sector than by mental health professionals (Manderschied, Rae, Narrow, Locke, & Regier, 1993), but that PCPs fail to treat 50–75% of patients suffering from common mental disorders (Borus, Howes, Devins, Rosenberg, & Livingston, 1988). The PRIME-MD was developed in reaction to such research by Spitzer et al. (1993) and underwritten by a grant from Pfizer Inc. It was designed to be flexible and user-friendly for PCPs.

Administration

The PQ is likely to take 5–10 minutes to complete, whereas the average time for physicians to complete the CEG in a study by Spitzer et al. (1994) was 8.4 minutes.

Scoring

Scoring follows the decision tree format and leads to diagnoses, not continuous scores.

Interpretation

Proper administration allows for accurate diagnosis of mental disorders.

Psychometric Properties

Norms.   Not applicable.

Reliability.   Index agreements between diagnoses of PCPs and mental health professionals regarding a sample of 431 patients yielded kappa coefficients of .71 regarding any diagnosis. For MDD, the coefficient was .61.

Validity.   PRIME-MD mood diagnoses were found to correlate (partial correlation) .58 with the Zung Depression Scale (p. 120). The sensitivity of the PRIME-MD concerning mood disorders was 67%, whereas the specificity was 92%. In addition, the positive predictive value for mood disorders was 78% and the overall accuracy rate was 84%.

Clinical Utility

High. The PRIME-MD appears user-friendly and a valid means of diagnosing depressive disorders in primary care populations.

Research Applicability

High. Initial research investigations are promising.

Source

Robert L. Spitzer, M.D., Biometrics Research Department, New York State Psychiatric Institute, 722 West 168th Street, Unit 74, New York, NY 10032.

Cost

None.

Alternative Forms

None.

PROFILE OF MOOD STATES (POMS)

Original Citation

McNair, D. M., Lorr, M., & Droppleman, L. F. (1992). *EdITS manual for the Profile of Mood States*. San Diego, CA: EdITS.

Purpose

To measure mood states and mood changes.

Population

Adults 18 years and older.

Description

The POMS is a self-report measure that contains 65 adjectives for which respondents are requested to rate the degree to which that adjective describes the way in which they have been feeling during the past week. Ratings range from 0 ("not at all") to 4 ("extremely"). Some adjectives are reflective of negative moods (e.g., sad, bushed, terrified), whereas others represent positive moods (e.g., alert, carefree, relaxed). The POMS can be scored according to six factor-analytically derived mood states: Tension-Anxiety; Depression-Dejection; Anger-Hostility; Vigor-Activity; Fatigue-Inertia; Confusion-Bewilderment. The Depression-Dejection scale contains 15 adjectives and represents a mood of depression accompanied by a sense of personal inadequacy. In addition, a Total Mood Disturbance Score can be calculated. The POMS short form consists of 30 items and the same six scales as measured by the long form.

Background

The POMS has a long history of use as an outcome measure to detect changes engendered by various therapeutic interventions, as well as to assess emotional distress in medical populations. For example, the POMS has been used to measure illness- and treatment-related factors regarding the psychological adjustment to cancer (e.g., A. M. Nezu, Nezu, Friedman, Faddis, & Houts, 1998; Taylor, Lichtman, & Wood, 1984). It has also been used to assess the change associated with time-limited psychotherapy (Haskell, Pugatch, & McNair, 1969).

Administration

The POMS usually takes about 3–5 minutes to complete.

Scoring

The score for each scale is derived by summing the responses to the relevant adjectives. The Total Mood Disturbance Score is calculated by summing the scores of the five negative mood scales and subtracting the Vigor scale.

Interpretation

Norms are provided based on a psychiatric outpatient sample of 1000 adults, as well as a sample of 856 college students. Using these norms, POMS raw scores can be converted into T-scores by sample and gender.

Psychometric Properties

Norms.   Substantial norms exist for comparison.

Reliability.   Internal consistency for the Depression scale was found to be .95 in two separate studies. Test–retest reliability of the Depression scale was estimated to be .74 in one study that included 100 patients entering treatment at a university-based psychiatry center.

Validity.   The POMS Depression scale was been found to correlate highly with other measures of depressive symptomatology. For example, the r value regarding its association with the BDI (p. 29) and MMPI-D scale (p. 73) was found to be .61 and .65, respectively.

Clinical Utility

High. The POMS has been used extensively to assess overall emotional distress in many investigations. It is likely, however, to be less sensitive and precise with regard to assessing depressive symptomatology as compared to measures designed solely for that purpose.

Research Applicability

High. The POMS has been used extensively in a variety of research studies.

Resource

EdITS, P.O. Box 7234, San Diego, CA 92167. Phone: 800-416-1666.

Cost

$9.00 for the manual and one copy of all forms (long and short forms); $9.50 for a package of 25 POMS inventories.

Alternative Forms

A short-form exists.

RASKIN THREE-AREA SEVERITY OF DEPRESSION SCALE

Original Citation

Raskin, A., Schulterbrandt, J. G., Reatig, N., & McKeon, J. J. (1970). Differential response to chlorpromazine, imipramine, and placebo: A study of subgroups of hospitalized depressed patients. *Archives of General Psychiatry, 23,* 164–173.

Purpose

To rate the severity of depressive symptoms in three general areas: verbal report, behavior, and secondary symptoms.

Population

Depressed adults in inpatient and outpatient settings.

Description

The Raskin Three-Area Scale is a three-item clinician-rated instrument that measures the severity of patients' depressive symptoms in the global areas of verbal report, behavior, and secondary symptoms of depression. Examples of symptoms are provided for the clinician in each area of depressive symptomatology (e.g., "Says he feels blue and talks of feeling helpless or worthless" is provided as an example of verbal report). Each of the three areas is rated along a 5-point scale ranging from 5 to 1 which represent descending severity of depressive symptoms.

Background

The Raskin Three-Area Scale was developed to provide a method for determining inclusion in a study examining the differential responses of depressed individuals to chlorpromazine, imipramine, and a placebo. Inpatients with a score of 9 or greater were determined to have at least moderate levels of depression and were included in the study. Later studies, which examined drug effects on outpatients, lowered the score for inclusion to 7.

Administration

Clinicians rate the severity of symptoms based on their observations of patient behavior and the cues provided for each area of depressive symptomatology; the instrument requires approximately 30 minutes.

Scoring

One simply adds the score for each of the three items in order to produce a total score. Scores range from 3 to 15.

Interpretation

A cutoff score of 9 has typically been used as the criterion for including inpatients in studies of psychopharmacological treatment effects; a cutoff score of 7 has been used for outpatients.

Psychometric Properties

Norms.   Not applicable.

Reliability.   Data on the reliability of the Raskin Three Area Scale are limited. According to Raskin (as cited in Bellack & Hersen, 1988), intraclass reliability coefficients developed from 880 depressed inpatients, 94 depressed outpatients, and 239 depressed patients in private practice were all in the high 80s.

Validity.   Similar to the reliability data, validity data on this instrument are also limited.

Clinical Utility

Limited. This instrument was developed to determine inclusion in drug trials. It was not intended for clinical use, and has not been tested for this purpose.

Research Applicability

Limited. Studies have shown that this instrument is a reliable screening instrument for entry into drug trials. According to Raskin (as cited in Bellack and Hersen, 1988), some studies have shown that this scale is sensitive to treatment effects. Although some studies have also used the Raskin Three-Area Scale as an outcome measure, the test was not developed for this purpose and its reliability and validity have not been examined in this capacity.

Source

The Raskin Three-Area Scale is reprinted in Appendix B. For additional information, contact Dr. Allen Raskin, Department of Psychiatry, University of Maryland School of Medicine, 645 West Redwood Street, Baltimore, MD 21201.

Cost

None.

Alternative Forms

None.

REVISED HAMILTON RATING SCALE FOR DEPRESSION (RHRSD): CLINICIAN RATING FORM

Original Citation

Warren, W. L. (1994). *Revised Hamilton Rating Scale for Depression (RHRSD): Manual.* Los Angeles: Western Psychological Services.

Purpose

To confirm a diagnosis of depression and to evaluate the significance of depressive symptoms in a patient's social environment.

Population

Adults.

Description

The RHRSD is available in two forms: the Clinician Rating Form and the Self-Report Problem Inventory (p. 101). The RHRSD is based on the original HRSD (p. 58), which was designed specifically as a clinician rating scale for use in evaluating individuals already diagnosed with a depressive disorder. The RHRSD was constructed around the original 17 items of the HRSD in order to preserve the applicability of the research previously conducted on that original version. Scores on the RHRSD are based on these 17 items (depressed mood, feelings of guilt, suicide, insomnia, nocturnal waking, early morning waking, work and activities, sexual symptoms, loss of insight, retardation, agitation, worry, somatic anxiety, gastrointestinal somatic symptoms, general somatic symptoms, hypochondriasis, loss of weight). Three items reflecting cardinal symptoms of depression were added, as well as 5 items designed to measure the significance of depressive symptoms in the social environment.

The Clinician Rating Form containing the above items can be completed by a trained clinician either during or after a clinical interview. General and specific instructions are included in the manual regarding how to conduct the interview. For each item, the clinician endorses a statement that best reflects the patient's condition (e.g., "Has no difficulty falling asleep"). Each statement, in turn, is associated with a score, some ranging from 1 to 2, whereas others range from 1 to 4.

Background

The original HRSD was designed to assess the severity of depressive symptoms among samples of patients already diagnosed as experiencing depressive illness. The RHRSD was constructed within the context of this original intent—to measure depression in psychiatric and medical populations. The HRSD is perhaps the most widely used clinician rating procedure to assess for depression. This version provides for the ability to confirm diagnoses in keeping with DSM-III-R and DSM-IV.

Administration

The form takes about 5–10 minutes to complete beyond the clinical interview.

Scoring

In addition to the total RHRSD score, which reflects the severity of depression, the Clinician Rating Form also provides for diagnostic confirmation of a Major Depressive Episode, an assessment of melancholic features based on DSM-III-R and DSM-IV criteria, and a Tricyclic Antidepressant Responsive (TCAR) cluster score that indicates the severity of those symptoms that have been shown to be particularly responsive to such antidepressant medication.

Interpretation

With regard to RHRSD total scores, the manual provides for the following descriptive categories: ≤ 10 = not depressed; 11–16 = minor depression; 17–25 = major depression; ≥ 26 = severe depression.

Psychometric Properties

To some degree, 30 years of use of the original HRSD provides for substantive support for its reliability and validity. With specific regard to this revised version by Warren, various psychometric properties were evaluated based on a verification sample of 202 psychiatric patients.

Norms.   Means and standard deviations by gender and setting (outpatient versus inpatient) are provided in the manual for the 202 patients in the verification sample.

Reliability.   Internal consistency, in the form of Cronbach's alpha, was found to be .79 for the verification sample. No estimates for the temporal stability of the RHRSD are provided in the manual.

Validity.   Strong correlations with other measures of depression and the original HRSD have been reported by Hedlund and Vieweg (1979). With regard to the verification sample, the RHRSD was found to correlate .67 with the MMPI-Depression score (p. 73). In addition, the Clinician Rating Form of the RHRSD correlated .66 with the Self-Report version of the RHRSD among inpatients, and .70 among outpatients.

Clinical Utility

High. This procedure provides both a means of confirming a diagnosis of major depressive disorder and a measure of the severity of depressive symptoms.

Research Applicability

High. The original HRSD is probably the most often used clinician rating procedure in outcome research.

Source

Western Psychological Services, 12031 Wilshire Blvd., Los Angeles, CA 90025-1251. Phone: 800-648-8857.

Cost

$72 for a manual, 10 clinician forms, and 10 self-report forms.

Alternative Forms

None.

REVISED HAMILTON RATING SCALE FOR DEPRESSION (RHRSD): SELF-REPORT PROBLEM INVENTORY

Original Citation

Warren, W. L. (1994). *Revised Hamilton Rating Scale for Depression (RHRSD): Manual.* Los Angeles: Western Psychological Services.

Purpose

To confirm a diagnosis of depression and to evaluate the significance of depressive symptoms in a patient's social environment.

Population

Adults.

Description

The RHRSD is available in two forms: the Clinician Rating Form (p. 99) and the Self-Report Problem Inventory. The RHRSD is based on the original HRSD (p. 58) which was designed specifically as a clinician rating scale for use in evaluating individuals already diagnosed with a depressive disorder. The RHRSD was constructed around the original 17 items of the HRSD in order to preserve the applicability of the research previously conducted on that original version. The self-report version provides for the same scores as the Clinician Rating Form in addition to two validity checks.

The self-report version contains 76 statements for which respondents are requested to indicate whether such statements are true or false as applied to themselves. These items cover the same symptom areas as that of the RHRSD Clinician Rating Form. Patients should be provided with the instructions to use the past 1–2 weeks as the time frame of interest. Sample items, reprinted with the permission of the publisher, include the following:

1. My mood is no different than usual.
5. I am aware of problems in my daily life that are caused by my moods.
10. I feel unusually sad.
20. I have thought about killing myself.
33. I am spending less time in my usual activities and am getting less done.
39. I am no longer interested in sex at all.
45. People say that I speak more slowly than usual.
56. Recently I've had some difficulty with my breathing, hearing, vision, or digestion.
71. Even though I have not been dieting, I've recently lost so much weight that my clothes no longer fit.
76. There are certain things I cannot stop thinking about or doing, no matter how hard I try.

Background

The original HRSD was designed to assess the severity of depressive symptoms among samples of patients already diagnosed as experiencing depressive illness. The RHRSD was constructed within the context of this original intent—to measure depression in psychiatric and medical populations. The HRSD is perhaps the most widely used clinician rating procedure to assess for depression. This version provides for the ability to confirm diagnoses in keeping with DSM-III-R and DSM-IV. This self-report version was written at a fourth-grade level for easy comprehension.

Administration

The form takes about 10–20 minutes to complete.

Scoring

In addition to the total RHRSD score, which reflects the severity of depression, the Self-Report version also provides for diagnostic confirmation of a Major Depressive Episode, an assessment of melancholic features based on DSM-III-R and DSM-IV criteria, and a Tricyclic Antidepressant Responsive (TCAR) cluster score that indicates the severity of those symptoms that have been shown to be particularly responsive to such antidepressant medication. In addition, two validity scales are included represented by cutoff scores to indicate whether the responses should be viewed cautiously or with confidence.

Interpretation

With regard to RHRSD total scores, the manual provides for the following descriptive categories: $\leqslant 10$ = not depressed; 11–16 = minor depression; 17–25 = major depression; $\geqslant 26$ = severe depression.

Psychometric Properties

To some degree, 30 years of use of the original HRSD provides for substantive support for its reliability and validity. With specific regard to this revised version by Warren, various psychometric properties were evaluated based on a verification sample of 202 psychiatric patients.

Norms.   Means and standard deviations by gender and setting (outpatient versus inpatient) are provided in the manual for the 202 patients in the verification sample.

Reliability.   Internal consistency, in the form of Cronbach's alpha, was found to be .81 for the verification sample. No estimates for the temporal stability of the RHRSD are provided in the manual.

Validity.   Strong correlations with other measures of depression and the original HRSD have been reported by Hedlund and Vieweg (1979). With regard to the verification sample, the RHRSD Self-Report version was found to correlate .80 with the MMPI-Depression score (p. 73). In addition, the Clinician Rating Form of the RHRSD correlated .66 with the Self-Report version of the RHRSD among inpatients, and .70 among outpatients.

Clinical Utility

High. This procedure provides both a means of confirming a diagnosis of major depressive disorder and a measure of the severity of depressive symptoms.

Research Applicability

High. The original HRSD is probably the most often used clinician rating procedure in outcome research. The self-report version provides a more efficient method of obtaining repeated measures of depressive severity in order to assess the effects of a given treatment.

Source

Western Psychological Services, 12031 Wilshire Blvd., Los Angeles, CA 90025-1251. Phone: 800-648-8857.

Cost

$72 for a manual, 10 clinician forms, and 10 self-report forms.

Alternative Forms

None.

REYNOLDS DEPRESSION SCREENING INVENTORY (RDSI)

Original Citation

Reynolds, W. M., & Kobak, K. A. (1998). *Reynolds Depression Screening Inventory: Professional manual*. Odessa, FL: Psychological Assessment Resources.

Purpose

To assess the severity of depressive symptomatology.

Population

Adults.

Description

The RDSI is a 19-item self-report measure that was developed to be an easy-to-use measure of depression severity. These items reflect specific symptoms as described in DSM-IV (e.g., dysphoric mood, loss of energy, feelings of worthlessness). The response format differs for individual items; some are scored 0 to 2, some 0 to 3, and some 0 to 4. Instructions to respondents ask them to endorse the statement within a group of statements that best describes their feelings or behavior over the past 2 weeks regarding a specific question. Sample items, reprinted with the permission of the publisher* (© 1991, 1995, 1998 by Psychological Assessment Resources, Inc.) appear below:

> 2. How does the future look to you?
> 0   OK
> 1   I feel a bit discouraged about the future.
> 2   I am somewhat discouraged and things seem hopeless to me.
> 3   I am very discouraged and do not think that things will ever get better.
> 4   The future is totally hopeless for me and I know things will never get better.

    6. Over the past 2 weeks, how often did you have trouble falling asleep at night?
        0 None.
        1 1 to 2 nights a week.
        2 3 to 5 nights a week.
        3 6 to 7 nights a week.

  12. How has your appetite been over the past 2 weeks?
        0 My appetite is fine.
        1 My appetite is not as good as usual.
        2 I have almost no appetite.
        1 My appetite has increased a bit.
        2 My appetite is much greater than usual.

  15. Have you noticed any change in your interest in or pleasure from sex?
        0 I have not noticed any change in my interest or pleasure from sex.
        1 I am less interested in or enjoy sex less.
        2 I don't enjoy or feel like having sex at all anymore.

  18. Over the past 2 weeks, how have you been feeling about yourself?
        0 I feel OK about myself.
        1 I feel that I am somewhat inadequate.
        2 I feel somewhat worthless as a person.
        3 I feel that I am a worthless person.
        4 I feel I am totally rotten and worthless as a person.

Background

The RDSI was derived specifically from the Hamilton Depression Inventory (HDI; p. 55), which is a self-report inventory developed to parallel the Hamilton Rating Scale for Depression (p. 58), which is a clinician rating scale. The RDSI items were drawn from the HDI, which in turn was based on the original interview questions of the 17-item version of the HRSD. It was created to be an easy-to-use measure based on DSM-IV symptoms of depressive disorders.

Administration

The RDSI requires approximately 5–10 minutes to complete.

Scoring

The total raw score of the RDSI is the numerical sum of item scores. No items are reverse-scored. Higher scores are indicative of more severe levels of depressive symptoms. The range of RDSI scores is 0–63.

Interpretation

A clinical raw score cutoff of 16 has been identified as useful in differentiating psychiatric outpatients with Major Depression from nonreferred community adults. In addition, there are tables included in the manual to help convert raw scores into T-scores broken down by gender. This should be used only as a screening device to be followed by a more comprehensive clinical interview in order to develop an accurate differential diagnosis.

Psychometric Properties

Norms.   Norms are provided for a group of 450 adults from a community sample. As noted above, standard scores are provided in tables.

Reliability.   Internal consistency estimates based on a sample of 855 adults yielded a coefficient of .93. The test–retest reliability of the RDSI was calculated on a sample of 190 adults who were retested 1 week after initial testing. This reliability coefficient was found to be .94.

Validity.   In the manual, evidence is provided indicating the RDSI to have acceptable validity properties in terms of content, criterion-related, construct, and factorial validity. For example, the RDSI has been found to correlate .93 with the HRSD (p. 58) and .94 with the BDI (p. 29).

Clinical Utility

High. The cutoff score of 16 is based on a very high hit rate (95%), sensitivity (95%), and specificity (95%).

Research Applicability

Unknown at present due to lack of studies using the RDSI.

Source

Psychological Assessment Resources, Inc., P.O. Box 998, Odessa, FL 33556. Phone: 800-331-TEST.

Cost

$44 for manual and 25 record forms.

Alternative Forms

None.

RIMON'S BRIEF DEPRESSION SCALE (RBDS)

Original Citation

Keltikangas-Järvinen, L., & Rimon, R. (1987). Rimon's Brief Depression Scale, a rapid method for screening depression. *Psychological Reports*, *60*, 111–119.

Purpose

To assess the severity of depressive symptoms

Population

Adults.

Description

The RBDS is a seven-item interview measure of depressive symptoms and is based on the criteria for diagnosing depressive disorders as delineated in the DSM-III. Areas assessed include suicidality, depressive mood, loss of interest, and various physical/health changes. The questions are asked in a fixed order by the interviewer. Each item is rated on a 4-point scale ranging from 0 to 3, representing ascending levels of severity (from absence to intense levels) of a given symptom.

Background

The RBDS was developed to provide a brief screening method that could be used by medical personnel without extensive psychiatric training. An early version of this measure had six questions; examining the early measure's results led to the division of one question concerning appearance, physical well-being, and sexual interest into two. The current version has one question on appearance, and one concerning health and well-being.

Administration

As noted earlier, this measure was designed specifically to be brief, and also to be administered by those without extensive psychiatric training.

Scoring

Each item is rated from 0 to 3, with the total score obtained by summing the ratings for the seven items. The maximum score is 21. Higher scores indicate higher levels of depressive symptomatology.

Interpretation

The following scores have been suggested as cutoffs for interpretation: 0–5, absence of depression; 6–9, mild depression; 10–13, moderate depression; and 14–21, severe depression.

Psychometric Properties

Psychometric properties for the six-item version are based on a sample of 103 patients (61 women, 42 men) admitted to the Department of Psychiatry at the University of Helsinki. The seven-item version has not been subjected to psychometric evaluation.

Norms. The mean score for the sample described above was 10.17, with a standard deviation of 4.32 and a range from 0 to 18.

Reliability. Internal consistency was estimated to be .85 for the total score, and .87, .83, .77, and .78, respectively for the four factors (Motivation, Guilt Feelings and Irritability, Consuming Alcohol, Vital Processes).

Validity. Concurrent validity was evaluated by correlating scores on this measure with those on the BDI (p. 29); the RBDS correlated .78 with the BDI. Construct validity was evaluated via correlation and factor analysis. Intercorrelations among the items, with the exception of one concerning alcohol consumption, indicate that they measure essentially the same concept, albeit along different dimensions. Based on the principal axis method and Varimax rotation, four major factors appear to underlie this scale's structure. These four factors also correlated with similar factors of the BDI.

Source

Liisa Keltikangas-Järvinen, Department of Psychology, University of Helsinki, Fabianinkatu 33, 01700 Helsinki 17, Finland.

Cost

None.

Alternate Forms

None.

SCHEDULE FOR AFFECTIVE DISORDERS AND SCHIZOPHRENIA (SADS) RESEARCH DIAGNOSTIC CRITERIA (RDC)

Original Citations

Endicott, J., & Spitzer, R. L. (1978). A diagnostic interview: The Schedule for Affective Disorders and Schizophrenia. *Archives of General Psychiatry*, *35*, 837–844.
Spitzer, R. L., Endicott, J., & Robins, E. (1978). Research Diagnostic Criteria. *Archives of General Psychiatry*, *35*, 773–782.

Purpose

To provide for a means for accurate diagnosis using relatively homogeneous diagnostic groupings.

Population

Adult psychiatric patients.

Description

There are multiple versions of the SADS. For instance, there is a standard version that is designed to assess severity of psychiatric symptoms, a version designed to measure change in psychiatric status, a lifetime version, and a variety of versions that have been modified to assess specific syndromes (e.g., bipolar mood disorders). The standard version is administered in two parts. The first part assesses severity of current psychopathology and the severity within the past week. Questions are organized in a progressive manner to aid in diagnostic decision-making. The second part contains interview questions that assess the frequency, intensity, and duration of previous episodes of psychopathology. The results of the interview can be summarized into groups of symptoms that relate to current functioning as well as functioning during the past week. The content of these symptom scales reflects major psychiatric constructs (e.g., formal thought disorders, endogenous features, manic syndrome).

The RDC provides guidelines for a specific set of psychiatric diagnoses. These diagnostic criteria are applied after the SADS is administered.

Background

Both the SADS and the RDC were developed as a comprehensive system for reducing variability in psychiatric diagnoses. Initial work on the RDC was based on the 15 Feighner criteria. The current version contains over 24 major psychiatric disorders (e.g., major depressive disorder), as well as disorder specific subtypes (e.g., recurrent major depressive disorder, endogenous major depressive disorder, and situational major depressive disorder). The manual also provides comparisons between RDC and DSM-IV diagnoses (APA, 1994).

Administration

The SADS requires sophisticated interviewers and takes between 90 and 120 minutes to complete. The protocol provides questions and follow-up prompts to obtain information about symptom severity. Although the interview is typically administered to patients, collateral information (e.g., from family members or client records) can also be used. Items are rated using either a Likert-type or a dichotomous format. A rating of 0 implies the item is not applicable or that there is no information available.

Scoring

Following the completion of the interview, scores are added together and organized according to clusters that reflect certain syndromes (e.g., major depressive disorder, delusions-hallucinations, anxiety). A table is available to help determine the percentage of points earned in each symptom cluster.

Interpretation

The SADS scale scores are interpreted based on the percentage of scale items scored in the pathological direction. Diagnoses are based on criteria specified in the RDC.

Psychometric Properties

Norms.   Although several large-scale epidemiological studies have evaluated the prevalence and incidence of psychiatric disorders in the general population, general normative data are not provided for the SADS or the RDC.

Reliability.   Coefficient alpha estimates for the SDAS scales ranged from .47 (Formal Thought Disorder) to .97 (Manic Syndrome). Interrater reliability estimates for the joint administration of the original version of the SADS ranged from .82 (Formal Thought Disorder) to .99 (Manic Syndrome). For the depression summary scales, interrater reliability was estimated at .95. Test–retest estimates ranged from .49 (Formal Thought Disorder) to .93 (Manic Syndrome).

With regard to the reliability of diagnoses made through SADS interviews, Spitzer et al. (1978) report a kappa value of .90 regarding the diagnosis of Major Depressive Disorder and .81 for Minor Depressive Disorder.

Interrater reliability for the diagnoses listed in the RDC was initially calculated in two separate studies and estimates ranged from .75 (Schizophrenia-Lifetime) to 1.00 (Obsessive Compulsive Disorder-Lifetime). Test–retest reliability estimates range from .40 (Bipolar I-Lifetime) to 1.00 (Alcoholism).

Validity.   Correlations between the SADS scales and the Symptom Checklist-90-R (p. 117) were moderate. Additional research has provided considerable support for both the SADS and the RDC.

Clinical Utility

High. The time and effort required for completing the SADS and the accompanying RDC are substantial. Nevertheless, clinical utility is high for situations where an accurate diagnostic picture is essential.

Research Utility

High. For research that is dependent on identifying relatively homogeneous groupings of psychopathology the research utility would be quite high. Additionally, there are videotapes and written instructions that can be implemented to insure acceptable levels of interrater reliability.

Source

Department of Research Assessment and Training, New York State Psychiatric Institute, Box 123, 722 West 168th Street, New York, NY.

Cost

A variety of options are available (interviewer booklets, scoring sheets, computer versions, training videos). Those interested should contact the people listed below for additional information.

- Permission for reproduction: Dr. Jean Endicott (212) 543-5536
- Training programs and videos: Jo Ellen Noth (212) 543-5528
- Computer programs: Dr. John Nee (212) 543-5514
- Shipment, order processing, and similar concerns: Renee Jarvis (212) 543-5270

Alternate Forms

The SADS has been adapted to meet a variety of clinical and research needs. For instance, Campbell and Cohn (1991) used a modified version to assess prevalence rates of postpartum depression among first-time mothers.

STATE TRAIT-DEPRESSION ADJECTIVE CHECKLISTS (ST-DACL)

Original Citation

Lubin, B. (1994). *State Trait-Depression Adjective Check Lists: Professional manual.* Odessa, FL: Psychological Assessment Resources.

Purpose

To measure feelings of dysphoria, sadness, and psychological distress.

Population

Adolescents and adults aged 14–89 years.

Description

The ST-DACL is a revision of the original DACL (Lubin, 1981), which contained seven different alternative checklists of 32 or 34 adjectives. The current version uses the same lists and adjectives, but now provides for an assessment of both state and trait mood. For the State version, respondents are requested to check words that describe how they feel "now—today." For the Trait forms, the frame of reference is "today and generally." Some adjectives represent positive feelings, such as "fine," "joyous," and "sunny," whereas others reflect a negative mood, for example, "tortured" and "sad" (items are reprinted with the permission of the publisher, Psychological Assessment Resources). Forms 1 and 2 are equivalent measures of both state and trait mood, whereas Forms A-B and C-D are equivalent measures of only state mood.

Background

The original DACL has been used extensively in empirical studies to assess depressed mood and feelings. The adjective checklist format was chosen for its ease of administration and high degree of acceptance by test takers. The task itself requires minimal cognitive sophistication, making it useful across various age groups (adolescents, adults, and the elderly). The DACL also meets the needs of researchers using repeated measures designs and contains various alternative forms.

Administration

The ST-DACL can be self-administered and generally requires about 3 minutes to complete each list.

Scoring

Scoring keys and profile sheets are available for each list. For Forms 1 and 2, the following scores can be derived: S-Neg (total number of negative adjectives endorsed), S-Pos (total number of positive adjectives endorsed) and State Mood-Total Score (summary score representing overall depressed mood calculated by the sum of S-Neg and the total number of positive adjectives that *were not endorsed*). A similar structure exists for trait mood. The higher the summary scores, the more state or trait depressed mood is present.

Interpretation

ST-DACL raw scores can be converted to both *T*-scores and percentile scores according to the respondent's age and gender. Norms are contained in the manual for the following three age groups: adolescents (14–18 years), adults (19–62 years), and elderly adults (63–89 years). These three groups are further broken down by gender. The manual suggests that a *T*-score of 65 and above represents a clinically elevated test score (i.e., indicative of depressed mood) and not in the range of normal limits.

Psychometric Properties

Norms.   The norms for the State version are based on a sample of over 3,000 adolescents and adults. For the Trait version, various nonreferred and referred samples were tested providing for data from hundreds of subjects (e.g., 308 subjects from a community mental health center, 67 subjects from a state hospital, 294 adults living in a midwestern city, 760 students in grades 8–12).

Reliability.   Internal consistency estimates for both versions were found to be relatively high. For example, coefficient alphas for the State measure ranged from .82 to .94. For the Trait scale, the same index was found to range from .79 to .91. Test–retest estimates for the State scale, due to the temporally specific nature of the scale, are expected to be low, but significant. Overall, the temporal reliability over short periods of time appears to be acceptable. For the Trait version, test–retest coefficients ranged between .44 and .84 over intervals of 5–7 weeks.

Validity.   Evidence is provided in the manual for the construct and factorial validity of both the State and Trait versions of the ST-DACL. For example, DACL scores correlate high with the BDI (p. 29), the POMS (p. 94), the CES-D (p. 39), and the MMPI-Depression scale (p. 73).

Clinical Utility

High. ST-DACL scores have been found to be related to psychiatric diagnoses. In addition, substantial norms are provided in the manual against which to compare specific patient scores.

Research Applicability

High. The DACL was been used extensively in research studies assessing the relationship between certain variables and depressed mood, as well as for an outcome measure to assess the effects of treatment for depression.

Source

Psychological Assessment Resources, Inc., P.O. Box 998, Odessa, FL 33556. Phone: 800-331-TEST.

Cost

$85 for an introductory kit which includes a manual, 25 copies of Forms 1 and 2, 25 copies of Form A-B, 25 copies of Form C-D, and 25 profile forms.

Alternative Forms

A variety of equivalent alternative forms exist.

STRUCTURED CLINICAL INTERVIEW FOR DSM-IV AXIS I DISORDERS (SCID)

Original Citation

First, M. B., Spitzer, R. L., Gibbon, M., & Williams, J. B. W. (1997). *User's Guide for the Structured Clinical Interview for DSM-IV Axis I Disorders*. Washington, DC: American Psychiatric Press.

Purpose

The Structured Clinical Interview for DSM-IV Axis I Disorders (SCID) is a semistructured interview designed to help clinicians and researchers make distinctions among various categories listed in the DSM-IV.

Population

The SCID was developed for use in clinical settings and may be administered to either psychiatric or general medical patients. It was designed for adults, ages 18 or older, but with slight modifications the measure can be used with adolescents.

Description

There is both a clinician and a research version of the SCID. The clinician version covers only diagnoses typically seen in clinical practice and excludes a majority of the subtypes and specifiers present in the research version. The research version is longer and includes some disorders that are not included in the clinician version, such as acute stress disorder, minor depressive disorder, mixed anxiety depressive disorder, and binge eating disorder. In addition, there is a different measure for evaluating personality disorders, the Structured Clinical Interview for DSM-IV Axis II Disorders.

Background

Initial work on developing a structured interview for the DSM began around 1983. In 1987, the Structured Clinical Interview for the DSM-III-R Axis I Disorders was published by the American Psychiatric Association. The goal was to assist clinicians with the differential diagnosis of a variety of conditions listed in the DSM-III. The current version, the Structured Clinical Interview for DSM-IV Axis I Disorders, reflects a modification of the previous version and was specifically designed to assist in the differential diagnosis of conditions described in the DSM-IV.

Administration

The clinician version of the SCID requires approximately 45–90 minutes to administer. It begins with an open-ended interview in which information is solicited regarding the present and past episodes of psychopathology. Patients are provided the opportunity to describe their presenting problem(s). The overview also provides the clinician with enough information to develop a working diagnosis. The clinician begins this section by asking the following: "I'm going to be asking you about problems or difficulties you may have had, and I'll be making some notes as we go along. Do you have any questions before we begin?"

Next, the clinician administers a series of questions and records the patient's responses verbatim. These questions elicit information about demographic and historical factors, the patient's current problem(s), environmental and contextual precipitants, course of the present illness, current social functioning and other relevant factors. The next step requires the clinician to administer a series of questions designed to help the clinician develop a differential diagnosis. This section is divided into six separate modules. The six modules are mood episodes, psychotic symptoms, psychotic disorders, mood disorders, substance use disorders, anxiety and other disorders. Each module contains items about a variety of related disorders. Responses to each item are rated using the following options: "inadequate information," "absent (or subthreshold)," or "present."

A rating of inadequate information is given in situations in which insufficient information is available, for instance, if the patient cannot remember or if the information is questionable. A rating of absent is given if the symptom described in the criterion is either absent or below diagnostic threshold. Finally, a rating of present is coded if the threshold for the criterion is reached.

The questions administered are based on the patient's responses. Directions for skipping or returning to previous items are clearly specified.

Scoring

After items have been scored, a Diagnostic Summary is completed by the clinician. The first determination is whether lifetime or current diagnostic criteria for the various Axis I disorders are met. A lifetime diagnosis is warranted if the criteria have ever been met, whereas a current episode is diagnosed if the criteria have been met within the past month.

A section is provided for completing Axis IV of the DSM-IV. The clinician checks off relevant psychosocial and environmental stress, and specifies other relevant problem areas.

Finally, the clinician completes Axis V of the DSM-IV by rating the patient's level of functioning according to criteria specified in the Global Assessment of Functioning Scale. This scale ranges from 0 (inadequate information) to 100 (superior functioning, no symptoms).

Psychometric Properties

Norms.   This version of the SCID is relatively new and normative data have not yet been published. Research conducted with its predecessors has mostly involved screening study participants to decrease sample heterogeneity. For these and other related reasons, normative data are not readily available.

Reliability.   The SCID is relatively new and reliability data have not yet been published. Because the current version reflects a modification of the previous version, reliability data are estimated from the previous version (Williams et al., 1992). Williams et al. (1992) used data collected at six different sites and estimated the levels of agreement for major categories using weighted kappa coefficients. For patient samples these estimates averaged .61 for current diagnosis and .68 for lifetime diagnosis. Diagnostic agreement was also assessed using a test-retest procedure. For major categories, the kappa coefficients ranged from .54 to .84. Intraclass estimates were used to assess ratings of patient functioning during the past month as measured by the Global Assessment of Functioning Scale; site estimates ranged from .47 to .82.

Validity.   Because there are no "gold standards" for determining psychiatric classification, validity of the Structured Clinical Interview for DSM-D Axis I Disorders is heavily dependent upon the validity of the DSM-IV.

Clinical Utility

High. The Structured Clinical Interview for DSM-IV Axis I Disorders provides a semi-structured interview with questions that target specific diagnostic criteria specified in the DSM-IV. The Administration Booklet and score sheet are easy to follow and score. However, this measure does require training and clinical judgment. Although clinicians interested in evaluating clients for depression are unlikely to spend the time required to administer the entire interview, a specific module can be administered and would require considerably less time (e.g., mood episodes, mood disorders).

Research Utility

High. The research version of the Structured Clinical Interview for DSM-IV Axis I Disorders is quite extensive and will prove helpful for studies that require a differential diagnosis for depression based on DSM-IV.

Source

First et al. (1997).

Cost

A starter kit (User Guide, Administration Booklet, and five score sheets) currently lists for $65.00. For information on recent product development and pricing contact American Psychiatric Press, Inc., 1400 K Street North West, Washington, DC 20005.

Alternative Forms

Information on the research version of the SCID can be obtained by contacting the Biometrics Research Department at New York State Psychiatric Institute, Unit 74, 722 West 168th Street, New York, NY 13002. Information on the SCID for Personality Disorders can be obtained by contacting the American Psychiatric Press, Inc., 1400 K Street North West, Washington, DC 20005.

SYMPTOM CHECKLIST-90-R (SCL-90-R)

Original Citation

Derogatis, L. R. (1994). *Symptom Checklist-90-R administration, scoring, and procedures manual* (3rd ed.). Minneapolis, MN: National Computer Systems.

Purpose

To assess psychological symptoms reported by psychiatric patients, medical patients, and nonpatients.

Populations

Adolescents and adults.

Description

The SCL-90-R is a self-report inventory, where each of the 90 symptoms listed is rated on a 5-point scale of distress ranging from 0 ("not at all") to 4 ("extremely"). In addition to three global distress indices (general severity index, positive symptom distress index, and positive symptom total), the SCL-90-R provides information on nine primary symptom dimensions. These include anxiety, depression, hostility, interpersonal sensitivity, obsessive-compulsive, paranoid ideation, phobic anxiety, psychoticism, and somatization. The Depression scale contains 13 items representing a range of symptoms of clinical depression (e.g., feeling blue, feeling lonely, feeling worthless).

Background

The SCL-90-R was developed from the Hopkins Symptom Checklist (Derogatis et al., 1974). The correlation between the primary symptom dimensions associated with the SCL-90-R and various MMPI subscales was used to determine concurrent validity. The SCL-90-R has been employed in a large number of studies that have assessed a wide range of psychopathology.

Administration

The SCL-90-R takes approximately 20 minutes to complete. Subjects are initially presented with a brief instructional set and the 90 items.

Scoring

Computer and hand scoring of the SCL-90-R are available. Hand scoring is completed using plastic scoring templates. A work sheet is also available for recording raw scores on the nine symptom dimensions and the three global indices. Raw scores are plotted on a profile sheet and T-score conversion allows for an analysis across scores. Profile sheets are available for patient and nonpatient samples.

Interpretation

High scores indicate more severe symptoms. The SCL-90-R manual suggests first evaluating the global indices to gain an understanding of the overall level of distress. The second step involves looking at the primary symptom dimensions. The manual suggests that such an analysis can provide information regarding specific concerns. Finally, the manual also suggests perusing the discrete items to identify specific symptoms that need to be addressed.

Psychometric Properties

Norms.   Data are available for psychiatric inpatients ($N = 423$), psychiatric outpatients ($N = 1002$), nonpatient respondents ($N = 974$), and adolescent nonpatients ($N = 806$).

Reliability.   Several samples have been used to derive coefficient alpha estimates for the nine primary symptom dimensions. Estimates range from .79 to .90; the estimate for the primary symptom dimension of depression is .90. Psychiatric outpatients were used to obtain stability estimates. One-week test–retest reliability estimates ranged from .78 to .90, whereas 2-week estimates ranged from .68 to .83. With specific regard to the primary symptom dimension of depression, 1-week test–retest reliability was estimated at .82, whereas 2-week test-retest reliability was estimated at .75.

Validity.   Several of the SCL-90-R scores correlate with related constructs measured using the MMPI. For instance, the primary symptom dimension of depression was significantly related to the Wiggins Content Scale ($r = .75$) and Tyron Depression Cluster Scale ($r = .68$). Unfortunately, the primary symptom dimension of depression was also related to various scales that are not typically conceptualized as depression-related (e.g., MMPI Scale 8, $r = .55$; MMPI Scale 7, $r = .48$; and Tyron Autism Cluster Scale, $r = .48$). Factor-analytic studies have also generally failed to identify nine primary symptom dimensions (e.g., Brophy, Norvell, Kiluk, 1988; A. Clark & Friedman, 1983; Strauman & Wetzel, 1992). The SCL-90-R is probably best thought of as a general screening device that measures global levels of psychopathology.

Clinical Utility

Limited. As a general measure of psychopathology the measure has high clinical utility. For instance, the measure possesses enough sensitivity that it can be used repeatedly to assess changes in psychiatric symptoms as a result of treatment. Unfortunately, the primary symptom dimension of depression has not been well validated and 86% of the items are not specifically related to depression.

Research Applicability

Limited. As a general measure of psychopathology the measure has high utility. For instance, the measure could clearly be used to equate samples for overall levels of psycho-pathology. Unfortunately, the primary symptom dimension of depression lacks the specificity and sensitivity that is often required in research instruments designed to quantify level of depressive symptoms. Therefore, the research utility of the SCL-90-R as a measure specifi-cally of depression is low (Choquette, 1994).

Source

National Computer Systems, Assessment Sales Dept., 5605 Green Circle Drive, Min-netonka, MN. Phone: 880-627-7271. Website: www.ncs.com.

Cost

A variety of options are available (e.g., Starter Kit, Preview Kit, Computer Generated Interpretative Reports, Audiocassette Version, Large Print Version, Hand Scoring Keys, etc.). The Hand Scoring Starter Kit costs $104. Contact National Computer Systems for additional prices.

Alternative Forms

Alternate forms are available in Spanish and 13 other languages.

ZUNG SELF-RATING DEPRESSION SCALE (ZUNG SDS)

Original Citation

Zung, W. W. K. (1965). A self-rating depression scale. *Archives of General Psychology*, *12*, 63–70.

Purpose

To assess symptoms of depression.

Population

Adults.

Description

The Zung SDS is a 20-item self-report measure of depression. Of the 20 items, half are worded positively ("I feel hopeful about the future") and half negatively ("I feel down-hearted and blue"). All items are rated on a 4-point scale with anchor points referring to the amount of time the item is currently experienced. These range from "a little of the time" to "most of the time."

Background

The Zung SDS was developed to assess depression quickly via self-report and to yield a quantifiable rating of current depression. It was specifically designed for patients with a primary depression diagnosis, targeting a wide range of related symptoms. Categories of items were selected based on factor analyses found in the literature that provided the most common types of symptoms associated with depression. Specific items within these categories were then developed from transcribed statements from patient records to select those statements that best represented the categories chosen.

Administration

Administration time is approximately 5 minutes or less.

Scoring

As amount of time endorsed increases, negatively worded items are scored from 1 to 4, with positively worded items reverse-scored from 4 to 1. Total scores are obtained by summing the ratings from the 20 items for a total score ranging from 20 to 80. Higher scores indicate higher levels of depression. An index score can also be obtained by dividing the obtained raw score by the maximum possible score of 80.

Interpretation

The following information on interpretive guidelines for the Zung SDS was provided by the GlaxoWellcome website (address provided below): below 50 = normal; 50–59 = mild depression; 60–69 = moderate to marked depression; 70 or higher = severe depression.

Psychometric Properties

Initial norms for the Zung SDS were developed on a sample of 56 patients admitted to an inpatient psychiatric service with a primary diagnosis of depressive disorder. Of these patients, 31 were treated for depressive disorders, whereas the other 25 received diagnoses of other (nondepressed) disorders following further evaluation. Within the depressed group, 22 patients completed the Zung SDS a second time following treatment for their depression. Finally, a control group of 100 hospital professional and nonprofessional staff, as well as medically hospitalized patients, all without a history and reports of depression, also completed the Zung SDS. Although the initial reference article refers to index scores, these have been converted back to raw scores for this handbook by multiplying the index score by 80.

Additional information regarding psychometric properties of the Zung SDS was provided in several later studies; the reliability and validity information provided below was obtained by Gabrys and Peters (1985), who administered the Zung SDS to a sample of 587 patients (218 nondepressed, 369 depressed) ranging in age from 12 to 69 years. Of these patients, 173 were accompanied by a family member; 109 family members also completed the Zung SDS (rating the patient) to provide independent ratings of patients' depression.

Norms.   The mean scores for the first sample described above were as follows: depressed, 59.2; nondepressed, 42.4; control, 26.4. The mean score for the depressed group posttreatment was 31.2. For the second sample, mean scores were 33.89 ($SD = 8.25$) for the family escort group, 36.05 ($SD = 4.41$) for the nondepressed clinical group, and 50.55 ($SD = 6.86$) for the depressed client group.

Reliability.   Split-half reliability was high, with $r = .94$. Internal consistency was also high, with alphas of .91 for family escorts, .88 for depressed clients, and .93 for nondepressed clients. For these three groups, mean item-total correlations were .80, .82, and .85 respectively.

Validity.   Examination of mean scores indicated that the Zung SDS adequately discriminated among family escorts, nondepressed clients, and depressed clients. All group differences were statistically significant. The comparison most likely to be of interest is that between depressed and nondepressed clients; this comparison yielded a t-score of 30.85 ($p < .001$). A cutoff score of 40 (index score = .50) was established to examine predictive validity. Of the nondepressed clinical group, 23% scored above the cutoff, yielding a successful prediction rate of 77%. Of the depressed clinical group, only 8% scored below the cutoff, yielding a successful prediction rate of 92%. Biggs, Wylie, and Ziegler (1978) reported a correlation of .80 between the Zung SDS and the Hamilton Rating Scale for Depression (p. 58). A lower correlation, .54, was found between the Zung SDS and the Beck Depression Inventory (BDI; p. 29) in a separate study (Kerner & Jacobs, 1983).

Clinical Utility

High. The Zung SDS is easily and quickly administered and scored, and can readily serve as an initial screen for depression. The Zung SDS is also suited for ongoing assessment, as repeated administrations are unlikely to be taxing to clients or clinicians.

Research Applicability

High. The Zung SDS has been used in numerous research studies as a brief measure of depression. Due to its brevity, it can be added to an assessment battery fairly easily.

Source

The Zung SDS can be downloaded free of charge from the following GlaxoWellcome website: http://www.wellbutrin-sr.com/eval/zung.htm.

Cost

None.

Alternate Forms

The Zung SDS has been translated into a number of languages, including Spanish, Chinese, Dutch, Japanese, and Iranian. In addition, a 10-item clinician-assisted version was developed by Tucker, Ogle, Davison, and Eilenberg (1986).

Chapter 5
Measures of Depression: Special Populations

INTRODUCTION

In this chapter, measures are included that can be used to measure depressive symptoms among a variety of special populations, including children and adolescents, the elderly, adults with mental retardation, adults with medical or physical problems, and adults with schizophrenia. As in the previous chapter, they are listed below by category, but given in this chapter in alphabetical order.

Adults with Physical Problems

- Medical-Based Emotional Distress Scale
- Visual Analog Mood Scales

Children and Adolescents

- Children's Depression Inventory
- Children's Depression Rating Scale-Revised
- Kiddie-SADS-PL
- Multiscore Depression Inventory for Children
- Reynolds Adolescent Depression Scale
- Reynolds Child Depression Scale
- Youth Depression Adjective Checklist

Elderly

- Cornell Scale for Depression in Dementia
- Depression Rating Scale
- Geriatric Depression Scale

Mentally Retarded Adults

- Psychopathology Inventory for Mentally Retarded Adults

Postpartum Depression

- Postpartum Depression Interview Schedule

Schizophrenia

- Calgary Depression Scale for Schizophrenia
- Visual Analog Mood Scales

CALGARY DEPRESSION SCALE FOR SCHIZOPHRENIA (CDSS)

Original Citation

Addington, D., Addington, J., & Maticka-Tyndale, E. (1993). Assessing depression in schizophrenia: The Calgary Depression Scale. *British Journal of Psychiatry*, *163*, 39–44.

Purpose

To assess depression in people with schizophrenia.

Population

Individuals diagnosed with schizophrenia.

Description

The CDSS is a nine-item clinician-rated measure that is completed following a semistructured, goal-directed interview. Each item contains a question that clinicians are instructed to ask as written (e.g., "How would you describe your mood over the last two weeks?"). Interviewers may follow up with probes or qualifiers at their own discretion. Then they choose the best score to represent respondent's answer based on a 4-point Likert-type scale ranging from 0 to 3. Respondents' answers represent their experience of each symptom during the past 2 weeks. The last question, number 9, is based on the participant's behavior during the interview as observed by the clinician. The authors recommend that the rater have experience working with schizophrenia and develop interrater reliability before administering the CDSS.

Background

The CDSS was developed in response to the observation that other assessment instruments for depression did not accurately represent depressive symptoms or syndromes in people with schizophrenia. It is often difficult to distinguish depressive symptoms from extrapyramidal symptoms or positive and negative symptoms of schizophrenia, and the authors could not find an instrument to address this distinction. Another problem was that people with more severe schizophrenic symptoms had difficulty completing self-report questionnaires. Items of the CDSS were taken from items of the Present State Examination (Wing, Birley, Cooper, Graham, & Issacs, 1967) and the HRSD (p. 58) by using factor and reliability analysis techniques.

Administration

It takes approximately 30 minutes to complete the CDSS interview and response scales. However, there may be some individual variability depending upon the communication skills of the participant.

Scoring

The CDSS is scored simply by adding the score for each item. Total scores range from 0 to 27.

Interpretation

Higher scores indicate greater degrees of depressive symptomatology.

Psychometric Properties

Norms. Norms for 50 acutely ill hospitalized people with schizophrenia and 100 outpatients with schizophrenia are reported in Addington et al. (1994).

Reliability. A measure of the internal consistency of the CDSS among 150 schizophrenics (100 outpatients and 50 inpatients) yielded a Cronbach's alpha score of .79 for the total sample (.78 for inpatients and .71 for outpatients). There was 86% agreement between raters for individual items, and the intraclass correlation was .895 (Addington et al., 1992).

Validity.   Construct validity of the CDSS was established by comparing this instrument to another well-established instrument for depression and by examining its ability to predict a major depressive episode. The correlation between the CDSS and the BDI (p. 29) was .73 (after outliers were excluded) for a sample of 150 schizophrenics. Using the CDSS, 93% of patients were correctly classified as having a major depressive episode.

Divergent validity of the CDSS was established by examining its ability to discriminate depression from extrapyramidal symptoms and negative symptoms of schizophrenia. The CDSS showed no correlation with a measure of extrapyramidal symptoms. The CDSS showed a weak correlation (.33) with negative symptoms among 50 inpatients and no correlation with negative symptoms among 100 inpatients. Negative symptoms were assessed with the Positive and Negative Symptom Scale (PANSS; Kay et al., 1987). None of the factors of the CDSS correlated with negative symptoms in a later study of 112 inpatients with schizophrenia where the PANSS was used to measure negative symptoms (Addington, Addington, & Atkinson, 1996).

Clinical Utility

High. Strong correlations with other depression instruments with established clinical utility, as well as its unique ability to differentiate depressive from negative extrapyramidal symptoms of schizophrenia, make this instrument a preferred depression instrument for this population.

Research Applicability

High. The high specificity, good reliability, and high construct validity of the CDSS make this a useful tool for research on depression in schizophrenia. Research has also demonstrated that the CDSS is sensitive to change.

Source

Dr. Donald Addington, Department of Psychiatry, Foothills Hospital, 1403 29th Street N.W., Calgary, Alberta, Canada T2N 2T9.

Cost

None.

Alternate Forms

French, Spanish, Dutch, Polish, and Swedish translations of the CDSS are available.

CHILDREN'S DEPRESSION INVENTORY (CDI)

Original Citation

Kovacs, M. (1992). *Children's Depression Inventory manual.* North Tonawanda, NY: Multi-Health Systems.

Purpose

To assess depressive symptoms.

Population

Children and adolescents aged 7–17 years.

Description

The CDI is a 27-item self-report measure of depressive symptoms in children and adolescents that was developed in response to a need for an economical, easy-to-administer, and readily analyzable measure of depression in children. The items represent symptoms and consequences particularly characteristic of depression in children and adolescents. These include disturbed mood, anhedonia, negative self-evaluation, ineffectiveness, and interpersonal problems. The 27 items are presented in groups of three statements, where the severity of each item is scored using a 3-point scale ranging from 0 (absence of the symptom) to 2 (definite symptom). A sample item, reprinted with permission of Multi-Health Systems, Inc., is as follows:

Item 20
☐ I do not feel alone
☐ I feel alone many times.
☐ I feel alone all the time.

The CDI was modeled after the BDI (p. 29) and constructed using 1,266 students aged 7 to 16 years. Factor analysis resulted in the identification of five factors: negative mood, interpersonal problems, ineffectiveness, anhedonia, and negative self-esteem. Respondents are requested to describe how they have been feeling during the past 2 weeks.

Administration

In general, the CDI requires 10–15 minutes to complete and can be administered individually or in small groups.

Scoring

Five factor scores and an overall score are obtained by summing over the ratings for relevant items. Higher scores indicate higher levels of depressive symptoms. The maximum score is 54.

Interpretation

Scores are converted to T-scores based on age range (7–12 or 13–17 years) and gender. T-scores are interpreted using the following guidelines: very much below average (below 30), much below average (30–34), below average (35–39), slightly below average (40–44), average (45–55), slightly above average (56–60), above average (61–65), much above average (66–70), and very much above average (above 70). Kovacs (1992) suggests that a T-score greater than 65 reflects a clinically significant elevation. Lower T-scores are recommended for general screening purposes. However, these are tentative cutoff points and should not be used as sole sources of information for diagnostic purposes.

Psychometric Properties

Norms. The normative sample was composed of a group of boys ($N = 592$, ages 7–15 years) and girls ($N = 674$, ages 7–16 years) in Florida public schools and a group of 134 clinically diagnosed children. Means, standard deviations, and T-score conversions are provided in the manual.

Reliability. Coefficient alpha estimates developed from the normative sample range from .59 to .68 for the five factors. A similarly derived estimate for the total score was .85. Stability estimates for 2- to 3-week intervals range from .74 to .83.

Validity. A discriminant functional analysis assessed the discriminant validity of the CDI when comparing clinical versus nonclinical samples. It was found to correctly classify nonclinical cases, but not the clinical cases. Results were similar when the five subscales were employed. In addition, factor analytic studies have rarely replicated the hypothesized five-factor structure of the CDI.

Clinical Utility

High. This measure is easy to administer, interpret, and score. It is a frequently used self-report measure of childhood depressive symptoms. Although there are some reservations when employing this measure to discriminate between clinical and nonclinical samples, the manual presents some tentative data that suggest the measure is sensitive to changes in depressive symptoms.

Research Applicability

High. A considerable body of research has employed the CDI as a self-report measure of childhood depressive symptoms.

Source

Multi-Health Systems, Inc., 908 Niagara Falls Boulevard, North Tonawanda, NY 14120-2060. Phone: 800-456-3003.

Cost

$55 for manual and 25 forms.

Alternative Forms

A 10-item short form has been developed as a quick screening device. Translations of the CDI are also available for research purposes. These are available in Arabic, Bulgarian, Italian, Hungarian, Hebrew, Spanish, German, French, and Portuguese.

CHILDREN'S DEPRESSION RATING SCALE-REVISED (CDRS-R)

Original Citation

Poznanski, E. O., & Mokros, H. B. (1996). *Children's Depression Rating Scale-Revised: Manual*. Los Angeles, CA: Western Psychological Services.

Purpose

To serve as a screening instrument, diagnostic, and severity measure of depression in children.

Population

Children aged 6–12 years.

Description

The CDRS-R is a semistructured interview for children. It assesses 17 symptom areas, including DSM-IV symptoms of depressive disorders. Of these 17 symptom areas, 14 (e.g., social withdrawal, appetite and sleep disturbances, suicidality, depressed feelings) are rated by the interviewer in response to the child's verbal responses to questions, with the other 3 (depressed facial affect, listless speech, and hypoactivity) evaluated by the interviewer based on the child's nonverbal behavior. Most symptom areas are rated on a 7-point scale, with 3 rated only on a 5-point scale. The interview includes a number of suggested topics and prompts to obtain the information necessary to score each symptom area, and sample responses and their corresponding ratings are provided in the manual as well.

Background

The CDRS was initially developed as a clinical instrument in response to growing recognition of the validity of children's depression. It was tailored to the age range of 6–12 years, since this age range was more likely to be homogeneous relative to adolescents who might express both adult- and child-related aspects of depression, yet were also old enough to respond verbally and report on their own emotional and behavioral states. Development of the CDRS was based on the Hamilton Rating Scale for Depression (HRSD; p. 58) widely used for adults, incorporating the concepts of symptom areas comprised of multiple items, clearly anchored rating scales, the use of multiple sources of information, and the use of an overall summary score. Over time, the CDRS was examined as a clinical research measure as well, and its use in pediatric and psychiatric inpatient settings led to its revision in the mid-1980s. Specifically, the revised version added and renamed several symptom areas, expanded the available rating scale anchors, and added suggested prompts for each symptom area. In addition, the CDRS-R provided separate ratings for each of multiple sources of information, whereas the earlier version had combined these into a single rating.

Administration

The CDRS-R generally takes 20–30 minutes, including both administration and scoring of the interview. The manual notes that it is to be administered by "properly trained professionals." Although specific training requirements are not described, the interview is sufficiently detailed in both administration and scoring instructions that well-trained mental health professionals should have no trouble with its use.

Scoring

Once information is gathered for each symptom area, the clinician rates that area using an anchored rating scale. As noted above, most of the 17 areas use a 7-point scale, whereas 3 use only a 5-point scale. After rating the child's interview, a summary score and a T-score are calculated. The summary score is a raw score ranging from 17 to 113, which is obtained by summing the individual ratings of all 17 symptom areas. Each scoring booklet includes a scale by which corresponding T-scores and percentiles are obtained for each summary score. A similar scoring procedure is used for additional information obtained by sources other than the child, with the clinician's determining ratings for the "Best Description of the Child" based on all available information. (When the clinician believes all rating sources provided equally valid information, this final rating consists of the highest score across the multiple sources.) A sample symptom area rating item is reprinted below, with permission of the publishers.

Instructions: Rate each symptom area for this child by writing only one number in the box. Write NR ("Not Rated") in the box if there is insufficient information to derive a rating.

1. IMPAIRED SCHOOLWORK   □
   Performance is consistent with ability   1
          2
   Decrease in school performance and/or ability to concentrate   3
          4
   Major interference with performance in most subjects   5
          6
   No motivation to perform   7

Comment   _____

Interpretation

Interpretive guidelines are provided for ratings for each symptom area, as well as for overall T-scores. For individual symptom areas, a 2 indicates that whereas problems may exist, they are not clinically significant, with ratings of 3–7 indicating increasing clinically significant problems within that area. Overall, T-scores between 55 and 64 indicate sufficient depressive symptoms likely to warrant further evaluation. T-scores above 65 are considered likely indicators of significant depressive disorder.

Psychometric Properties

Psychometric properties are based on two samples: a clinical sample ($N = 78$) of children drawn from a depression research clinic, and a nonreferred sample ($N = 223$) of children drawn from a magnet school in Chicago. Within the clinical sample, 60 children met DSM-III criteria for a depressive disorder and 15 of the remaining children met criteria for another psychiatric diagnosis.

Norms. The mean T-score for the clinical sample meeting criteria for depressive disorders was 71, and for the nonclinical sample was 53. For the nonclinical sample, means are also available for individual symptom areas, broken down across a number of variables. Within the nonclinical sample, these ranged from 1.2 ($SD = 0.6$) to 2.1 ($SD = 1.0$) for those children not reporting suicidality, and from 1.6 ($SD = 0.9$) to 3.2 ($SD = 1.3$). In both cases, appetite disturbance was the area of least severity, and morbid ideation, the most. Similar means are available for a subset of the clinical sample for which both child and parent interviews were conducted ($N = 34$). Individual symptom area means for the child interviews in this sample ranged from 1.5 ($SD = 1.0$; appetite disturbance) to 3.7 ($SD = 1.7$; low self-esteem).

Reliability. Interrater reliability was established using a clinical sample of children ($N = 25$). Four child psychiatrists conducted the interviews, with each interview corated by two of the psychiatrists. Summary scores showed excellent interrater reliability ($r = .92$). Test–retest reliability was also established with a clinical sample ($N = 52$) based on intake and 2-week postintake interviews conducted by two different clinicians, with the second rater blind to initial ratings. These findings indicated very good stability over the 2-week interval ($r = .80$).

The CDRS-R also showed good internal consistency for the nonclinical sample (alpha = .85). Internal consistency was not reported for the clinical sample. Item-total correlations ranged from .28 (impaired schoolwork) to .78 (depressed feelings) in the clinical sample, and from .36 (appetite disturbance) to .71 (depressed facial affect) in the nonclinical sample.

Validity. CDRS-R Summary Scores were compared with independently assigned Global Ratings of Depression and summary scores from a modified version of the HRSD ($N = 36$). Correlations between the CDRS-R scores and these measures indicated moderate to good convergence (.87 for Global Ratings, .48 for HRSD). The CDRS-R was also compared with Dexamethasone Suppression Test (DST) scores to provide a comparison with a measure not relying on clinical judgment. Results indicated that CDRS-R scores were significantly higher among cortisol-nonsuppressors (nonsuppression being widely considered a biological marker of depression) than among cortisol-suppressors.

Discriminant validity of the CDRS-R was examined by comparing the CDRS-R Summary Scores for psychiatrically referred children diagnosed with depressive disorders ($N = 60$), psychiatrically referred children diagnosed with difficulties other than depression ($N = 18$), and children from the nonclinical sample ($N = 223$). Results indicated that children diagnosed with depressive disorders ($M = 53.68$; $SD = 15.70$) scored higher on the CDRS-R than either the other psychiatric disorder group ($M = 34.12$; $SD = 8.4$) or the nonclinical group ($M = 27.8$; $SD = 8.9$).

Clinical Utility

High. The CDRS-R is a relatively efficient structured procedure with which to gather a significant amount of information regarding children's depression. The ability to glean information from multiple informants and integrate that information increases its utility especially in clinical settings.

Research Applicability

High. The semistructured nature of the CDRS-R allows for more standardized results than would be available through general clinical interviews, and the interview provides quantified data that have been shown to have acceptable psychometrics.

Source

Western Psychological Services, 12031 Wilshire Boulevard, Los Angeles, CA 90025-1251. Phone: 310-478-2061; Fax: 310-478-7838.

Cost

Specimen kits (includes manual and 25 administration booklets) are $57 each; packages of 25 administration booklets only are $16.50 each ($13.90 each in quantities of two or more).

Alternative Forms

None.

CORNELL SCALE FOR DEPRESSION IN DEMENTIA (CORNELL SCALE)

Original Citation

Alexopoulos, G. S., Abrams, R. C., Young, R. C., & Shamoian, C. A. (1988). Cornell Scale for Depression in Dementia. *Biological Psychiatry, 23*, 271–284.

Purpose

To assess depression among people with dementia.

Population

Dementia patients. Specifically, the Cornell Scale was developed with a population of individuals with primary degenerative dementia, multiinfarct dementia, or mixed primary degenerative dementia and multiinfarct dementia who could communicate their basic needs.

Description

The Cornell Scale is a 19-item clinician-rated instrument. Clinicians obtain the information necessary to complete this instrument from both the caregiver and the patient. The clinician begins by first interviewing a caregiver of the person with dementia in order to obtain sufficient information to complete all 19 items. Then the clinician interviews the patient to obtain the same information. If caregiver and patient responses are discrepant, then the clinician repeats the interview with the caregiver, attempts to understand the discrepancy, and chooses the best response based on all of the interviews. Each item contains a symptom of depression (e.g., "sadness," "appetite loss") and is rated on a 3-point scale where 0 = absent, 1 = mild or intermittent, and 2 = severe. A response of "999" is also available to indicate symptoms which the clinician was unable to evaluate. Responses represent symptoms observed during the week prior to interview.

Background

The Cornell Scale was developed to address the special problems inherent in the assessment of depression in people who are also diagnosed with dementia. A clinician-rated response format was selected because people with dementia often have difficulty describing their own experience of depressive symptoms. Furthermore, the questions of the Cornell Scale were designed to detect the unique presentation of depression, which is often complicated by the cooccurring symptoms of dementia in this population.

Administration

The time frame for administering the Cornell Scale is approximately 30 minutes.

Scoring

Scores range from 0 to 38.

Interpretation

Higher scores indicate greater severity of depressive symptoms.

Psychometric Properties

The psychometric properties of the Cornell Scale were assessed in a population of 83 demented participants. The developers used nonparametric statistical analysis because the rating scales used for comparison yielded ordinal data.

Norms.   Means and standard deviations for a sample of 83 people with dementia are reported in Alexopoulos et al. (1988).

Reliability.   The interrater reliability of the Cornell Scale was assessed in a group of 26 demented participants. Correlations between the scores for each item ranged from .64 to .99. Regarding internal consistency, the mean intercorrelation among items was .24 ($SD = .15$) and Cronbach's alpha was estimated to be .84 for a sample of 48 demented participants.

Validity.   Scores on the Cornell Scale were compared to the rank ordering of depression subtypes described by the Research Diagnostic Criteria (p. 108) and significant correlations ($r = .83$) supported the instrument's concurrent validity.

The sensitivity of the Cornell Scale was demonstrated by its ability to distinguish each diagnostic category from the other categories in a sample of 20 hospitalized patients. Studies also demonstrated that scores on the Cornell Scale increased with more severe depression in demented patients.

Clinical Utility

High. The ability to differentiate varying degrees of depression provided by the Cornell Scale is helpful in clinical settings with this specific population. Preliminary data also supported the Cornell Scale's utility for observing change in depressive symptoms over time.

Research Applicability

High. The demonstrated sensitivity of the Cornell Scale makes this a useful instrument for measuring response to psychological or pharmacological interventions for depression in patients with dementia.

Source

The Cornell Scale is reprinted in Appendix B.

Cost

None.

Alternative Forms

The Cornell Scale has been translated into German, French, and Chinese.

DEPRESSION RATING SCALE (DRS)

Original Citation

Cohen-Mansfield, J., & Marx, M. S. (1988). Relationship between depression and agitation in nursing home residents. *Comprehensive Gerontology. Section B, Behavioral, Social, and Applied Sciences*, 2, 141–146.

Purpose

To assess social functioning and depressed affect in nursing home residents.

Population

Elderly individuals who are frail, cognitively impaired, and reside in nursing homes.

Description

The DRS is a six-item, caregiver-rated instrument that measures depressive symptoms in the areas of sad mood, social functioning, and activity level. The informants for most of the validity tests of the DRS were nurses and social workers. Caregivers rate each of the items based on a 7-point Likert-type scale ranging from 1 to 7. The time frame for which the answers should be based is not specified.

A factor analysis reveals that the items load on two factors. The first factor is described as "social functioning," the second as "depressed affect."

Background

The DRS was developed in order to examine the dimensions of depression, as defined by DSM-III criteria, in nursing home residents. The author was interested in gaining a better understanding between the aggressive behavior observed in nursing home residents and either dementia or depression. However, the depression instruments that existed at the time were deemed inadequate for this purpose because many individuals in the population of interest were incapable of completing self-report questionnaires or providing the verbal self-reports necessary to complete most clinician-rated instruments. Therefore, the DRS was developed to provide an alternative method of assessing depression when participants are incapable reporting their own experience.

Administration

Caregivers familiar with the participants read the questions and circle the appropriate answers.

Scoring

Scores range from 6 to 42, where high scores represent greater symptom severity.

Psychometric Properties

Norms.   None.

Reliability.   In order to examine the interrater reliability of the DRS, scores provided by two daytime charge nurses were compared for each of nine depression questions in a sample of 31 nursing home residents. Correlations averaged .73.

Validity.   Tests of the construct validity of this instrument are not reported. However, higher scores were found among the more verbally agitated participants, bringing into question the ability of the DRS to detect depressive symptoms in nonverbal patients, a shortcoming that was criticized in the other depression instruments.

Comparison between the DRS and the agitation subscales of the Cohen–Mansfield Agitation Inventory showed that the depressed affect subscales of the DRS significantly correlated with verbally agitated behavior, whereas the social functioning subscale significantly negatively correlated with aggressive behavior.

Clinical Utility

Limited. The ability of the DRS to identify symptoms that correlate with agitation is promising. However, its ability to correctly label affect among nonverbal patients needs to be further examined and possibly refined.

Research Applicability

Limited. Few studies have been conducted using the DRS and additional examinations of its reliability and validity are required.

Source

The DRS is reprinted in Appendix B. For additional information, contact Jiska Cohen-Mansfield, Ph.D., Research Institute of the Hebrew Home of Greater Washington, 6121 Montrose Road, Rockville, MD 20852.

Cost

None.

Alternative Forms

None.

GERIATRIC DEPRESSION SCALE (GDS)

Original Citation

Yesavage, J. A., Brink, T. L., Rose, T. L., Lum, O., Huang, V., Adey, M., & Leirer, V. O. (1983). Development and validation of a geriatric depression screening scale: A preliminary report. *Journal of Psychiatric Research, 17*, 37–49.

Purpose

To measure depression in older adults.

Population

Adults over 65 years old. Some studies support its reliability and validity in younger adults as well.

Description

The GDS is a 30-item self-report questionnaire that may be administered orally or in written format. Each item contains a yes/no response. When administered orally, interviewers are allowed to repeat a question until the response is clearly "yes" or "no." When administered in written format, the words "yes" and "no" are written after each question and respondents are instructed to circle the better response for each question. Although an exact time reference is not included in the instructions, each question is worded in the present tense to imply recent experience of depressive symptoms.

Background

A number of difficulties arise in the assessment of depression among elderly populations. For example, it is often difficult to differentiate between symptoms of depression and symptoms of dementia. In addition, several somatic symptoms of depression, such as decreased sleep and decline in sexual functioning, are more prevalent among normal elderly populations than among younger groups. Long or complicated depression questionnaires are too difficult for some patients who are physically or cognitively impaired, and clinicians have observed that some elderly individuals become offended by questions about sexuality. The GDS was designed to measure depressive symptoms among elderly populations while accounting for the special problems inherent in such an assessment. The GDS places less emphasis on the somatic symptoms of depression. It is also designed to be easy to use and acceptable to most patients.

Administration

The GDS can be administered in written format or orally. It takes at least 30 minutes to complete and may take longer among patients who are hearing or cognitively impaired.

Scoring

Each depressive answer is counted as 1 point and each nondepressive answer is counted as 0 points. After the instrument is completed, the points are added to compose a total score. Scores range from 0 to 30 with higher scores indicating greater depression.

The guidelines for scoring and administration are provided in Appendix B, and the authors recommend that they not be altered.

Interpretation

Brink et al. (1982) describes scores from 0 to 10 as being in the normal range, scores from 11 to 20 as the mild depression range, and scores from 21 to 30 as the moderate to severely depressed range.

Psychometric Properties

Norms. Means and standard deviations for the GDS measured among 51 depressed and 20 nondepressed elderly individuals are reported in Brink et al. (1982).

Reliability. One study of the internal consistency of the GDS found Cronbach's alpha to be .94. The same study also demonstrated a split-half reliability of .94, a mean intercorrelation between items of .36, and a median correlation between items of .56 (Yesavage et al., 1983).

Another study examined the reliability of the GDS among 193 younger adults (ages 17–55 years) because younger samples sometimes serve as control groups in studies of geriatric depression. Results yielded an alpha coefficient of .82, a median correlation with the total score of .38, a mean inter-item correlation of .15, and a split-half reliability of .80 (Rule, Harvey, & Dobbs, 1989).

Validity. Comparisons of the ability to differentiate depressed from nondepressed elderly individuals yielded superior results for the GDS ($t = 8.51$) as compared to the Zung SDS (p. 120; $t = 5.38$) and the HRSD (p. 58; $t = 6.77$) (Brink et al., 1982). A later comparison of the ability to differentiate non-depressed, mildly depressed, and severely depressed individuals showed the GDS to be comparable to the HRSD (F-scores of 99.48 and 110.63, respectively) and superior to the Zung SDS (44.75) (Yesavage et al., 1983). The GDS also has high sensitivity (84%) as well as specificity (95%).

The GDS has adequate construct validity among younger participants, with one study demonstrating a correlation of .66 between the GDS and the CES-D (p. 39).

Clinical Utility

High. The guidelines for interpretation are useful for gauging the severity of depression in elderly populations.

Research Applicability

High. Numerous studies confirm the sound psychometric properties of the GDS for geriatric populations. Some results also support its applicability even when age-matched control groups are not feasible. The authors suggest that researchers start with a clinically depressed sample when trying to show a treatment effect (T. L. Brink, personal communication, December 1998). Brink also recommends using nonparametric statistics such as the Fisher exact, Mann–Whitney, sign test, Friedman, or Kolmogorov–Smirnov with small samples.

Source

The GDS is reprinted in the appendix. It can also be downloaded by accessing the following website: http://www.stanford.edu/~yesavage/GDS.html.

Cost

None.

Alternate Forms

The GDS has been translated into numerous languages including Chinese, Danish, Dutch, French, German, Greek, Hebrew, Hungarian, Italian, Japanese, Korean, Portugese, Rumanian, Russian, Spanish, Swedish, Thai, Vietnamese, and Yiddish. Updated information about alternate forms is available on the website listed above, and many of these translations can be downloaded from that site as well.

KIDDIE-SCHEDULE FOR AFFECTIVE DISORDERS AND SCHIZOPHRENIA FOR SCHOOL-AGE CHILDREN-PRESENT AND LIFETIME VERSION (K-SADS-PL)

Original Citation

Kaufman, J., Birmaher, B., Brent, D., Rao, U., Flynn, C., Moreci, P., Williamson, D., & Ryan, N. (1997). Schedule for Affective Disorders and Schizophrenia for School-Age Children-Present and Lifetime Version: Initial reliability and validity data. *Journal of the American Academy of Child and Adolescent Psychiatry, 36*, 980–989.

Purpose

To assess current and lifetime history of childhood psychiatric disorders and to obtain symptom severity ratings.

Population

Children aged 6–17 years.

Description

The K-SADS-PL is a semistructured interview based on the DSM-IV criteria (APA, 1994). The instrument evaluates the presence of 32 Axis I child psychiatric diagnoses, assesses current and past episodes of psychopathology, and includes scales for rating symptom severity and level of functioning.

The K-SADS-PL is a recent revision of the Present Episode Version (Chambers et al., 1985), a diagnostic interview for children modeled after the SADS (p. 108). Similar to previous versions, the K-SADS-PL yields diagnostic information based on parent–child interviews. The interview is actually conducted twice, once with the parent and again with the child. Detailed questions and probes are provided to guide the interview.

The interviewer initially elicits background information and then administers a screen interview that assesses 82 symptoms across 20 diagnostic areas. This allows the interviewer to skip subsequent segments of the interview if a threshold is not reached. Based on results of the screen interview, the interviewer may move on to the five diagnostic supplements, which include affective disorders, psychotic disorders, anxiety disorders, behavioral disorders, and substance abuse, tic, and eating disorders. The final segment allows the interviewer to rate global impairment.

Background

The original K-SADS was developed by Puig-Antich and Chambers (1978), and has been periodically updated with changes in newer editions of the DSM. There are a number of published versions of the K-SADS available as well as a number of unpublished versions.

Administration

The K-SADS-PL must be administered by a sophisticated interviewer familiar with diagnostic classification and differential diagnosis and who has been trained in the use of the instrument. The time it takes depends on the symptom picture. In the absence of any threshold level psychopathology, parent and child interviews each takes 35–45 minutes. Psychiatric patient interviews are likely to run 75 minutes.

Scoring

Most symptoms assessed during the screen interview and diagnostic supplements are rated using a 4-point scale where a score of 0 indicates no information available to make the rating, a score of 1 suggests the symptom is not present, a score of 2 indicates subthreshold levels of symptomatology, and a score of 3 represents symptom presence at threshold criteria. Some symptoms are more simply rated on a 0- to 2-point scale. The score for global impairment is based on a clinical anchored rating of level of functioning, ranging from a low of 0 ("needs constant supervision") to a high of 100 ("superior functioning in all areas"). Item scoring is facilitated by detailed probes and scoring criteria provided with the protocol.

Interpretation

A symptom picture and a DSM-IV diagnosis are derived by synthesizing parent and child data. Interviewers are instructed to use their best clinical judgment when integrating information.

Psychometric Properties

Norms.   Items contained in the K-SADS-PL are operationalized DSM criteria. The authors note that they simplified the scoring to reduce unreliability in rating symptom severity seen in earlier versions (Kaufman et al., 1997).

Reliability.   The authors report excellent interrater reliability. Agreement for the use of the screen interview skipout criteria across diagnostic areas was 100% for past diagnoses and ranged from 93% to 100% for current diagnoses. The percentage agreement in assigning present and lifetime diagnoses ranged from 93% to 100% (Kaufman et al., 1997). Kappa coefficients ranged from .50 to .70 across a number of the diagnostic areas associated with the screen interview and ranged from .63 to 1.00 for various current and past diagnoses (Kaufman et al., 1997).

Validity.   Kaufman et al. (1997) report data which support the concurrent validity of the skipout criteria and diagnoses generated with the K-SADS-PL. Children who met criteria for a specific diagnostic category (e.g., depressive disorder, anxiety disorder, behavior disorder) scored significantly higher than the other children on rating scales assessing the related symptoms (e.g., Children's Depression Inventory; p. 127).

Clinical Utility

High. The K-SADS-PL is a direct assessment of DSM-IV diagnoses, the primary diagnostic manual in clinical use. This version also remedies limitations of its predecessors by (a) assessing a wider range of current and lifetime child psychiatric disorders, (b) providing global and diagnosis-specific impairment ratings, and (c) including revised probes and the scoring criteria to improve symptom identification and diagnosis.

Research Utility

High. The K-SADS-PL generates reliable and valid psychiatric diagnoses and is consistent with the DSM-IV, which provides uniform standards for diagnoses in clinical research. However, test administration is time-consuming, involves lengthy interviews with both child and adult caretaker, and must be administered by highly trained, sophisticated clinical interviewers.

Source

Dr. Joan Kaufman, Western Psychiatric Institute and Clinic, Division of Child and Adolescent Psychiatry, University of Pittsburgh School of Medicine, 3811 0'Hara Street, Pittsburgh, PA 15213.

Cost

The K-SADS-PL is copyrighted, but usage is freely permitted without further permission for not-for-profit institutions and/or Institutional Review Board-approved research protocols. All other uses require written permission of the principal author, Dr. Joan Kaufman. The latest version of the instrument, a pointer to the author's electronic mail address, and other useful information can be found at www.wpic.pitt.edu/ksads.

Alternate Forms

None.

MEDICAL-BASED EMOTIONAL DISTRESS SCALE (MEDS)

Original Citation

Overholser, J. C., Schubert, D. S. P., Foliart, R., & Frost, F. (1993). Assessment of emotional distress following a spinal cord injury. *Rehabilitation Psychology, 38,* 187–198.

Purpose

To assess emotional reactions to severe physical illness or disability that are not the direct result of a physical condition or problem.

Population

Adults with physical illnesses or disabilities.

Description

The MEDS is a 60-item clinician-administered questionnaire that is completed following a structured interview. This instrument measures distress along seven subscales: Dysphoria, Irritability, Anhedonia, Social Withdrawal, Ruminations over Past Events, Cognitive Perspective in the Present, and Expectations for the Future. Each item provides a question (e.g., "How has your mood been this past week; have you been feeling fairly depressed or fairly cheerful … or equal amounts of both?") and is followed by a range of responses that are on a 5-point scale for either intensity (ranging from not present at all to very much present) or frequency (ranging from never to always present). The questions are organized by subscale and the interview is structured such that a denial of problems in a certain area allows the interviewer to skip to the next subscale.

Background

Similar to other instruments developed to measure distress in medical patients, the MEDS was developed in order to provide a more valid assessment of distress so that results are not biased by physical symptoms of the cooccurring medical disorder. This instrument measures several different types of distress and differentiates among them. Accurate diagnosis of emotional disorders has numerous implications for quality of life, as well as recovery or rehabilitation from the medical disorder. The MEDS focuses on the cognitive and psychological factors of distress rather than the physical factors and measures distress as it has been experienced during the past week. This instrument was developed on a group of adults with spinal cord injuries.

Administration

Clinicians begin by reading the first question of the first category. If the participant endorses symptoms pertaining to this subscale, then the clinician proceeds with follow-up questions. If the participant denies symptoms, then the clinician skips to the first question in the next category. The same procedure is followed for each category. The MEDS can take as long as 45 minutes to complete depending upon the amount of distress experienced by the patient.

Psychometric Properties

Norms.   Limited information is available on the norms for this instrument.

Reliability.   Coefficient alpha for the total MEDS was .92. Internal consistency for the subscales ranged from .60 to .86. The subscales were derived logically and they have a high degree of intercorrelation.

Validity.   Scores on the MEDS were compared to scores on the Beck Hopelessness Scale (BHS; p. 175), the SCL-90-R (p. 117), and the Zung Self-Rating Depression Scale (p. 120). Numerous significant correlations were found among the subscales of the various scales to demonstrate the instrument's convergent validity. However, the correlations demonstrate the poor divergent validity of the MEDS. The specific correlations are reported in Overholser et al. (1993).

Clinical Utility

High. The MEDS provides a useful screening tool for distress in medical patients. It is easy to administer and is less biased by the physical symptoms of medical conditions.

Research Applicability

Limited. Further research is needed to demonstrate the utility of the MEDS in other medical populations in addition to patients with spinal cord injuries. However, its high correlation with other frequently used instruments is promising.

Source

The MEDS is reprinted in Appendix B. For additional information, contact James C. Overholser, Ph.D., Case Western Reserve University, Department of Psychology, 10900 Euclid Avenue, Cleveland, OH 44106-7123.

Cost

None.

Alternative Forms

None.

MULTISCORE DEPRESSION INVENTORY FOR CHILDREN (MDI-C)

Original Citation

Berndt, D. J. & Kaiser, C. F. (1996). *Multiscore Depression Inventory for Children manual.* Los Angeles, CA: Western Psychological Services.

Purpose

To assess depressive and related symptoms.

Population

Children ages 8–17 years.

Description

The MDI-C is a self-report inventory that contains 79 items designed to evaluate depression-related symptoms in children and adolescents. The manual describes eight subscales: Anxiety, Defiance, Instrumental Helplessness, Low Energy, Pessimism, Sad Mood, Self-Esteem, and Social Introversion. Respondents read self-descriptive statements and indicate whether each statement is true or false as applied to themselves. Items from the Instrumental Helplessness subscale are reprinted below with the permission of the publisher:

> I get punished for no reason.
> I don't have much fun.
> I don't get much attention.
> People don't treat me fairly.
> No one would care if I died.
> No one listens when I complain.
> My friends are never there when I need them.

Background

The MDI-C was derived from the Multiscore Depression Inventory for Adolescents and Adults (MDI; p. 84). A 120-item version was administered to 1,465 children. Items that were endorsed by less than 5% of the sample were discarded. The 79 items contained in the final version were selected based on their relationship to the hypothesized MDI-C subscales and other measures. A unique feature of this inventory is that children contributed to the wording of the directions and the items.

Administration

The MDI-C requires 15–20 minutes to complete and can be administered in individual or group format.

Scoring

Raw scores are obtained by counting the number of items endorsed in the keyed direction. Raw scores are then plotted on gender- and age-related (8–10, 11–13, 14–17 years) profile grids. These grids provide T-scores for each of the eight subscales and the total score. Double-marked items are considered a missing response. More than eight missing responses cause the profile to be invalid.

Interpretation

All scales are scored so that higher T-scores represent greater severity: T-scores from 56 to 65 indicate mild to moderate symptoms, T-scores from 66 to 75 indicate moderate to severe symptoms, and T-scores over 75 indicate severe symptoms. An Infrequency Index, composed of rarely endorsed items, is available to aid in evaluating potential response bias (e.g., malingering).

Psychometric Properties

Norms. The normative sample consisted of 1,465 children (710 girls and 755 boys). The sample was both geographically and ethnically diverse. A table in the manual, as well as profile sheets, can be used to convert raw scores to T-scores.

Reliability. Coefficient alpha for the total score was estimated at .94, whereas estimates for the eight subscales ranged from .66 to .85. Four-week test–retest stability for the total scale score was estimated at .92, with subscale estimates ranging from .77 to .86.

Validity. Concurrent validity was established by correlating the MDI-C with the Children's Depression Inventory (p. 127), the BDI (p. 29), and the MDI (p. 84). Moderate to strong correlations were reported for these measures. Construct validity was established by factor analysis conducted on a sample of 1,114 children and a cross-validation sample of 250 children. As opposed to the eight subscales that were developed on the basis of content analysis, the results supported the existence of a four-factor structure.

Clinical Utility

High. The MDI-C appears to be a useful tool for screening depression and depression-related constructs. The instrument is easy to administer to individuals and/or groups. The Infrequency Index may also prove to be useful in helping clinicians to identify individuals who present themselves in an overly negative manner.

Research Applicability

High. Coefficient alpha estimates and preliminary validity data for the total score are acceptable. Data available for the reliability and the validity of the hypothesized subscales are more variable.

Source

Western Psychological Services, 12031 Wilshire Boulevard, Los Angeles, CA 90025-1251. Phone: 800-648-8857.

Cost

$105 for 25 test forms, 25 profile forms, a manual, and two prepaid mail-in answer sheets for computer scoring and interpretation.

Alternative Forms

None.

POSTPARTUM DEPRESSION INTERVIEW SCHEDULE (PDIS)

Original Citation

Campbell, S. B., & Cohn, J. F. (1991). Prevalence and correlates of postpartum depression in first-time mothers. *Journal of Abnormal Psychology*, *100*, 594–599.

Purpose

To assess depression during the postpartum period.

Population

Postpartum women.

Description

The PDIS is a semistructured clinical interview that consists of several general questions about demographics, pregnancy and delivery complications, and the baby's health. Women are asked about their mood during the postpartum period. They are also asked about major symptoms of depression, such as sleep disturbances, appetite loss, loss of interest in usual activities or lack of interest in the baby, feelings of guilt or self-reproach, and suicidal thoughts. Questions also address the duration of the depressed mood and whether the woman is currently depressed. An effort is made to differentiate between normal changes during the postpartum period and actual symptoms of depression. A diagnosis is made with a modification of the Research Diagnostic Criteria (p. 108). To meet criteria for depression, the woman has to report a period of at least 2 weeks during the postpartum period when she felt sad, tearful, or blue. She must also report at least three additional symptoms.

Background

The PDIS is a slightly modified and shortened version of the Schedule for Affective Disorders and Schizophrenia (SADS; p. 108). It was developed to study prevalence rates of postpartum depression in a large sample of primiparous women. The sample was rather homogeneous, consisting of married White women over 18 years old who were delivering their first infant. The PDIS was developed to give a more accurate measure of prevalence rates of postpartum depression. Prevalence rates using semistructured interviews were found to be lower than rates found in studies that relied solely on self-report symptom checklists. Self-report symptom checklists measure somatic symptoms that are endorsed by many postpartum women regardless of depression status and assess a range of symptoms that are not specific to a depressive disorder.

Administration

The PDIS can be administered over the telephone or in person. Interviewers require some training.

Scoring

The SADS symptoms are rated as present or absent; to qualify as present, symptoms had to be reported as severe enough to interfere with functioning. Women who do not report depressed mood lasting at least 2 weeks and a minimum of three additional symptoms are considered nondepressed.

Interpretation

An endorsement of at least a 2-week period of depression during the postpartum period and five or more symptoms indicates major depression. A report of sad mood and four additional symptoms must be reported to qualify for a diagnosis of probable major depression, and report of sad mood and three symptoms is considered minor depression.

Psychometric Properties

Norms. Norms are based on a sample of 1,033 women. Ninety-six (9%) of the women met depression criteria (i.e., depressed mood and at least three symptoms) for at least a 2-week period during the postpartum period.

Reliability. The reliability of the PDIS was determined by comparing the diagnosis derived from the telephone interview with the diagnosis made independently by a home visitor who administered a full SADS. Agreement on diagnosis was 100% for 32 women who were interviewed at home by an independent clinical interviewer who had not administered the telephone interview.

Validity. At the time of the telephone interview, the 21 items from the Center for Epidemiological Studies-Depression Scale (CES-D; p. 39) were read to 1,007 of the women. More than half of the women (77 of 132 or 58%) with elevated CES-D scores did not meet modified Research Diagnostic Criteria for depression on the SADS; conversely, 37 (40%) of the 92 women who met criteria for depression did not receive elevated CES-D scores; thus, concordance between measures was obtained for only 60% of the depressed women. Prevalence rates of postpartum depression based on the PDIS were similar to those reported in other studies of postpartum women in the United States, Canada, and Great Britain (Cooper et al., 1988; Gotlib et al., 1989; O'Hara et al., 1990). Rates were also similar to those reported by investigators who studied women in the general population (e.g., Myers et al., 1984). This supports O'Hara et al. (1990), who concluded that depression is not more common in postpartum women than in non-child-bearing women of similar age and demographics.

Clinical Utility

High. The PDIS is fairly brief and easily administered. However, some training is required for administration.

Research Utility

High. The PDIS appears more accurate in diagnosing postpartum depression than self-report questionnaires.

Source

Campbell and Cohn (1991).

Cost

The PDIS is a modified version of the SADS. Information regarding the use of the SADS appears elsewhere in this volume (p. 108). Additional information regarding the modifications employed can be obtained from the reference listed above or by contacting Susan B. Campbell, Department of Psychology, University of Pittsburgh, Pittsburgh, PA 15260.

Alternative Forms

None.

PSYCHOPATHOLOGY INVENTORY FOR MENTALLY RETARDED ADULTS (PIMRA)

Original Citation

Matson, J. L. (1988). *The PIMRA manual.* New Orleans, LA: International Diagnostic Systems.

Purpose

To assess the presence and severity of a variety of psychopathology behaviors of persons who are dually diagnosed (both mentally retarded and mentally ill).

Population

Adults with mental retardation.

Description

The PIMRA contains 56 items that cut across eight clinical scales: schizophrenia, affective disorder, psychosexual disorder, adjustment disorder, anxiety disorder, somatoform disorder, personality disorder, and inappropriate adjustment. Each item can be answered "yes" or "no." The Affective Disorder scale includes seven symptoms (e.g., mood swings, sadness, insomnia). The PIMRA consist of two structured interviews: "other" and "self-report." The first involves a trained interviewer asking questions based on these items with a parent, caretaker, teacher, or work supervisor who knows the patient well. The "self-report" version involves an actual interview with the individual. The manual strongly suggests that only professionals who are trained to work with mentally retarded persons should use the PIMRA.

Background

Although the prevalence of psychopathology in mentally retarded persons typically is significantly greater than among persons of normal intellectual functioning (C. M. Nezu, Nezu, & Gill-Weiss, 1992), there are few psychometrically sound instruments that are geared to assess these problems. The PIMRA was developed to meet this need and is based on DSM-III categories and symptom pictures. Items representing key features of each of the diagnoses were selected and stated in a manner appropriate for this population.

Administration

The entire PIMRA, conducted with a parent or caretaker, takes about 30–45 minutes to complete. Depending on the language skills of a given mentally retarded subject, additional time may be needed when conducting the "self-rating" interview. The Affective Disorder scale takes about 10 minutes to complete, barring communication problems.

Scoring

The presence of each psychopathology symptom is rated as 1, where each scale score is the numerical sum of these scores regarding the items on a scale. A total score is possible, summing across the seven clinical scales (some items are reverse-scored, as they represent the lack of psychopathology). Thus, the higher the overall total score, the higher the subject's level of general psychopathology.

Interpretation

Subjects can be considered as depressed if they were rated as sad on that one item and were also rated positive for four or more additional symptoms. Caution is noted, however, that the PIMRA is intended to be but one part of an overall assessment procedure. For additional guidelines regarding the assessment of depression among this population, see Kazdin, Matson, and Senatore (1983) and C. M. Nezu et al. (1992).

Psychometric Properties

Norms.   Not available.

Reliability.   Based on a population of 209 mentally retarded adults, support for the PIMRA's high level of internal consistency was obtained. Specifically, coefficient alpha for the total score was .83, and the Spearman–Brown split-half reliability was .88. Test–retest reliability for the PIMRA total score was found to be .68 and .91 for the "self-report" and "other" versions, respectively. Such estimates for the Affective Disorder scale were .69 and .74, respectively. Time between testings was 5 months.

Validity.   Evidence is provided only with regard to concurrent validity. Specifically, using the above Affective Disorders scale guidelines to designate a sample of mentally retarded adults as depressed versus nondepressed, depressed subjects also reported high scores on both the BDI (p. 29) and the Zung SDS (p. 120).

Clinical Utility

High. Few instruments exist to assess depression and other forms of psychopathology among this population.

Research Applicability

High. The PIMRA has been used in various research studies as a validated measure of dual diagnosis, as well as a dependent variable to assess changes in mental health status relating to treatment.

Source

Johnny Matson, Ph.D., Department of Psychology, Louisiana State University, Baton Rouge, LA 70803.

Cost

None.

Alternative Forms

Two versions exist: "self-report" and "ratings-by-others."

REYNOLDS ADOLESCENT DEPRESSION SCALE (RADS)

Original Citation

Reynolds, W. M. (1987). *Reynolds Adolescent Depression Scale: Professional manual.* Odessa, FL: Psychological Assessment Resources.

Purpose

To assess depressive symptomatology in adolescents.

Population

Adolescents aged 13–18 years.

Description

The RADS is a 30-item self-report measure of depressive symptoms that uses a 4-point Likert-type response format. The inventory given to respondents is actually entitled "About Myself," in order to minimize the likelihood of a mood induction if it were identified as a depression inventory. Adolescents are requested to read each of the items and to indicate whether a given statement has occurred almost never, hardly ever, sometimes, or most of the time. Items are worded in the present tense in order to elicit respondents' current feelings and symptom status. Twenty-three items represent positive psychopathological signs of depressive disorder (e.g., "I feel upset"), whereas the remaining 7 items are feelings inconsistent with depression (e.g., "I feel happy") and are reverse-scored. Additional items, reprinted with the permission of the publisher, Psychological Assessment Resources,* include the following: "I feel important," "I feel worried," and "I like eating meals."

Background

Item selection for the RADS was based on symptoms included in the DSM-III for major depression and dysthymic disorder, as well as those areas delineated by Research Diagnostic Criteria. The construction, standardization, and validation process involved over 10,000 adolescents.

Administration

The hand-scored version of the RADS (RADS-HS) requires between 5 and 10 minutes to complete.

Scoring

The RADS-HS is scored by using a scoring template. Item scores range from 1 to 4; reverse-score items range from 4 to 1. The total RADS score involves the sum of the scores, allowing for a range of 30–120. Higher scores represent more severe depression.

Interpretation

The manual suggests that a score of 77 and above on the RADS represents a level of symptom endorsement associated with clinical depression.

Psychometric Properties

Norms.   A series of tables are provided in the manual to allow the user to convert raw scores into percentile ranks for various subsamples (e.g., age, sex, grade) based on a validation sample of 2,460 adolescents.

Reliability.   Estimates for internal consistency yielded a range of alpha coefficients of .91–.94. Split-half reliability, as measured by the Spearman–Brown correction formula, was found to be .91. Test–retest reliability coefficients provided in the manual for the time intervals 6 weeks, 3 months, and 1 year are .80, .79, and .63, respectively.

Validity.   Evidence of the content, criterion, and construct validity of the RADS is provided in the manual. For example, the RADS was found to be correlated .83 with the HRSD (p. 58), .73 with the BDI (p. 29), .75 with the CES-D (p. 39), .72 with the Zung SDS (p. 120), and .73 with the CDI (p. 127).

Clinical Utility

High. Strong associations with clinician rating scales and formal diagnostic interview procedures support its clinical efficacy.

Research Applicability

High. The RADS has been shown to be sensitive to the effects of treatment for depressed adolescents (e.g., Reynolds & Coats, 1986).

Source

Psychological Assessment Resources, Inc., P. O. Box 998, Odessa, FL 33556. Phone: 800-331-TEST.

Cost

$89.00 for manual, scoring key, and 50 hand-scorable answer sheets.

Alternate Forms

None.

REYNOLDS CHILD DEPRESSION SCALE (RCDS)

Original Citation

Reynolds, W. M. (1989). *Reynolds Child Depression Scale: Professional manual*. Odessa, FL: Psychological Assessment Resources.

Purpose

To assess depressive symptomatology in children.

Population

Children in grades 3–6 (ages 8–12 years).

Description

The RCDS is a 30-item self-report measure of depressive symptoms in children that can be administered in individual or group formats. Of the 30 items, 29 use a 4-point Likert-type response format, whereas the remaining item consists of five faces depicting emotions ranging from happy to sad. The child, in completing the RCDS, is asked to fill in a circle that best describes the frequency of how he or she has been feeling for the past 2 weeks regarding these statements. Sample items, reprinted with the permission of the publisher, Psychological Assessment Resources,* include "I feel sad," "I feel that the other kids don't like me," "I feel loved," "I feel bored," "I feel like nothing I do helps anymore." Responses include almost never, sometimes, a lot of the time, or all the time.

Background

The item content of the RCDS was based on symptoms delineated by DSM-III and by the Research Diagnostic Criteria. Items were written to require only a second-grade reading level and to be relevant to a child population. A greater weight is given to dysphoric mood and anhedonia in the RCDS as they are the primary inclusion criteria in DSM-III-R for major depression and dysthymia. A major use of the RCDS is large-scale screening in school settings for childhood depression.

Administration

The RCDS can be administered in individual, small group, or classroom formats. The hand-scored form (Form HS) takes about 10 minutes to complete. Similar to the Reynolds Adolescent Depression Scale, the title of inventory, as seen by the children, is "About Me."

Scoring

Scoring is conducted using a scoring key, as several items are reverse-scored. The possible range of total RCDS scores is 30–121. High scores are indicative of more depressive symptomatology.

Interpretation

Although not a diagnostic measure, a cutoff score of 74 and above is offered as the benchmark to identify a child as in need of further evaluation aimed at a more formal

*Adapted and reproduced by special permission of the Publisher, Psychological Assessment Resources, Inc., 16024 North Florida Avenue, Lutz, Florida 33549, from the Reynolds Depression Screening Inventory, by William M. Reynolds, Ph.D., Copyright, 1980 by PAR, Inc. Further reproduction is prohibited without permission of PAR, Inc.

diagnosis. Scores can also be used to compare against a normative sample of 1,620 children broken down by grade and gender. In addition, six items are noted as critical items (e.g., "I feel like hurting myself") and were selected on the basis of their ability to discriminate between clinically depressed and nonclinically depressed children.

Psychometric Properties

Norms.   Normative tables are provided to allow for conversion of raw scores into percentile ranks according to gender and grade.

Reliability.   The alpha reliability coefficient for the overall sample of 1,620 children was .90. In a sample of 24 fifth-grade children, test–retest reliability was found to be .82 over a 2-week period. In another sample of 220 children from grades 3–6, test–retest reliability was found to be .85 over a 4-week period.

Validity.   In the RCDS manual, evidence is provided to support its validity properties regarding content validity, concurrent validity, construct validity, and factorial validity. For example, with regard to convergent validity, as part of an overall assessment of the construct validity of the RCDS, it was found to correlate .73 with the CDI (p. 127) and −.63 with a measure of self-esteem.

Clinical Utility

High. Research estimates using the RCDS cutoff score to classify children as depressed versus nondepressed yields a specificity ratio of 97%, a sensitivity rating of 73%, and a hit rate of 94%.

Research Applicability

High. The RCDS has been shown to be sensitive to the effects of a cognitive-behavioral treatment protocol in a research investigation (Stark, Reynolds, & Kaslow, 1987).

Source

Psychological Assessment Resources, Inc., P.O. Box 998, Odessa, FL 33556. Phone: 800-331-TEST.

Cost

$89.00 for manual, scoring key, and 50 hand-scorable answer sheets.

Alternate Forms

None.

VISUAL ANALOG MOOD SCALES (VAMS)

Original Citation

Stern, R. A. (1997). *Visual Analog Mood Scales: Professional manual.* Odessa, FL: Psychological Assessment Resources.

Purpose

To measure depression and anxiety symptoms in persons with difficulties completing more verbally or cognitively demanding instruments, such as neurological patients.

Population

Adults.

Description

The VAMS is a self-report instrument that contains eight individual scales representing the following mood states: afraid, confused, sad, angry, energetic, tired, happy, tense. All eight items are unipolar in nature, where the anchors include a "neutral" face, as well as a face depicting a specific mood (e.g., sad). These anchors are at ends of a 100-mm vertical line allowing the respondent to place a mark across the line at a point that best describes "How you are feeling right now." Examples are given in the test booklet to illustrate these instructions.

Background

The VAMS was specifically developed for use with neurologically impaired patients with primary or concomitant visuospatial problems. Additional uses include assessment with people with limited cognitive abilities, as well as to screen for mood disorders in primary care medical settings. Although similar scales have been used in psychiatric and medical settings, the VAMS provides for a standardized set of instructions and stimulus material.

Administration

The VAMS can be self-administered or conducted by an examiner using a set of specific instructions. The usual amount of time to complete the VAMS is 5 minutes.

Scoring

A ruler capable of measuring 100 mm is included in conjunction with VAMS materials. Scoring is rather straightforward: A scale's raw score is the distance in millimeters from the neutral pole. Tables are included in the manual to convert these raw scores into *T*-score values by gender and age group (18–54 years and 55–94 years).

Interpretation

The inclusion of normative data providing *T*-score conversions allows for a statistical interpretation of a given respondent's scores. For example, a *T*-score of 70 and above represents 2 standard deviations above the mean, connoting a pronounced deviation from "typical" responses of the comparison group. Based on a subsample of the normative group, a Sad scale raw score of 50 was identified as a useful cutoff score to screen for the presence or absence of abnormal mood states. This cutoff score yielded a sensitivity value of 78%, a specificity value of 88%, and an overall correct classification value of 83%. The manual cautions, however, that this information should only be used as part of an overall assessment procedure.

Psychometric Properties

Norms.   Norms are based on a sample of 579 adults and broken down by gender and age. In addition, the manual also contains means and standard deviations for a sample of 290 psychiatric patients including the following four DSM-IV-based subgroups: major depression, minor depression, anxiety disorder, and other.

Reliability.   An estimate of the test–retest reliability of the Sad scale of the VAMS that included a sample of university students was found to be .49 (15 minutes between test administrations). A second study was conducted with a group of 27 acute stroke patients using the same time period. This estimate was found to be .83.

Validity.   Investigations focused primarily on the construct validity of the VAMS. For example, the Sad scale of the VAMS was found to correlate .72 with the Depression scale of the POMS (p. 94) and .53 with the BDI (p. 29), indicating strong convergent validity properties.

Clinical Utility

High. As noted above, the sensitivity and specificity of the Sad scale cutoff score was found to be strong, making it clinically useful as a screening procedure.

Research Applicability

High. The VAMS has been found to be sensitive to the effects of treatment in a study of psychiatric patients receiving electroconvulsive therapy (Arruda, Stern, & Legendre, 1997).

Source

Psychological Assessment Resources, Inc., P.O. Box 998, Odessa, FL 33556. Phone: 800-331-TEST.

Cost

$49.00 for an introductory kit containing a manual, 10 response booklets, and a metric ruler.

Alternative Forms

None.

YOUTH DEPRESSION ADJECTIVE CHECKLIST (Y-DACL)

Original Citation

Carey, M. P., Lubin, B., & Brewer, D. H. (1992). Measuring dysphoric mood in pre-adolescents and adolescents: The Youth Depression Adjective Checklist (Y-DACL). *Journal of Clinical Child Psychology*, *21*, 331–338.

Purpose

To assess dysphoric mood in preadolescents and adolescents.

Population

Late childhood and adolescent age range (i.e., approximately 11–17 years of age).

Description

The Y-DACL is a 22-item adjective checklist designed to measure dysphoric mood in preadolescents and adolescents. The measure consists of 14 depressive adjectives (e.g., "wilted," "lifeless") and 8 nondepressive adjectives (e.g., "jolly," "strong"). Respondents are asked to endorse those adjectives that correspond to their current mood.

Background

The Depression Adjective Checklist (DACL; Lubin, 1981; p. 111) was the introductory instrument designed for use as a brief instrument for assessment of changes in dysphoric mood for both clinical and research settings. The subsequent Children's Depression Adjective Checklist (C-DACL) was constructed for use with younger populations. Limitations of the preliminary study of this measure, such as the inclusion of adjectives from inappropriate reading levels, led the researchers to modify their adjective list, resulting in the Y-DACL.

Administration

When self-administered, the Y-DACL takes 5–10 minutes to complete.

Scoring

Y-DACL scores are obtained by summing the number of negative adjectives that *are* endorsed and the number of positive items that *are not* endorsed. Scores range from 0–22; higher scores represent higher levels of dysphoric mood.

Interpretation

Cutoff scores for the Y-DACL are not provided; however, scores can be compared with the norms referred to below.

Psychometric Properties

Psychometric properties were based on seven samples of youths from larger ongoing studies in the southern and midwestern United States. The samples consisted of 234 non-referred participants drawn from school populations and 195 emotionally disturbed participants drawn from inpatient psychiatric facilities and from residential treatment facilities.

Norms.   Means and standard deviations for the nonreferred samples, grouped by age, are outlined in table format in the reference article. The means ranged from 3.20 ($SD = 2.99$) for 12-year-old children to 6.14 ($SD = 6.0$) for 16-year-old respondents, with an overall mean of 4.92 ($SD = 4.59$).

Reliability.   The median internal consistency coefficient (Cronbach's alpha) for the Y-DACL was .89 (range = .85–.94) and the median split-half coefficient was .87 (range = .86–.94). Test–retest estimates, based on two administrations 1 week apart in two separate samples, were low (.17 in one sample, .16 in the other).

Validity.   A variety of measures, including the BDI (p. 29), the RADS (p. 152), the BHS (p. 175), and the Automatic Thoughts Questionnaire (ATQ; p. 172), were administered along with the Y-DACL in both clinical and nonreferred samples to determine construct validity. For example, the Y-DACL had low to moderate correlations with the BDI ($r = .60$) and the RADS ($r = .48$).

Additional analysis of construct validity consisted of a series of principal-component analyses for the emotionally disturbed and nonreferred samples. Factor groupings were similar for populations resulting in two factors: Negative Affect and Positive Affect. The adjective "good" loaded for both positive and negative affect factors in the referred sample.

Clinical Utility

High. The Y-DACL can be used for multiple clinical purposes including monitoring of treatment effects, quick screening measures of psychological distress, and recording daily fluctuations in mood.

Research Applicability

High. The Y-DACL can be quickly administered and is cost-efficient.

Source

The 22 adjectives comprising the Y-DACL can be found in the source article listed above. For additional information, contact Michael P. Carey, Ph.D., Medical College of Ohio, Department of Psychiatry, Kobacker Center, 3130 Glendale Avenue, Toledo, OH 43614.

Cost

None.

Alternate Forms

The Y-DACL is available in both state and trait versions. Spanish translations are also available.

Chapter 6
Measures of Depression-Related Constructs

INTRODUCTION

In this last chapter of measures, we include a variety of assessment tools that address various depression-related constructs. As noted earlier in Chapter 1, we limited this section to those constructs that have been empirically linked to depression, either as a causal variable, a mediator, or a related clinical phenomenon. Assessment of such factors has major treatment implications. For example, data from a coping inventory that suggest a particular client is characterized by ineffective coping ability can help shape treatment decisions for that patient. In addition, the vast majority of the measures included in this section have been used in research investigations, underscoring not only their potential psychometric soundness, but also their applicability to the research community.

We did not include every possible measure per construct, as this is far beyond the scope of this book. However, we wished to increase the breadth of our coverage, and again apologize if we left out any important measure. As in the previous two chapters, the measures are listed below by category, but are given in this chapter in alphabetical order.

Activities and Behavior

- Actigraphy
- Depression Check Questionnaire
- Pleasant Events Schedule
- Pleasant Events Schedule-AD
- Unpleasant Events Schedule

Bereavement and Grief

- Revised Grief Experience Inventory

Cognitive Variables

- Anticipatory Cognitions Questionnaire
- Attributional Style Questionnaire
- Automatic Thoughts Questionnaire-Revised
- Beck Hopelessness Scale
- Children's Attributional Style Questionnaire-Revised
- Cognitive Bias Questionnaire
- Cognitive Error Questionnaire
- Cognitive Triad Inventory
- Cognitive Events Schedule
- Depression Beliefs Questionnaire
- Divorce Dysfunctional Attitudes Scale
- Dysfunctional Attitude Scale
- Goal Orientation Inventory
- Positive Automatic Thoughts Questionnaire

Coping

- Coping Inventory for Stressful Situations
- Coping Resources Inventory
- Ways of Coping
- Ways of Responding

Interpersonal/Social Factors

- Interpersonal Events Schedule
- Social Adjustment Scale
- Social Resourcefulness Scale

Personality/Self-Esteem

- Depressive Personality Disorder Inventory
- Depression Proneness Rating Scale
- Self-Esteem Worksheet
- Sociotropy Autonomy Scale

Problem Solving

- Problem-Solving Inventory
- Social Problem-Solving Inventory-Revised

Self-Control and Self-Reinforcement

- Frequency of Self-Reinforcement Questionnaire
- Self-Control Questionnaire for Depression
- Self-Control Schedule

Suicide

- Beck Scale for Suicide Ideation
- Life Attitudes Schedule
- Suicide Ideation Questionnaire
- Suicide Probability Scale

ACTIGRAPHY (MODEL 7164)

Original Citation

Tyron, W. W., & Williams, R. (1996). Fully proportional actigraphy: A new instrument. *Behavior Research and Methods, Instruments, and Computers, 28*, 392–403.

Purpose

The actigraph is a physiological assessment that directly measures activity level, including both frequency and intensity of movement.

Population

Children, adolescents, and adults.

Description

The actigraph is an ambulatory monitor of activity level. It can be worn around the wrist, waist, or ankle, and is slightly larger than a U.S. quarter. It collects approximately 10 measurements per second, with up to 1,440 measurements over the course of a 24-hour period, and can be used continuously for up to 22 days before the computer memory fills.

Background

Activity level is a component of a variety of psychological and physiological constructs. Tyron and Williams (1996) noted that a need for a direct measurement of activity level that included both frequency and intensity was the impetus for their development of the Model 7164 actigraph reviewed here; other actigraphs are also available.

Disturbances in activity level are reflected in several of the DSM-IV symptoms of depression, most notably psychomotor agitation/retardation and sleep disturbances. Therefore, the actigraph may assist in more directly measuring these symptoms.

Administration

The actigraph weighs approximately 1.5 ounces and is approximately $2 \times 1.5 \times 0.6$ inches. The actigraph can be strapped in a pouch on the subject's wrist, ankle, or waist, and is powered by a lithium battery for 4–6 months.

Scoring

Data storage capacity is from 8K to 64K RAM. Data can be downloaded into an IBM-compatible computer, desktop, or portable. Data are written in ASCII file and have the option to be converted into spreadsheets such as Microsoft Excel. Tyron and Williams (1996), in addition to manufacturers' instructions, offer in-depth, step-by-step instructions for this procedure.

Interpretation

Thus far there are no interpretation guidelines relating actigraph output to depression levels, although it can be compared either between or within subjects.

Psychometric Properties

Norms.   Norms for specific disorders such as depression are not yet available. Some norms are available for sleep disorders, although these vary according to the type of actigraphy employed.

Reliability.   Tyron and Williams (1996) evaluated the calibration of 40 different Model 7164 activity monitors. Between-device agreement in laboratory tests was adequate from 0 to 5 Hz. Individual devices were also tested against data obtained from a pendulum, so that variability in scores could be attributed correctly to either instrument error or to differences in movement; these tests showed a maximum mean count difference of 6.78 (0.56% of 1,208 counts). Because of the wide variability in movement levels outside of laboratory settings, instrumental reliability in relation to movement outside of the laboratory has not been established.

Validity.   Pendulum data, as described above, have also been used to establish the concurrent validity of actigraphy. The actigraph performed well in such tests.

Tyron and Pinto (1994) reviewed the output of an actigraph with ratings by teachers on various standardized measures of activity. There was a significant correlation between these measures and measured activity by the actigraph over a 2-week period. Actigraphy was also validated against polysomnography in the assessment of sleep disorders, and demonstrated adequate agreement for this purpose (for a full review of such studies, see Tyron, 1996).

Clinical Utility

Limited. Requires significant client adherence.

Research Applicability

High. Actigraphy can provide objective activity measurements that currently are obtained primarily through self-reported behavior, thus increasing the accuracy of such information. Given the relevance of activity level to depression, this instrument can aid in collecting and quantifying data likely to be of interest to depression researchers.

Source

The Model 7164 actigraph reviewed in Tyron and Williams (1996) can be purchased from Computer Science and Applications, Inc., 2 Clifford Drive, Shalimar, FL 32579.

Cost

Contact the manufacturer for prices.

Alternative Forms

None.

ANTICIPATORY COGNITIONS QUESTIONNAIRE (ACQ)

Original Citation

Légeron, P., Rivière, B., Marboutin, J.-P., & Rochat, C. (1993). The Anticipatory Cognitions Questionnaire (ACQ): Presentation and validation. *L'Encéphale*, *19*, 11–16.

Purpose

To investigate depression-related cognitive disturbances focusing specifically on anticipation abilities.

Population

Adults.

Description

The ACQ is an eight-item self-report questionnaire that assesses anticipatory cognitions by presenting the patient with a simple cognition (e.g., "I have trouble performing a task which used to be easy to perform") and a cognitive reply (e.g., "I couldn't bear it if I failed"). Respondents indicate how well the cognitive reply represents their own thinking by choosing one of four possible answers on a Likert-type scale. Scores for each item represent the responses "true," "rather true," "rather false," and "false." Responses represent the subject's current thought processes.

Background

The ACQ is based on research demonstrating that anticipatory cognitions are impaired in depressed individuals (Sutter, 1990; Sutter & Berta, 1991). This research was based on the cognitive model of depression, which describes depressive thinking in terms of negative views of the self, the outside world, and the future (A. T. Beck, 1967). Although instruments measuring depressive thought processes had previously been created (e.g., the Dysfunctional Attitude Scale, p. 212; the Beck Hopelessness Scale, p. 175), and others had been developed to measure anticipation, an instrument measuring the cognitive dimension of anticipation did not exist. Hence, the ACQ was developed.

Administration

The ACQ takes approximately 20 minutes to complete.

Scoring

Scores on the ACQ range from 0 to 24, where higher scores indicate more highly depressive cognitions. Six items represent depressed cognitions, a "true" response indicates a score of 3, "rather true," a score of 2, "rather wrong," a score of 1, and "wrong," a score of 0. The remaining two items represent nondepressed cognitions and are reverse-scored.

Interpretation

A cutoff score of 7 or higher has been demonstrated to be the most highly sensitive, as well as specific, diagnostic indicator of depression using the ACQ.

Psychometric Properties

Norms.   None.

Reliability.   Tests of the reliability of the ACQ are not reported and the authors identify this as a current drawback of this instrument.

Validity. In order to assess the construct validity of the ACQ, this instrument was compared to the Montgomery–Asberg Depression Rating Scale (p. 75). Results showed the ACQ to have a sensitivity of 89%, specificity of 67%, accuracy of 82%, and likelihood ratio of 2.7.

Clinical Utility

High. With its high sensitivity and specificity, the ACQ is a useful tool for measuring depressed cognitions.

Research Applicability

Limited. Without results on its reliability, there is no evidence to suggest that research results using the ACQ would be reproducible or applicable to other groups. Other aspects of the instrument's validity need to be examined as well.

Source

A copy of the ACS is printed in Legéron et al. (1993).

Cost

None.

Alternative Forms

The original ACQ is in French and an English translation is available.

ATTRIBUTIONAL STYLE QUESTIONNAIRE (ASQ)

Original Citation

Peterson, C., Semmel, A., von Baeyer, C., Abramson, L. Y., Metalsky, G. I., & Seligman, M. E. P. (1982). The Attributional Style Questionnaire. *Cognitive Therapy and Research, 6,* 287–300.

Purpose

To assess the causal ascriptions people use when explaining the cause of positive and negative life events.

Population

Adults.

Description

Causal judgements are assessed using six positive and six negative events. The content of these life events relates to either affiliation (e.g., meeting a friend who offers a compliment) or achievement (e.g., becoming rich) concerns. The measure provides an analysis of the dimensions of internality (i.e., whether the cause is due to the person or some external event), stability (i.e., whether the cause is stable or variable over time), and globality (i.e., whether the cause is specific to this situation or relevant to other life areas) associated with attributions people use for explaining these life events. A rating of the importance of each event can also be obtained.

Background

Various theories view cognitive processes as important for explaining the etiology, maintenance, and treatment of depression. Within this framework, considerable empirical research has identified a relationship between explanatory styles regarding life events and depressive symptoms. Abramson, Seligman, and Teasdale (1978) developed a Reformulated Learned Helplessness theory of depression, which asserts a relationship between attributional style and depressive symptoms. The ASQ was developed to measure various components they posited as being related to level of depression.

Administration

The ASQ can be administered in individual or group formats. The first step requires the person to read a brief description of an event (e.g., "You have been looking for a job unsuccessfully for some time"). The second step requires the person to list one major cause for the event. The third step directs the person to use a 7-point Likert-type scale to rate the event according to the dimensions of internality, stability, and globality. The final step requires rating the personal importance of the event.

Scoring

Four ratings (internality, stability, globality, and importance) are obtained for each of the 12 items. These item-level ratings can be aggregated to produce a score for positive events, negative events, achievement-related events, affiliation-related events, and combinations thereof.

Interpretation

High scores are associated with ratings of increasing internality, stability, globality, and importance.

Psychometric Properties

Norms.   A sample of 130 undergraduate students was used to develop the questionnaire. Means and standard deviations for the three attributional dimensions are contained in Peterson et al. (1982). Additional data are available for a community-based sample of adult volunteers and sales personnel (Whitley, 1991), agoraphobic patients (Michelson, Bellanti, Testa, & Marchione, 1997) and depressed patients (Levitan, Rector, & Bagby, 1998).

Reliability.   Using the same sample of 130 undergraduate students, Peterson et al. reported coefficient alpha estimates of .75 and .72 for the six positive and the six negative items, respectively. Five-week test–retest reliability estimates were .70 for the positive items and .64 for the negative items. Test–retest estimates for the dimensions of internality, stability, and globality ranged from .58 to .69. The results for the content dimensions of achievement and affiliation were unimpressive and the authors suggest considerable caution is warranted when organizing scores based on those content areas.

Validity.   Both quantitative and qualitative reviews have provided support for the construct validity of the ASQ (e.g., Reivich, 1995; Gladstone & Kaslow, 1995). Moreover, preliminary data found that undergraduate students, even when provided with coaching and a monetary incentive, were unable to produce reliable fake good profiles (Schulman, Seligman, & Amsterdam, 1987).

Clinical Utility

Limited. Few idiographic designs have used the ASQ, although it can be used to probe for a patient's attributional style.

Research Applicability

High. The ASQ is a commonly used research instrument. Considerable data exist on the nomothetic use of this measure. For instance, a search using the *Psych Info* component of the *First Search* database resulted in over 280 citations.

Source

M. E. P. Seligman, Ph.D., Department of Psychology, University of Pennsylvania, 3815 Walnut Street, Philadelphia, PA 19104 (also contained in Peterson et al., 1982).

Cost

None.

Alternate Forms

Several versions of the ASQ have been developed for adults (e.g., Dykema, Bergbower, Doctora, & Peterson, 1996) and children (e.g., Thompson, Kaslow, Weiss, & Nolen-Hoeksema, 1998). Versions of the ASQ have also been used cross-culturally (e.g., China: Lee & Seligman, 1997; Japan: Sakamoto & Kambara, 1998; and West Africa: Fox, 1997).

AUTOMATIC THOUGHTS QUESTIONNAIRE-REVISED (ATQ-R)

Original Citation

Kendall, P.C., Howard, B.L., & Hays, R.C. (1989) Self-referent speech and psychopathology: The balance of positive and negative thinking. *Cognitive Therapy and Research*, *13*, 583–598.

Purpose

To assess the frequency of negative and positive self-statements.

Population

Adults.

Description

The ATQ-R is a 40-item self-report measure. Each item consists of a self-statement (e.g., "I'm worthless," "I wish I were somewhere else"), which is rated on a 5-point scale of frequency of how often the thought occurred to the person in the previous week. Ratings range from 0 ("not at all") to 4 ("all the time").

Background

The ATQ-R is a revised version of the Automatic Thoughts Questionnaire (ATQ; Hollon & Kendall, 1980). The original ATQ consisted of 30 self-statements, all of which were negative. Based on recent theories such as the States of Mind model (Schwartz & Garamoni, 1989), in which both positive and negative self-statements are thought to play a role in depression and other forms of psychopathology, the authors revised the ATQ to include 10 positive self-statements, as well as the original negative ones. Using the ATQ-R, for example, Kendall et al. (1989) found that a psychologically healthy internal dialogue is a 1.6 to 1.0 ratio of positive to negative thinking.

Administration

The ATQ-R may be completed either in individual or group self-report administration, requiring 5–10 minutes to complete.

Scoring

ATQ-R scores are obtained by summing all responses, for a range of total scores of 30–150.

Interpretation

Cutoff scores are not available, but scores can be compared with norms listed in the reference article for the ATQ. To compare scores on the ATQ-R, add 10 to each value for the ATQ.

Psychometric Properties

Psychometric properties of the ATQ-R are not yet available; however, the authors note that they are comparable to those of the ATQ, as the only difference between the two measures is the addition of the 10 positive items. Several studies have examined the psychometric properties of the ATQ. Hollon, Kendall, and Lumry (1986), for example, examined a sample of 138 subjects who were classified into nine clinical groups based on the Schedule for the Affective Disorders and Schizophrenia (SADS-L; p. 108) and Research Diagnostic Criteria (RDS; Spitzer, Endicott, & Robins, 1978). These included bipolar depressed ($N = 12$), unipolar depressed ($N = 16$), substance abuse depressed ($N = 12$), substance abuse nondepressed ($N = 17$), general psychiatric disorder ($N = 12$), medical control ($N = 12$; selected from outpatient medical service), normal control ($N = 32$; selected from university classes), remitted bipolar ($N = 12$), and remitted unipolar ($N = 13$).

Norms.   Means for each of the groups noted above were as follows: bipolar depressed = 91.75 ($SD = 36.65$); unipolar depressed = 85.00 ($SD = 23.62$); substance abuse depressed = 95.75 ($SD = 25.37$); substance abuse nondepressed = 60.25 ($SD = 22.82$); general psychiatric disorder = 46.83 ($SD = 12.59$); medical control = 44.83 ($SD = 8.80$); normal control = 45.12 ($SD = 11.02$); remitted bipolar = 41.25 ($SD = 10.47$); and remitted unipolar = 45.77 ($SD = 10.91$).

Reliability.   In a sample of 114 outpatient mental health and medical clients (Harrell & Ryon, 1983), split-half reliability (odd versus even items) was calculated at .96. Coefficient alpha within this sample was calculated at .98. Split-half reliability and coefficient alphas were calculated for the three subsamples of depressed, nondepressed medical, and nondepressed mental health clients as well: depressed = .91 and .94; nondepressed medical = .87 and .91; nondepressed mental health = .59 and .89, indicating generally adequate reliability.

Validity. ATQ scores were examining across the groups described above, using the Beck Depression Inventory (BDI, p. 29) as a measure of depression. The ATQ was closely associated with depression level, supporting its use as a measure of depressive cognitions. Further, the three clinical groups that included current depression demonstrated significantly higher ATQ scores than did the nondepressed or depression-in-remission groups.

Clinical Utility

High. The ATQ-R is brief and easy to complete. Self-statements have been shown to play an important role in depression, and thus a quick way to assess such self-statements can be readily used in a clinical practice. As a predictor measure, the ATQ-R might be used clinically to identify persons potentially at risk for relapse, who might benefit from additional treatment targeting depressive thoughts.

Research Applicability

High. The assessment of cognitions has been an important part of depression research, and the assessment of positive, as well as negative, cognitions is supported by a number of theories of depression. The ATQ has been used widely in depression research already; as the revised version shows increased predictive power relative to the original, it should thus be even more useful.

Source

The ATQ-R is reprinted in Appendix B. For additional information, contact Phillip C. Kendall, Ph.D., Department of Psychology, Weiss Hall, Temple University, Philadelphia, PA 19122.

Cost

None.

Alternate Forms

None.

BECK HOPELESSNESS SCALE™ (BHS™)*

Original Citation

Beck, A. T., & Steer, R. A. (1988). *Manual for the Beck Hopelessness Scale*. San Antonio, TX: The Psychological Corporation.

Purpose

To measure the extent of negative attitudes, pessimism, or hopelessness about the future.

Population

Adults and adolescents.

Description

The BHS is a 20-item self-report inventory geared to assess one's negative expectancies about the immediate and long-term future. Respondents are requested to read each statement and indicate whether it is true or false regarding their attitudes during the past week. Of these 20 items, 9 are keyed false (e.g., "I look forward to the future with hope and enthusiasm") and 11 are keyed true (e.g., "I can't imagine what my life would be like in ten years").

Background

The construct of hopelessness is tied to A. T. Beck's (1967) model of depression, whereby a depressed individual is hypothesized to endorse the following negative triad of cognitions: negative view of oneself, negative view of the future, and negative view of the world. Hopeless persons believe that their attempts to achieve important goals and solve difficult problems would be unsuccessful, and that nothing will turn out right for them in general. Research has provided support for the significant association between hopelessness and depression among adults (A. T. Beck, Kovacs, & Weissman, 1975), as well as among children (Kazdin, French, Unis, Esveldt-Dawson, & Sherick, 1983).

The BHS is based on an earlier 20-item inventory, called the Generalized Expectancy Scale (Minkoff, Bergman, Beck, & Beck, 1973), that was developed to measure hopelessness in suicide attempters and patients expressing suicide ideation.

Administration

When self-administered, the BHS takes between 5 and 10 minutes to complete.

Scoring

Items are scored either 0 or 1, yielding a total score range of 0–20. Higher scores indicate higher levels of pessimism and hopelessness.

Interpretation

Scores of 9 or greater have been shown to be predictive of eventual suicide in depressed suicide ideators. However, the authors of the BHS caution the test user to address other aspects of a patient's functioning in concert with BHS scores, particularly levels of depression and suicide ideation within a comprehensive assessment.

Psychometric Properties

Norms.   Means and standard deviations are provided in the manual for seven patient samples: suicide ideators ($N = 165$), suicide attempters ($N = 437$), alcoholics ($N = 105$), heroin addicts ($N = 211$), patients diagnosed with major depression-single episode ($N = 72$), patients diagnosed with major depression-recurrent episode ($N = 134$), and patients diagnosed with dysthymic disorder ($N = 177$).

Reliability.   Internal consistency estimates (Kuder-Richardson scores) for the above seven samples were found to be .92, .93, .91, .82, .92, .92, and .87, respectively. Test-retest estimates of a group of 22 patients who took the BHS twice, 1-week apart, were .69. In a second outpatient sample ($N = 99$), the correlation was .66 (time between tests was 6 weeks).

Validity.   Information regarding six aspects of validity are presented in the manual (content, concurrent, discriminant, construct, predictive, and factorial). For example, with regard to concurrent validity, correlations between clinical ratings of hopelessness and the BHS among two patient samples (general medical practice; psychiatric inpatients who made recent suicide attempts) was .74 and .62, respectively. With regard to discriminant validity, a study by Topol and Reznikoff (1982) indicated that BHS scores were higher in a group of adolescent suicide attempters than either a group of adolescent psychiatric inpatients or a sample of suburban high school students.

Clinical Utility

High. The BHS manual provides for several clinical scenarios highlighting its use with patients.

Research Applicability

High. The BHS is a frequently used measure in research studies assessing depression and suicide ideation.

Source

The Psychological Corporation, 555 Academic Court, San Antonio, TX 78204-2498. Phone: 800-211-8378.

Cost

$53.00 for manual, scoring key, and 25 record forms.

Alternative Forms

A Spanish version is available.

BECK SCALE FOR SUICIDE IDEATION™ (BSS™)*

Original Citation

Beck, A. T., & Steer, R. A. (1991). *Beck Scale for Suicide Ideation: Manual.* San Antonio, TX: The Psychological Corporation.

Purpose

To assess suicidal ideation as an indicator of suicide risk.

Population

Adults and adolescent psychiatric patients (both outpatient and inpatient groups) 17 years and over.

Description

The BSS is a self-report measure consisting of 21 items, the first 19 of which focus on three gradations of suicidal wishes, attitudes, and plans. These gradations are associated with scores of 0, 1, and 2. The last two items ask about the number of previous suicide attempts and the seriousness of the intent to die regarding the last attempt. These two items are included to provide additional clinical information, but are not part of the actual BSS score. In addition, the test is structured such that "0" answers to Items 4 and 5, which focus on current desires to kill oneself (0 = no desire), as well as the desire to save oneself if in a life-threatening situation

(0 = strong desire to save one's life), lead the respondent to skip the subsequent 17 items and go to Questions 20 and 21 (see above). If a respondent does reply to Items 4 and 5 with a 1 or 2, then he or she is instructed to continue with Item 6.

Two sample items, reprinted with permission of the publisher, The Psychological Corporation, are as follows:

> 2   0   I have no wish to die.
>   1   I have a weak wish to die.
>   2   I have a moderate to strong wish to die.
>
> 9   0   I can keep myself from committing suicide.
>   1   I am unsure that I can keep myself from committing suicide.
>   2   I cannot keep myself from committing suicide.

Background

The BSS was developed to parallel the content of the Scale for Suicide Ideation (SSI; A. T. Beck, Kovacs, & Weissman, 1979), which is a clinician rating scale that measures suicidal ideation in psychiatric patients. It also is able to identify specific suicidal characteristics which may require additional clinical scrutiny (e.g., actual suicidal plan).

Administration

The BSS can be self-administered and takes approximately 5–10 minutes to complete. Instructions are also provided in the manual for oral administration by an examiner.

Scoring

If a respondent completes all items, given that he or she did in fact respond with a 1 or 2 to either Items 4 or 5, then the severity of suicidal ideation is calculated by summing the ratings for the first 19 questions. Total BSS scores can range from 0 to 38, where higher scores reflect more-suicidal ideation.

Interpretation

Various cautions are noted throughout the manual regarding the appropriate use of the BSS. For example, Beck and Steer underscore the idea that the BSS scores should be perceived as indicators of suicide risk, rather than as predictors of eventual suicide in a specific case. In addition, as the BSS was developed with adult psychiatric outpatients and inpatients, appropriate use with other populations is questionable. The BSS is also to be considered as one part of a larger comprehensive clinical evaluation.

Psychometric Properties

Norms.   Means and standard deviations for 126 inpatient and 52 outpatient suicidal ideators are provided in the manual.

Reliability.   Cronbach alpha estimates of .90 and .87 (inpatient and outpatient samples, respectively) suggest that the BSS has high internal consistency. Test–retest coefficients on a different sample of 60 inpatient adults was found to be .54 (time between testing was 1 week). The low level of reliability is considered to be due to a significant decrease in suicidal ideation for this sample as a function of treatment.

Validity.   A moderate amount of data is included in the manual suggesting that the BSS is valid regarding content, concurrent, construct, discriminant, factorial, and predictive validity dimensions.

Clinical Utility

High. Provides for means to detect systematically the presence and severity of suicidal ideation.

Research Applicability

Unknown. The SSI, the clinician rating procedure that the BSS is based on, has been used in a variety of research studies. The BSS is relatively new and its research utility remains to be evaluated.

Source

The Psychological Corporation, 555 Academic Court, San Antonio, TX 78204-2498. Phone: 800-211-8378.

Cost

$53.00 for manual and 25 record forms.

Alternative Forms

A Spanish version and computer scoring are available.

CHILDREN'S ATTRIBUTIONAL STYLE QUESTIONNAIRE-REVISED (CASQ-R)

Original Citation

Thompson, M., Kaslow, N. J., Weiss, B., & Nolan-Hoeksema, S. (1998). Children's Attributional Style Questionnaire-Revised: Psychometric evaluation. *Psychological Assessment*, *10*, 166–170.

Purpose

To assess explanatory styles for positive and negative events in children.

Population

Children aged 8–18 years.

Description

The CASQ-R consists of 24 forced-choice items, each listing a specific outcome (e.g., getting an "A" on a test) and two possible explanations for this outcome (e.g., being smart versus being good in the specific subject that the test was in). Half of the items refer to positive outcomes and half to negative outcomes, with the choices reflecting the three dimensions of attributional style (i.e., internal versus external, stable versus unstable, global versus specific).

Background

Attributional style is the key element in the reformulated learned helplessness theory of depression (Abramson et al., 1978). Abramson et al. (1978) describe this style as existing along three dimensions: internal–external, stable–unstable, and global–specific. According to their theory, which has been supported by considerable research, an attributional style in which negative events are ascribed to internal, stable, and global causes is associated with increased depression. Increased depression is also associated with the opposite end of each dimension (i.e., external, unstable, and specific) to explain the causes of positive events. The original CASQ, a 48-item self-report measure, was developed to assess attributional styles in children (Seligman et al., 1984). The briefer CASQ-R was developed due to the shortened attention span of children, with items from the original CASQ selected on the basis of psychometric analyses of CASQ data from a sample of 449 children.

Administration

The CASQ-R can be administered in both individual and group formats. Children can complete the measure on their own or the items can be read aloud by the tester. When self-administered, the CASQ-R takes approximately 10 minutes to complete; when read aloud by an adult, it takes between 10 and 15 minutes to complete.

Scoring

The CASQ-R includes three composite scales, positive, negative, and overall, with the overall score comprised of the positive minus the negative composites. One of the choices for each item is indicated for scoring, and scores are obtained by summing the number of items on which the response matched the indicated choice. This yields scores for internality, stability, and globality for positive and negative events, and the three scores for each are then summed to provide the composite positive and negative scores. Lower overall composite scores are associated with higher levels of depressive attributional styles.

Interpretation

Cutoff scores were not provided, but scores can be compared with norms of a community sample, as noted below.

Psychometric Properties

Psychometric properties were developed in a sample of children aged 9–12 years, drawn from nine public elementary and middle schools. The sample included 515 boys and 570 girls, and was 56% African American and 44% White. An additional 118 children from other ethnic groups were included in the original sample, but were excluded from data analyses due to insufficient numbers per cell for other ethnic groups. Approximately half of the participants completed the CASQ-R twice, with a 6-month interval between administrations.

Norms.   The mean overall composite score was 4.87 (SD = 3.39). Means were compared across gender, ethnic, and age groups, all of which are included in the reference article. No statistically significant gender differences were found on any of the scales, but on the CASQ-R negative scale, African American children scored slightly lower than did White children (M = 2.62 versus 2.87), and 9- to 10-year-old children scored slightly higher than did 11- to 12-year-old children (M = 2.86 versus 2.57).

Reliability.   Test–retest reliabilities indicated low to moderate stability over the 6-month interval for the overall, positive, and negative composite scores (rs = .53, .53, and .38, respectively). No differences in stability were observed based on gender, ethnicity, or age group. Internal consistencies were also moderate at both administrations, with alphas ranging from .45 (negative composite score, Time 1) to .61 (overall composite score, both Time 1 and Time 2). No differences in internal consistency were observed based on gender or age group, but the CASQ-R was significantly more internally consistent in the White sample (alpha = .66) than in the African American group (alpha = .55).

Validity.   The three composite scores of the CASQ-R were compared with the Vanderbilt Depression Inventory (VDI; Weiss & Garber, 1995), with each yielding statistically significant correlations in the expected directions with VDI scores (rs = −.40, −.31, and .35 for the overall, positive, and negative composite scores, respectively). Thus, depressive attributional styles, as defined by the endorsement of internal–stable–global causes for negative events and external–unstable–specific causes for positive events, were associated with higher levels of depression in this sample. As with internal consistencies, no differences were observed based on gender or age, but intercorrelations between composite scores and VDI scores were higher, indicating greater criterion-related validity, for White (r = −.46) than for African American children (r = −.31).

Clinical Utility

High. The CASQ-R is quick to administer and provides valuable information regarding attributional style, which has consistently been associated with depression. CASQ-R results might be used by the clinician to suggest particular areas of vulnerability that might be targeted in treatment.

Research Applicability

High. Considerable research has amassed regarding the role of attributional style in depression, and this line of research is likely to continue. The authors suggest that for research purposes especially, the original 48-item CASQ might be preferable if time constraints allow for its use, due to its superior psychometric properties over the CASQ-R.

Source

The measure is reprinted in its entirety in the reference article. For permission to use, contact Nadine J. Kaslow, Ph.D., Department of Psychiatry and Behavioral Sciences, Grady Health System, Emory University School of Medicine, 80 Butler St., Atlanta, GA 30335.

Cost

None.

Alternative Forms

None.

COGNITIVE BIAS QUESTIONNAIRE (CBQ)

Original Citation

Krantz, S., & Hammen, C. (1979). The assessment of cognitive bias in depression. *Journal of Abnormal Psychology*, *88*, 611–619.

Purpose

To assess the degree of cognitive distortion associated with depression.

Population

Adults.

Description

The CBQ was designed to examine cognitive distortions associated with depression. It contains six short scenarios that are 8–12 sentences long and are written in the third person. Each scenario has an accompanying list of 3 or 4 questions, resulting in a total of 23 questions. Subjects read each vignette and choose the response option that best represents how they would react to the event described in the scenario. The response options within each question are classified as depressed and distorted, nondepressive and distorted, depressive and non-distorted, and nondepressive and distorted. A modified sample item is presented below, with permission of the author.

> Peggy (Paul) is a member of an organization and was encouraged by her (his) friends to run for the presidency. She (he) has lost the election. Place yourself in Peggy's (Paul's) place and try to imagine as vividly as you can how she (he) felt.
> 1. When you first heard you lost you immediately:
>   a. Feel bad and imagine I've lost by a landslide.
>   b. Shrug it off as unimportant.
>   c. Feel sad and wonder what the total counts were.
>   d. Shrug it off, feeling I tried as hard as I could.

Background

The CBQ was developed to evaluate and demonstrate a relationship between cognition and depression. More specifically, this measure was designed to assess A. T. Beck's (1967) argument that depressed individuals interpret situations in a distorted manner and make negatively biased interpretations of events. Specifically, Beck proposed that an essential component of a depressive disorder is a negative cognitive set—the tendency to view the self, the future, and the world in a dysfunctional, negative context. As such, depressed persons are hypothesized to regard themselves as unworthy and incapable, to expect failure and rejection, and to perceive most experiences as confirming these beliefs. The major symptoms of depression are viewed as a direct consequence of this negative triad. Therefore, interventions aimed at changing these views should lead to changes in such symptoms.

Administration

The CBQ requires approximately 15 minutes to complete and can be administered in individual or group formats.

Scoring

Five of the vignettes are followed by 4 questions. The sixth vignette is followed by 3 questions. Each of the 23 questions is followed by four response options, characterized as (a) depressive and distorted, (b) nondepressive and distorted, (c) depressive and nondistorted, and (d) nondepressive and nondistorted. Scores are obtained by summing the number of items endorsed within each of the four categories.

Interpretation

Interpretations can be understood from the pattern of options an individual has selected to the various scenarios. According to Krantz and Hammen (1979), these dimensions can be used to evaluate dysphoric content, both with and without cognitive distortions, and vice versa. An analysis of the response pattern provides information about an individual's tendency to endorse response options associated with depression.

Psychometric Properties

Norms. The original normative group consisted of two samples of college students ($N = 527$), as well as a sample of outpatient ($N = 29$) and inpatient ($N = 20$) psychiatric patients. Krantz and Hammen (1979) provide means and standard deviations for the depressive distortions as well as BDI (p. 29) scores for all samples.

Reliability. Test–retest reliability indicates that subjects who scored high on the BDI and high on the CBQ continued to have high levels of depression 8 weeks later. The test–retest correlation coefficient of depressive-distortion scores was .60. With regard to internal consistency of the depressive-distorted responses within the two college samples, coefficient alpha estimates were found to be .62 and .69, respectively.

Validity. There is a modest correlation between the CBQ and the BDI. In addition, Krantz and Hammen's (1979) results indicate that the CBQ reliably distinguishes depressed and nondepressed individuals, with the depressed individuals having significantly higher depressive-distortion scores. The CBQ also appears sensitive to changes in mood level within individuals.

Clinical Utility

High. This measure is easily administered during the initial evaluation. The results can be used as an aid to treatment planning.

Research Utility

High. There are videotapes and written instructions on interrater reliability. This measure has been used in previous research studies.

Source

Permission to reproduce this instrument can be obtained by contacting Constance L. Hammen, Ph.D., Department of Psychology, University of California, 401 Hilgard Avenue, Los Angeles, CA 90024.

Cost

None.

Alternative Forms

None.

COGNITIVE ERROR QUESTIONNAIRE (CEQ) (GENERAL AND LOWER BACK PAIN VERSIONS)

Original Citation

Lefebvre, M. F. (1981). Cognitive distortion and cognitive errors in depressed psychiatric and low back pain patients. *Journal of Consulting and Clinical Psychology*, *49*, 517–525.

Purpose

To measure overall cognitive distortion and cognitive distortion along four specific cognitive errors: catastrophizing, overgeneralization, personalization, and selective abstraction.

Population

The General-CEQ is intended for all adults and the Lower Back Pain (LBP)-CEQ is intended for adults with lower back pain.

Description

Both the General-CEQ and the LBP-CEQ are 24-item self-report questionnaires. Each item presents a brief vignette that reflects a cognitive error. Respondents reply to each item by indicating how well the cognition represents their own thinking on a scale of 0 to 4, where 0 = "not at all like I would think," 1 = "a little like I would think," 2 = "somewhat like I would think," 3 = "a lot like I would think," and 4 = "almost exactly like I would think."

Sample items, reprinted with the permission of the author, Mark LeFebvre, include the following:

2. You are a manager in a small business firm. You have to fire one of your employees who has been doing a terrible job. You have been putting off this decision for days and you think to yourself, "I know that when I fire her, she is going to raise hell and will sue the company."

10. You and your spouse recently went to an office party at the place where your spouse works. You didn't know anybody there and had a terrible time. When your

spouse asks you if you want to go to the neighbors to visit, you think, "I'll have a terrible time just like that office party."

21. Your friends are all going to ride their snowmobiles. Last time you went, you ran out of gas, and you think to yourself, "What if I run out of gas again; I'll freeze to death."

Background

The General-CEQ was designed to measure the specific cognitive errors described in A. T. Beck's (1967) cognitive model of depression. The LBP-CEQ was designed to measure not only depressive cognitive errors, but how those errors are evident in LBP-related cognitions and how depressed cognitions compare between generally depressed groups and groups of LBP patients with comorbid depression. Studies showed that both groups had distorted cognitions consistent with Beck's theory, and that LBP patients' LBP-related cognitive distortions were even stronger than their general distortions. This led Lefebvre to conclude that the presence as well as the content of cognitive distortions are important.

Administration

The CEQ is self-administered and takes about 15 minutes to complete.

Scoring

Overall scores for the General-CEQ and LBP-CEQ are obtained by adding the scores for each of the items. Scores range from 0 to 96 for each version. The author also provides a CEQ scoring key that delineates which items represent each of the four types of cognitive distortions so that a score ranging from 0 to 24 can be obtained for each individual cognitive error (e.g., overgeneralization).

Interpretation

Higher scores indicate more frequent and intense depressive cognitive distortions. Cutoff scores are not provided.

Psychometric Properties

Norms. Norms for nondepressed individuals ($N = 23$), depressed psychiatric patients ($N = 18$), and nondepressed and depressed LBP patients ($N = 29$ and $N = 19$, respectively) are reported for both the General-CEQ and LBP-CEQ in Lefebvre (1981).

Reliability. Test–retest reliability of the two versions was .80 and .85 in the original validation of the instrument. Parallel form correlations were significant (.87 and .88 overall and ranged from .55 to .79 for each item). Cronbach's alpha values ranged from .62 to .94.

Validity. The concurrent validity, tested by comparing both versions to the Depressed-Distorted scale (Hammen and Krantz, 1976), was found to be .53 for the General-CEQ and .60 for the LBP-CEQ.

Clinical Utility

High. The CEQ is based upon the cognitive model of depression, so it would be most applicable to clinical situations where cognitive therapy is employed.

Research Applicability

High. The author suggests that the instruments can be used to measure change in cognitive distortions or monitor process variables in cognitive therapy.

Source

Mark Lefebvre, Ph.D., 4505 Meadow Lane, Suite 211, Raleigh, NC 27607.

Cost

None.

Alternate Forms

None.

COGNITIVE EVENTS SCHEDULE (CES)

Original Citation

Muñoz, R. F., & Lewinsohn, P. M. (1975). *Cognitive Events Schedule*. University of Oregon, Eugene, OR (see also Muñoz, 1977).

Purpose

To assess thoughts related to A. T. Beck's (1967) negative cognitive triad.

Population

Adults.

Description

The CES contains 160 items (e.g., "I am worthless," "I have good self-control," "I am ugly," "I can't express my feelings") for which respondents are requested to rate the frequency of occurrence (3-point scale) and impact (5-point scale ranging from "very disturbing" to "very pleasant") of various thoughts hypothesized to operationalize Beck's cognitive triad. The CES contains eight *a priori* scales: Self Present Positive; Self Future Positive; Self Present Negative; Self Future Negative; World Present Positive; World Future Positive; World Present Negative; and World Future Negative.

Background

The CES was developed to operationalize A. T. Beck's (1967) negative triad, which is one of the basic ingredients of the cognitive theory of depression. Specifically, Beck proposed that an essential component of a depressive disorder is a negative cognitive set—the tendency to view the self, the future, and the world in a dysfunctional, negative context. As such, depressed persons are hypothesized to regard themselves as unworthy and incapable, to expect failure and rejection, and to perceive most experiences as confirming these beliefs. The major symptoms of depression are viewed as a direct consequence of this negative triad. Therefore, interventions aimed at changing these views should lead to changes in such symptoms.

Administration

The CES should take about 30 minutes to complete.

Scoring

Scores can be computed for each scale, as well as for general positive and negative thoughts.

Interpretation

In its present format, no norms exist for comparison, making interpretation difficult clinically. However, it can be used descriptively to develop a finer analysis of patients' negative thoughts about themselves, the future, and the world.

Psychometric Properties

Norms.   None.

Reliability.   Among a group of 74 normal control adults, test–retest reliability was assessed across the eight scales. These correlations ranged from .40 (Self Future Negative) to .86 (World Present Negative), where the mean $r = .67$.

Validity. Data addressing differences between depressed and nondepressed adults revealed that depressed individuals reported lower frequencies of positive thoughts and higher frequencies of negative thoughts than nondepressed controls. Impact scores were significant in the predicted direction for all four positive scales and two negative scales (Self Present and Self Future).

Clinical Utility

Limited due to the absence of norms.

Research Applicability

High. The CES has been used in several investigations addressing negative cognitions and depression.

Source

Peter M. Lewinsohn, Ph.D., Oregon Research Institute, 1715 Franklin Blvd., Eugene, OR 97403-1983.

Cost

None.

Alternative Forms

A 64-item short form version is available.

COGNITIVE TRIAD INVENTORY (CTI)

Original Citation

Beckham, E. E., Leber, W. R., Watkins, J. T., Boyer, J. L., & Cook, J. B. (1986). Development of an instrument to measure Beck's cognitive triad: The Cognitive Triad Inventory. *Journal of Consulting and Clinical Psychology, 54*, 566–567.

Purpose

To measure the three aspects of the cognitive triad as espoused by a cognitive model of depression (e.g., A. T. Beck, Rush, Shaw, & Emery, 1979).

Population

Adults.

Description

The CTI is a 36-item self-report inventory. Each item provides a statement that represents a possible view of oneself, the world, or the future (e.g., "The world is a very hostile place.") Respondents indicate how well each statement represents their own thinking *during the moment of test-taking* on a 7-point Likert-type scale ranging from "totally agree" to "totally disagree."

Background

The CTI was developed to operationalize A. T. Beck's (1967) negative triad, which is one of the basic ingredients of the cognitive theory of depression. Specifically, Beck proposed that an essential component of a depressive disorder is a negative cognitive set—the tendency to view the self, the future, and the world in a dysfunctional, negative context. As such, depressed persons are hypothesized to regard themselves as unworthy and incapable, to expect failure and rejection, and to perceive most experiences as confirming these beliefs. The major symptoms of depression are viewed as a direct consequence of this negative triad. Therefore, interventions aimed at changing these views should lead to changes in such symptoms. The CTI was designed to be sensitive to small changes in these cognitions so that such treatment effects could be measured.

Administration

The CTI takes approximately 10 minutes to complete.

Scoring

Six items of the CTI are filler items and are not scored. Sixteen items are reverse-scored. Scores for the Total View, which range from 30 to 210, are obtained by adding the scores of each item. Self, World, and Future subscale scores can also be obtained. Each subscale is comprised of 10 items and scores are obtained by adding item scores. Scores for each subscale range from 10 to 70. An SAS computer scoring package is available.

Interpretation

High scores indicate negative views and low scores indicate positive views. Further information on the meaning of the scores is not yet available, except to compare scores to the limited normative data that have been reported.

Psychometric Properties

Norms.   An SAS scoring package provided by the authors includes means, standard deviation, and *T*-scores for a sample of 28 depressed patients.

Reliability.   With regard to internal reliability, the coefficient alpha in a sample of 28 depressed patients was .95. Alpha scores for the subscales ranged from .81 to .93.

Validity.   The convergent validity was tested by comparing the CTI to related measures, including the Beck Hopelessness Scale (p. 175), and the cognitive subset of the BDI (p. 29), as well as by dividing the items of the BDI into subscales and comparing them to the CTI subscales. Correlations ranged from .61 to .80.

The validity of the factors of the CTI was partially supported by a principal components factor analysis with Varimax rotation by Anderson and Skidmore (1995). Five factors were identified and labeled as "positively phrased future items," "negatively phrased future items," "positively phrased world items," "negatively phrased world items," and "positively phrased self items." The negatively phrased self items did not form a strong factor. Although the wording of the items contributed to the factor loadings, factors representing each of the three dysfunctional thought patterns did emerge.

Clinical Utility

Limited. Without further information on its interpretation, the meaning of the CTI results are unclear at this time.

Research Applicability

Limited. However, with more research, the CTI can provide valuable information about the process of cognitive changes in cognitive therapy for depression. The developers hope it may be so sensitive as to detect changes after only one therapy session. The CTI may also be useful in gaining a better understanding of the relationships among the three areas of the cognitive triad, and whether one of them is more valuable in facilitating changes in depression.

Source

The CTI is reprinted in Appendix B. For additional information, contact Edward Beckham, Ph.D., Psychiatric Associates, Inc., 6406-A North Santa Fe, Oklahoma City, OK 73116.

Cost

None.

Alternative Forms

None.

COPING INVENTORY FOR STRESSFUL SITUATIONS (CISS)

Original Citation

Endler, N., & Parker, J. (1990). *Coping Inventory for Stressful Situations manual.* North Tonawanda, NY: Multi-Health Systems.

Purpose

To measure the coping responses endorsed for dealing with stressful situations.

Population

Adolescent (age 13–18 years) and adult (18 years and older) versions are available.

Description

The CISS is a 48-item self-report questionnaire. Items represent coping reactions to stressful events. Both the adult and adolescent versions are similar in content: six of the items associated with the adult version were reworded for use with a younger population. Both versions measure emotion-oriented, task-oriented, and avoidance-oriented coping. The Avoidance-Oriented scale is divided into a Distraction and a Social Diversion component. Respondents use a Likert-type scale to rate how often they participate in each of the 48 activities. Examples, reprinted with permission of the publisher, Multi-Health Systems, Inc., include "try to go to sleep," "watch TV," "phone a friend," "spend time with a special person," and "try to be with other people." Ratings range from 1 ("Not at All") to 5 ("Very Much").

Background

Substantial research in the area of stress points to the significant relationship between stressors and depressive reactions, i.e., the experience of a stressful negative life event, chronic stressors, or a traumatic event can lead to depression (A. M. Nezu & Ronan, 1985). In addition, researchers and clinicians have also identified various mediators of this stressor–depression relationship, a primary one being coping resources and skills (Cronkite & Moos, 1995). Coping, then, may be an area of interest for clinicians and researchers alike when working with depressed individuals.

The CISS was developed from an interactional model of anxiety, stress, and coping (Endler, 1988). An initial pool of 120 items was developed and a subsequent analysis resulted in a 70-item inventory labeled the General Reaction Inventory IV. A series of factor analytic studies and some logical ratings of the items resulted in the final 48-item adult version. The wording of 6 of the adult items was simplified to make the adolescent version of the CISS.

Administration

The CISS requires 10 minutes to complete.

Scoring

Raw scores are derived from summing the 16-item scores associated with each of the scales (i.e., Emotion-Oriented, Task-Oriented, and Avoidance-Oriented). Raw scores for the Distraction (8 items) and Social Diversion (5 items) components of the Avoidance-Oriented subscale are derived in a similar manner. Raw scores are plotted on profile sheets that provide *T*-score conversions.

Interpretation

T-scores between 45 and 55 are considered average. The higher the *T*-score, the greater the degree of coping activity. Interpreting scores on the CISS involves first evaluating the individual scale scores to determine strengths and weaknesses, and then conducting an analysis of the pattern created by plotting the five scores.

Psychometric Properties

Norms.   Normative data for the adult version were based on general adults (249 males and 288 females), undergraduates (471 males and 771 females), and psychiatric inpatients (164 males and 138 females). Data are also available for male factory workers (185) and male prisoners (124). Normative data for the adolescent version are based on a sample of 13- to 15-year-old adolescents (152 males and 161 females) and a sample of 16- to 18-year-old adolescents (270 males and 234 females).

Reliability.   Coefficient alpha estimates for the adult version, across a variety of samples, range from .72 to .91. Six-week test–retest reliability estimates range from .51 to .73. Similar results were found for the adolescent version.

Validity.   For the adult version, a significant relationship emerged between the Emotion-Oriented scale and the Marlowe–Crowne Social Desirability Scale (Crowne & Marlowe, 1964). The manual presents concurrent validity data for the adult version based on the relationship with the Ways of Coping Scale (p. 262). Factor-analytic studies conducted on both the adult and adolescent versions have generally supported the existence of the hypothesized three-factor model (i.e., Emotion-Oriented, Task-Oriented, and Avoidance-Oriented).

Clinical Utility

High. The CISS could serve as an initial evaluation of coping strategies and as an aid for treatment planning. It assesses a construct that is likely to be relevant for many clients who experience stress-related depressive symptoms.

Research Applicability

High. The scales of the CISS possess several useful characteristics. The scales are relatively short (16 items) and easy to administer. The three major sales have adequate internal consistence, test–retest reliability, and validity data. More recent findings have also been generally supportive (Endler & Parker, 1994; Kurokawa & Weed, 1998).

Source

Multi-Health Systems, 908 Niagara Falls Boulevard, North Tonawanda, NY 14120-2060. Phone: 800-456-3003.

Cost

$28 for a specimen set, which includes a manual, three adult forms, and three adolescent forms.

Alternate Forms

Spanish versions are available. The manual presents data on a sample of Mexican undergraduates (71 males and 94 females).

COPING RESOURCES INVENTORY (CRI)

Original Citation

Hammer, A. L. (1988). *Manual for the Coping Resources Inventory*. Palo Alto, CA: Consulting Psychologists Press.

Purpose

To assess coping resources currently available to individuals for managing stress.

Population

Adolescents and adults aged 14–83 years.

Description

The CRI is a 60-item self-report measure that requests respondents to indicate, according to a 4-point scale, how often they engaged in a particular behavior described in each item during the past 6 months. Sample items include, "I can cry when sad," "I exercise vigorously 3–4 times a week," and "I know what is important in life." The CRI contains the following five scales: Cognitive (the degree to which individuals maintain a positive sense of self-worth); Social (the degree to which individuals have a social network that provides support during times of stress); Emotional (the degree to which people are able to express a range of emotions); Spiritual/Philosophical (the degree to which individuals' behaviors are guided by certain religious, familial, or philosophical values); and Physical (the degree to which people engage in health-promoting behaviors).

Background

Substantial research in the area of stress points to the significant relationship between stressors and depressive reactions, i.e., the experience of a stressful negative life event, chronic stressors, or a traumatic event can lead to depression (A. M. Nezu & Ronan, 1985). In addition, researchers and clinicians have also identified various mediators of this stressor–depression relationship, a primary one being coping resources and skills (Cronkite & Moos, 1995). Coping, then, may be an area of interest for clinicians and researchers alike when working with depressed individuals.

Administration

The CRI usually requires 10 minutes to complete.

Scoring

Scores for each of the five scales are the sums of the item responses for each scale. Six items, however, are reverse-scored. In addition, a Total Resource score is possible by adding the five scale scores. The higher the scale score, the higher the particular resource.

Interpretation

Norms are provided in the manual where raw scores can be converted into standard scores for comparison.

Psychometric Properties

Norms. The sample making up the norm group consisted of 818 adults (327 men, 491 women). In addition, the means and standard deviations for several reference groups (e.g., high school students, bereaved caregivers) are included in the manual.

Reliability.   Internal consistency, as estimated by Cronbach's alpha, was found to be .91 for the Total Resource Scale regarding a sample of 749 adults. Test–retest reliability was calculated using a sample of 115 high school students where the time between testings was 6 weeks. This correlation was .73 for the Total Resource Scale.

Validity.   The CRI was found to be a significant predictor of stress symptoms beyond that accounted for by stressful life events. It has also been found to discriminate between healthy and ill college students, as well as healthy and ill adults. It correlated low (.16) with a measure of social desirability, but high with the BDI (−.66; p. 29), thus supporting its construct validity.

Clinical Utility

High. The CRI can be used to identify strengths and weaknesses regarding a patient's coping resources, and thus help guide treatment decisions.

Research Applicability

High. The CRI has been used in various research investigations.

Source

Consulting Psychologists Press, 577 College Avenue, Palo Alto, CA 94306. Phone: 800-624-1765.

Cost

$26 for a preview kit (item booklet, answer sheet, manual).

Alternative Forms

None.

COPING RESPONSES INVENTORY (CRI)

Original Citation

Moos, R. H. (1993). *Coping Responses Inventory-Adult Form, professional manual.* Odessa, FL: Psychological Assessment Resources.

Purpose

To assess styles of coping with life stressors.

Population

Adults.

Description

The CRI is a 48-item self-report measure. Eight types of coping styles are assessed with scales of six items each; individual items are rated on a 4-point scale ranging from "not at all" to "fairly often." Ten additional items assess aspects of a particular current stressor, such as whether it has occurred before and whether it has been resolved.

Background

The authors of the CRI note that coping responses have generally been categorized by either the focus or method of coping; the CRI was developed to assess both these aspects of coping responses. The categories of coping responses assessed are broken into approach styles (i.e., Logical Analysis, Positive Reappraisal, Seeking Guidance and Support, and Problem Solving scales) and avoidance styles (i.e., Cognitive Avoidance, Acceptance or Resignation, Seeking Alternative Rewards, and Emotional Discharge scales). CRI items were initially derived conceptually, and were later refined via empirical studies.

Substantial research in the area of stress points to the significant relationship between stressors and depressive reactions, i.e., the experience of a stressful negative life event, chronic stressors, or a traumatic event can lead to depression (A. M. Nezu & Ronan, 1985). In addition, researchers and clinicians have also identified various mediators of this stressor–depression relationship, a primary one being coping resources and skills (Cronkite & Moos, 1995). Coping, then, may be an area of interest for clinicians and researchers alike when working with depressed individuals.

Administration

The CRI may be completed as self-report, either in individual or group administration, or as a structured interview. When self-administered, the CRI takes about 15 minutes to complete; as an interview it takes between 15 and 30 minutes.

Scoring

Each answer sheet includes a template for scoring in which the eight scales noted earlier are automatically scored. Scores are tabulated by assigning number values of 0 to 3 to each of the four answer choices (e.g., 0 = "not at all" and 3 = "fairly often") and summing the values in each scale. A profile on the scoring sheet includes a T-score conversion as well. Using the scoring template and profile, scoring of the CRI takes approximately 5 minutes.

Interpretation

An IBM-compatible software program is available to provide analyses of the CRI results. In addition, the manual provides general criteria for interpreting CRI scores, listing the T-score range, equivalent percentile ranking, and general description. These seven cutoff categories range from $T < 34$ ("considerably below average") to $T > 66$ ("considerably above average"), with T-scores between 46 and 54 considered "average."

Psychometric Properties

Psychometric properties for the CRI are based on two field trials, one including alcoholic, depressed, and arthritic patients as well as normal controls; and the other including problem-drinking and normal-drinking adults. The combined field trials consisted of 1,194 men and 722 women; data are provided separately by gender.

Norms. The mean scores for the sample described above ranged from 3.37 ($SD = 3.27$) to 11.01 ($SD = 3.97$) for the men, and from 4.08 ($SD = 3.24$) to 11.48 ($SD = 3.87$) for the women. Both groups had the lowest scores on Emotional Discharge and the highest on Logical Analysis.

Reliability. Internal consistencies (Cronbach's alpha) were moderate, ranging from .61 to .74 for men, and from .58 to .71 for women among the eight subscales. Test–retest reliabilities, based on 12-month lapse showed an average r of .45 for men and .43 for women.

Validity. Differences on CRI responding were compared across the various groups included in the field trials, with depressed patients generally demonstrating higher levels of avoidance-based coping strategies than controls. Information on specific validity tests was not available. The CRI does not appear to be strongly affected by social desirability.

Clinical Utility

High. The CRI assesses a variety of coping styles in a relatively brief time, and also provides for specific information regarding coping with a particular recent life stressor, which may be important information for clinicians to gather.

Research Applicability

High. The CRI has been used in a variety of research studies.

Source

Psychological Assessment Resources, P.O. Box 998, Odessa, FL 33556. Phone: 800-331-TEST.

Cost

$66 for an introductory kit, which includes a manual, 10 reusable test copies, and 25 answer sheets. The CRI Software System, including administration and interpretation for both the adult and youth versions of the CRI, costs $325.

Alternate Forms

A CRI-Youth version, for ages 12–18 years, is also available. Both the adult and child versions are available in computerized administration and interpretation format; the computerized format takes approximately 10–15 minutes to complete.

DEPRESSION BELIEFS QUESTIONNAIRE-VERSION I (DBQ-I)

Original Citation

Moras, K., Newman, C., & Schweizer, E. (1995). *Depression Beliefs Questionnaire-Version I (DBQ-I)*. Unpublished manuscript, University of Pennsylvania School of Medicine, Philadephia, PA. Development of measure funded by NIMH Grant R21 MH52737.

Purpose

To identify depressed patients' beliefs about the causes of depression, as well as their expectations regarding psychotherapeutic and pharmacological treatments.

Population

Adolescents and adults.

Description

The DBQ-I is a 41-item self-report instrument. Respondents are requested to indicate their agreement with a given statement along a 6-point Likert scale (range = "Totally Agree" to "Totally Disagree"). "No Opinion" is an additional response option. Items are grouped into five rationally derived scales: attitudes/beliefs toward medication (positive and negative), attitudes/beliefs toward psychotherapy (positive and negative), beliefs about the causes of depression (e.g., hereditary, environmental stressors), predictors of responsiveness to treatment (e.g., hopelessness versus hopefulness, secondary gains of being depressed), and belief that depression is socially stigmatizing. Sample items per such scales are reprinted below with the permission of the first author, Kayla Moras.

> *Negative Attitudes Toward Medication*
>> Taking antidepressant medication will change my personality in ways I don't want it to.
>> 12. The side-effects of antidepressant medication are more trouble than they're worth.
> *Negative Attitudes Toward Psychotherapy*
>> Most therapists can't really understand what it is to be truly depressed.
>> My self-esteem and self-confidence would go down if I had to see a therapist and talk about my depression.
> *Positive Predictors of Treatment Response*
>> Depression is something that can be overcome with the proper treatment.
>> I have confidence that there exists some form of treatment that can help me with my depression.
> *Depression is Stigmatizing*
>> Being depressed is something to be embarrassed or ashamed of.
>> People would view me more negatively if they knew I was depressed.

Background

The DBQ-I was developed as part of an effort to develop an efficacious combined medication and cognitive-behavioral psychotherapy treatment for medication-resistant depression. The item pool for the DBQ-I was derived from the clinical observations of an experienced research psychopharmacologist (E.S.) and an experienced cognitive therapist (C.N.). Items reflect beliefs about depression and attitudes toward medication and psychotherapy that commonly are expressed by depressed outpatients, particularly those who manifest a negative reaction to either psychopharmacology or psychotherapy while in treatment. Hypotheses based on clinical observation led to the development of the DBQ-I. The hypotheses were as follows: (1) Individuals with treatment-resistant depression are likely to (a) require combined medication and psychotherapeutic interventions, (b) have personal, specific beliefs about the causes of their depression, (c) expect negative consequences from alternative interventions for depression, and (d) in some cases, have negative expectations about potential benefits of alternative treatments for their depression. (2) If a depressed individual's biases against medications and/or psychotherapy (e.g., unrealistic fears) can be identified and addressed at the outset of treatment, the potential efficacy of a combined treatment will be enhanced.

Administration

In general, the DBQ-I takes 10–15 minutes to complete. It was designed for completion *before* the first treatment session or initial evaluation appointment.

Scoring

For clinical use, scoring is not necessary. Rather, item responses can be inspected for strong endorsement (e.g., "Totally Agree," "Totally Disagree," "Very Much Agree"). Strong endorsement of any item that involves a negative belief or expectation about medication or psychotherapy, or about one's ability to benefit from treatment for depression, can then be explored during the initial evaluation or therapy session. Unrealistic or unfounded negative views can be addressed by the therapist (e.g., using standard therapist responses to the negative DBQ items, see Description above).

For research purposes, scale scores can be created by summing scale items and weighting the sums. Weighting is needed to compare scale scores because the number of items per scale varies.

Interpretation

See Scoring above.

Psychometric Properties

The DBQ-I is in the initial phase of development. Responses have been obtained from a relatively large sample of treatment-seeking outpatients ($N = 300$) with DSM-IV diagnoses of major depression and/or dysthymia at a cognitive psychotherapy clinic and at a psychopharmacology clinic, both of which are in a university-affiliated medical center in the northeastern United States. No refinement of the original version of the instrument (e.g., dropping items from scales) has been done yet.

Norms. Preliminary means (and standard deviations) are as follows: Negative Attitudes Toward Medication = 3.84 ($SD = 1.05$); Negative Attitudes Toward Psychotherapy = 4.18 ($SD = .97$); Depression is Stigmatizing = 3.46 ($SD = 1.23$); Positive Predictors of Treatment Response = 2.12 ($SD = .81$).

Reliability. Internal consistency reliabilities (coefficient alpha) for some of the DBQ-I scales as they were rationally constructed were found to be in the acceptable range in preliminary analyses: Negative Beliefs About Medication (.81, $n = 96$); Negative Beliefs About Psychotherapy (.67, $n = 102$); Depression is Stigmatizing (.80, $n = 104$); Positive Predictors of Treatment Response (.62, $n = 136$). Others were lower, (e.g., Negative Predictors of Treatment Response [.34, $n = 97$]), suggesting possible directions for shortening and modifying the DBQ. The internal consistency of the DBQ scales, however, is not necessarily an indication of the clinical utility of specific items.

Test–retest reliability has been computed for DBQ-I total scores for two time intervals: ≤ 14 days; and ≥ 14 to ≤ 30 days. Pearson correlation coefficients were .81 ($n = 28$) and .92 ($n = 21$), respectively.

Validity. No validity estimates are available yet. Construct validity data currently are being collected.

Clinical Utility

High. The DBQ-I was designed to help mental health professionals identify and address depressed patients' unrealistic biases against medication and/or psychotherapeutic interventions that could impede patients' ability to benefit from them. Thus, it can also be used to assist in formulating a treatment plan more likely to be effective for a given patient and with which the patient will comply.

Research Applicability

High. Given the increased emphasis on effectiveness and on matching treatments to patients, the DBQ-I may be a particularly useful measure for treatment research on depression.

Source

Karla Moras, Ph.D., Clinical Research Center for the Study of Psychotherapy, Room 641, 3535 Market Street, Philadelphia, PA 19104. Phone: 215-349-5219. morask@landru.cpr.upenn.edu

Cost

None.

Alternative Forms

None.

DEPRESSION CHECK QUESTIONNAIRE (DCQ)

Original Citation

Tan, J. C. H., & Stoppard, J. M. (1994). Gender and reactions to dysphoric individuals. *Cognitive Therapy and Research*, *18*, 211–224.

Purpose

To measure the behaviors indicative of depression.

Population

Adults.

Description

The DCQ is a 13-item observer-reported questionnaire that involves rating depressive behavior on a 7-point Likert-type scale. The first 7 items represent the interpersonal impression of the depressed person (e.g., "friendly," "active"). The last 6 items represent the rater's observation of the depressed person's overt behaviors (e.g., "eye contact," "facial expression").

Background

The DCQ was designed to measure nonverbal depressive behavior in a study examining Coyne's (1976) interpersonal model of depression. Coyne's model proposes that the interpersonal behavior of a depressed persons leads others to reject them, thus perpetuating the depressive syndrome. Depressed individuals are viewed as creating a negative social environment by relating to others in such a manner whereby support is withdrawn. The depressed person's behavior becomes more demanding and aversive and eventually begins to elicit feelings of resentment and anger. In this light, a measure of nonverbal behavior tied to depression allows for an important assessment.

Administration

The DCQ is administered after a 15-minute face-to-face interaction between a nondepressed rater and a depressed person. In the Tan and Stoppard (1994) study, the two participants were strangers. This instrument has not been used with acquaintances, people in intimate relationships, or those in therapeutic relationships.

Scoring

Separate scores for the interpersonal impression and overt behaviors can be obtained by adding the scores of the first seven items and the last six items, respectively.

Interpretation

Higher scores indicate more-depressive behavior.

Psychometric Properties

Norms.   Means and standard deviations of the overt behavior component were reported in Tan and Stoppard (1994) for a sample of 95 pairs divided into eight groups matched by gender and presence of dysphoria.

Reliability.   The internal consistency reliability of the overt behavior component was measured in a sample of 95 pairs. The internal consistency of the entire scale was estimated to be .84 (alpha) and the two components correlate with each other; $r = .63$ (J. C. H. Tan, personal communication, December 1998).

Validity.   Although the authors plan to conduct specific tests of the validity of the DCQ, none have been conducted to date.

Clinical Utility

Limited. At this point, the DCQ has not been widely used in clinically settings.

Research Applicability

Limited. Further research on the reliability and validity of the DCQ is needed.

Source

The DCQ is reprinted in Appendix B. For additional information, contact Josephine Tan, Ph.D., C. Psych., Psychology Department, Lakehead University, Thunder Bay, Ontario, P7B 5E1 Canada.

Cost

None.

Alternative Forms

None.

DEPRESSION PRONENESS RATING SCALE (DPRS)

Original Citation

Zemore, R., Fischer, D. G., Garratt, L. S., & Miller, C. (1990). The Depression Proneness Rating Scale: Reliability, validity, and factor structure. *Current Psychology: Research and Reviews*, *9*, 255–263.

Purpose

To measure depression-proneness, defined as "the tendency to experience relatively frequent, long-lasting, and severe depression" (Zemore et al., 1990, p. 255).

Population

Adults.

Description

The DPRS is a 13-item self-report questionnaire that is comprised of two parts. The first part, the DPRS-3, asks respondents to compare their own experiences of depression to the experiences of most people they know according to the frequency, length, and severity of depressive episodes. Respondents are requested to indicate their ratings on 9-point scales that range from "much less often," "much shorter," or "much less deeply," to "much more often," "much longer," or "much more deeply." The second part, the DPRS-10, asks respondents to compare their experience of 10 commonly assessed depressive symptoms to the symptoms experienced by other people they know. Responses are indicated according to a 9-point frequency scale. All questions on the DPRS pertain to the participant's experience during the past 2 years.

Background

This instrument was developed in order to measure a person's tendency to become depressed, while improving upon some of the drawbacks of other instruments designed for this purpose. The authors sought to design an instrument that would assess the propensity toward depression without relying on current symptom severity or past history of depressive episodes as the sole criterion. The DPRS treats depression as a continuous variable, can be used to quickly assess large samples, and can be applied with a variety of nonclinical samples. In addition, the DPRS can be used along with a measure of current depressive severity to partial out the influence of current symptoms on the rating of depression-proneness.

Administration

The DPRS takes approximately 10 minutes to complete.

Scoring

There are two options for scoring the DPRS. Investigators can obtain sums of the individual item scores. In this case, scores range from 13 to 117. Investigators can also compute scores by obtaining the mean of the item scores.

Interpretation

Higher scores indicate greater vulnerability toward depression.

Psychometric Properties

Norms.   Means and standard deviations for each item of the DPRS are reported in Zemore et al. (1990). Means and standard deviations for the subscales, tested in a sample of female university students, are also reported in Zemore and Veikle (1989).

Reliability.   The test–retest reliability of the DPRS, measured in a sample of 100 undergraduates with a 9-week interval between administrations, was found to be .82. This correlation showed greater stability than current symptom severity measured by the BDI (p. 29) in the same sample. Internal consistency was measured in a sample of 1,101 undergraduates. Cronbach's alpha was .90 and correlations between each item and the total score ranged from .39 to .76.

Validity.   One test of the validity of this instrument involved comparing scores on the DPRS to a person's history of depression. Results showed a significant correlation, .41, in a group of 440 university students. This correlation was significantly greater than the relationship between current symptom severity measured by the BDI (p. 29) and history of depression.
Other investigations showed positive correlations between the DPRS and parent and peer ratings of depression-proneness (Zemore, 1983), and negative correlations between the DPRS-3 and interpersonal problem-solving skill (Zemore & Dell, 1983).

Clinical Utility

High. The DPRS can provide for meaningful information about a particular client's proneness or vulnerability to depression.

Research Applicability

High. This instrument accounts for more of the variance in proneness toward depression than an instrument of symptom severity. The DPRS is particularly useful in studies examining cognitive theories of depression (see Zemore & Veikle, 1989, for an example).

Source

The DPRS is reprinted in Appendix B.

Cost

None.

Alternative Forms

None.

DEPRESSIVE PERSONALITY DISORDER INVENTORY (DPDI)

Original Citation

Huprich, S. K., Margrett, J., Bathelemy, K. J., & Fine, M. A. (1996). The Depressive Personality Disorder Inventory: An initial examination of its psychometric properties. *Journal of Clinical Psychology, 52,* 153–159.

Purpose

To assess thoughts related to the DSM-IV provisional category of depressive personality disorder.

Population

Adults.

Description

The DPDI is a 41-item self-report measure of thoughts related to the proposed category of depressive personality disorder (e.g., "My mood could frequently be described as gloomy"). Each item is rated on a 7-point Likert-type scale ranging from 1 ("totally agree") to 7 ("totally disagree").

Background

The DPDI was developed to assess attitudes and beliefs thought to be representative of a depressive personality disorder, which was included as a category warranting further consideration in the DSM-IV. The authors of the DPDI note that personality disorders are characterized by pervasive maladaptive thoughts, and that if depressive personality disorder may be included in future editions, measures of the disorder would be needed. It should also be noted that a number of theorists have emphasized the role of maladaptive cognitions in the development and maintenance of depression, although depression itself is not the construct directly of interest for this measure. The initial version of the DPDI contained 42 items, with 1 dropped following psychometric studies to improve internal consistency.

Administration

No time frame was provided regarding the length of time required; however, the scale appears to take approximately 15–20 minutes to complete when self-administered.

Scoring

Each item is rated from 1 to 7, with the total score obtained by summing the ratings for the 41 items. Higher scores indicate greater agreement with cognitions related to depressive personality disorder.

Interpretation

Guidelines for interpretation were not provided, beyond the note that higher scores are indicative of endorsement of greater numbers of depressive personality disorder-related items.

Psychometric Properties

Psychometric properties for the DPDI are based on a sample of 32 male and 57 female undergraduate students at a private midwestern Catholic university. The mean age of the sample was approximately 19, and 95.5% of the sample was White.

Norms.   The mean score for the sample described above was 127.1, with a standard deviation of 33.8. For males, the mean was 124.8 with *SD* of 35.9; females had a mean of 128.7 and *SD* of 32.4. Psychometric tests using clinical populations, as well as those yielding separate norms based on psychiatric status or other factors, were not conducted.

Reliability.   Internal consistency (Cronbach's alpha) was estimated to be .94. Principal components analyses suggested the DPDI yields a single construct.

Validity.   Construct validity was evaluated by comparing the DPDI with two other measures of depressive thoughts, the Automatic Thoughts Questionnaire-Revised (ATQ-R; p. 172) and the Dysfunctional Attitude Scale (DAS; p. 212). These tests yielded significant correlations with both the ATQ-R ($r = .85$) and the DAS ($r = .57$). The authors noted that they purposely did not validate the DPDI against measures of depressive symptoms themselves, as that would not aid in establishing the DPDI as a measure of depressive personality disorder. The DPDI was recently compared with the Diagnostic Interview for Depressive Personality (Gunderson, Phillips, Triebwasser, & Hirschfeld, 1994), where the corelation was found to be .81 (Huprich & Nelson-Grey, 1998). In a separate study (Huprich & Nelson-Gray, 1998), the DPDI was compared with the Diagnostic Interview for Depressive Personality (Gunderson et al., 1994), with results indicating good convergent validity ($r = .81$).

Clinical Utility

High. The DPDI is among the only measures assessing the construct of depressive personality disorder, and thus might be especially useful for clinicians who wish to track progress with clients potentially meeting this diagnosis.

Research Applicability

High. If depressive personality disorder may indeed be included in future editions of the DSM, additional research on the disorder will be needed and thus related measures will be important.

Source

Scale is located in Huprich et al. (1996). For more information, contact Steven K. Huprich, Ph.D., Department of Psychology and Neuroscience, Baylor University, P.O. Box 97334, Waco, TX 76798-7334.

Cost

None.

Alternate Forms

None.

DIVORCE DYSFUNCTIONAL ATTITUDES SCALE (DDAS)

Original Citation

Lakey, B., Drew, J. B., Anan, R. M., Sirl, K., & Butler, C. *Dysfunctional attitudes, social support, and stress vulnerability: Global vs. stressor-specific approaches.* Unpublished manuscript.

Purpose

To measure dysfunctional attitudes specifically related to divorce.

Population

Adult men and women who are divorced or contemplating getting divorced.

Description

There is a 50-item version of the DDAS, as well as a shorter 39-item version of this instrument. Both are self-report questionnaires which provide the instructions, "This questionnaire lists some of the things that people might think about the subject of divorce. For each one, circle the letters which best fit whether you agree or disagree with the statement." The instructions are followed by the statement "Getting divorced means that ...," which is followed by 39 or 50 statements (e.g., "It is difficult to be happy if you're not married"). Respondents choose from the following five possible answers: strongly agree; agree; unsure; disagree; and strongly disagree.

Background

The DDAS was developed in keeping with the body of literature that suggests that stressor-specific approaches are more predictive of vulnerability to stress vulnerability than global approaches (Swindle et al., 1988). Lakey and his colleagues followed up on this hypothesis by examining how stressor-specific dysfunctional attitudes may predict an even greater amount of distress than global dysfunctional attitudes. The relationship between global dysfunctional attitudes and depression is well established, its roots based in the cognitive model for depression (A. T. Beck, 1967) and the relationship between dysfunctional attitudes and schema content (Gotlib and Hammen, 1992). Divorce was selected as the specific stressor because of its high prevalence, its well-established relationship with stress and distress, and the accessibility to potential subjects through public records. Therefore, although divorce was identified as the specific stressor to be investigated, the greater goal leading to the development of the DDAS was to examine specific stressors in general.

The DDAS is a new instrument. The article describing its psychometric properties is currently under review.

Administration

The 50-item questionnaire takes approximately 30 minutes to complete.

Scoring

Scores for this instrument represent varying degrees of depressive cognitive distortions.

Interpretation

Higher scores indicate greater severity of divorce-related dysfunctional attitudes.

Psychometric Properties

Norms.   Means and standard deviations are reported for a group of individuals filing for or being sued for divorce ($N = 62$), as well as a group having been granted divorce ($N = 97$).

Reliability.   The internal consistency of the 50-item DDAS was tested on a sample of 60 men and women who had filed for or were being sued for divorce and was found to have an alpha value of .92. The internal consistency of the 39-item version tested on a sample of 97 divorced men and women was estimated to have an alpha value of .91. The internal consistency, tested on a sample of 90 married adults, was $\alpha = .84$.

Validity.   One of the primary goals of the DDAS was to add incremental validity above and beyond the validity of measuring general dysfunctional attitudes. This was tested by examining the added prediction of emotional distress by DDAS while controlling for global dysfunctional attitudes as well as social desirability. The change in R^2 was .10 ($p < .001$). To further support the incremental validity, the relationship between the DDAS and emotional distress was compared for divorced and married groups. Two hierarchical multiple regressions were conducted for two separate samples with DDAS by group interaction terms. Both analyses showed that the DDAS–distress relationship was significant for the divorced group and nonsignificant for the married group.

With regard to construct validity, Lakey et al. purport that a relationship between dysfunctional attitudes and information-processing effects would demonstrate that dysfunctional attitudes are organized schematically. One study lends some evidence to this by demonstrating a relationship between DDAS and negative interpretation of social situations ($r = .24$, $p < .05$).

Clinical Utility

Limited. The DDAS is a promising new instrument, but it has not yet been widely studied. The authors hope that it will be useful for "identifying at-risk individuals, the specific beliefs that underlie their distress, and for guiding the course of cognitive interventions" once it has been studied in greater detail.

Research Applicability

Limited. Again, the DDAS is only newly developed and information about its psychometric properties is limited. Information about its ability to detect treatment effects is not reported and may not have been studied yet.

Source

The DDAS is reprinted in Appendix B. For additional information, contact Brian Lakey, Ph.D., Department of Psychology, Wayne State University, 71 West Warren Avenue, Detroit, MI 48202.

Cost

None.

Alternate Forms

A 39-item short form is available.

DYSFUNCTIONAL ATTITUDE SCALE (DAS)

Original Citation

Weissman, A. N., & Beck, A. T. (1978). *Development and validation of the Dysfunctional Attitude Scale: A preliminary investigation.* Paper presented at the meeting of the Association for the Advancement of Behavior Therapy, Chicago.

Purpose

To assess maladaptive thinking patterns and dysfunctional cognitions.

Population

Adults.

Description

The original DAS is a 100-item self-report measure developed to assess dysfunctional cognitions related to depression (e.g., "I must be a useful, productive, creative person or life has no purpose," "It is difficult to be happy unless one is good-looking, intelligent, rich, and creative"). Currently, the DAS is available in two 40-item inventories. Respondents are requested to rate items using a Likert-type scale ranging from a score of 1 (totally agree) to 7 (totally disagree).

Background

A. T. Beck (1967) hypothesized that depressed people maintain a negative view of themselves, their world, and their future. This self-report measure was specifically designed to measure these constructs, especially the "silent assumptions" or schemas hypothesized to make individuals vulnerable to depression. The content of the items contained in the DAS reflects the negative or dysfunctional attitudes depressed people harbor toward the self, the outside world, and the future.

Administration

The DAS requires approximately 10–15 minutes to complete and can be administered in an individual or a group setting.

Scoring

A total score results from summing item scores.

Interpretation

Total score results can range from 100 to 700 (100-item version). Higher scores indicate more distorted thinking.

Psychometric Properties

Norms.   Initial norms were provided for a college student sample. Since then, the measure's psychometric properties have been more widely examined with clinically depressed populations (A. T. Beck, Brown, Steer, & Weissman, 1991; Nelson, Stern, & Cicchetti, 1992). For example, Nelson et al. (1992) examined depressed psychiatric inpatients ($N = 72$) and a nondepressed group of patients ($N = 61$) using the DAS. Oliver and Baumgart (1985) administered the DAS and the BDI (p. 29) to 275 hospital employees and their spouses.

Reliability.   Correlations between the DAS parallel forms and the total test score ranged from .84 to .97. Coefficient alpha estimates ranged from .88 to .97 (Nelson et al., 1992). Oliver and Baumgart (1985) used 45 subjects to evaluate the 6- week test–retest reliability and found a correlation of .73. These authors also found modest item-total correlations and a lack of factorial equivalence between the two forms of the DAS. They suggest that the DAS is best treated as a whole. A correlation of .41 was obtained between the DAS and the BDI (p. 29).

Validity.   Nelson et al. (1992) demonstrated support for the discriminate validity of the DAS, as 73% of the subjects scoring high on the test received an independent Research Diagnostic Criteria diagnosis of clinical depression, whereas only 36% of the low test scorers were so diagnosed. A. T. Beck et al. (1991) studied the responses of a large clinical sample ($N = 2,023$) and factor-analyzed all 100 items of the DAS. The scale was reduced to 80 items, 66 of which loaded on nine first-order factors. These factors included vulnerability, need for approval, success-perfectionism, need to please others, imperatives, need to impress, avoidance of appearing weak, control over emotions, and disapproval-dependence. It has also been found to be sensitive to the positive effects of cognitive therapy.

Clinical Utility

High. The DAS is easily administered. Scores are available for a variety of samples.

Research Utility

High. The DAS has been used in a large number of research projects. It can be administered in individual or group formats. This self-report inventory provides for a useful assessment of depression-related cognitive distortions.

Source

ERIC Document Reproduction Service, 7420 Fullerton Road, Suite 110, Springfield, VA, 22153-2852.

Cost

Contact ERIC for information concerning cost.

Alternative Forms

Several alternative forms are available. For instance, a Swedish version has been developed (Ohrt & Thorell, 1998), as has a version for medically ill elders (Koenig et al., 1994).

FREQUENCY OF SELF-REINFORCEMENT QUESTIONNAIRE (FSRQ)

Original Citation

Heiby, E. M. (1983). Assessment of frequency of self-reinforcement. *Journal of Personality and Social Psychology*, *44*, 1304–1307.

Purpose

To measure self-control skills deemed relevant to the etiology, maintenance, and alleviation of depression as well as other behaviors with delayed natural consequences (e.g., health behaviors).

Population

Adolescents and adults.

Description

The FSRQ is a 30-item self-report questionnaire. Each item provides a statement concerning people's beliefs or attitudes (e.g., "I seem to blame myself when things go wrong and am very critical of myself"). Respondents are instructed to indicate how well each statement represents their own attitudes in a true/false format. For 15 of the items, "true" responses represent nondepressed attitudes, and for 15 of the items, "false" responses represent nondepressed attitudes.

Background

The FSRQ was developed in concert with behavioral formulations of depression which hypothesize that a low frequency of self-reinforcement predicts and may contribute to the etiology and maintenance of depression (e.g., Lewinsohn, 1974; Rehm, 1977). Heiby defines self-reinforcement as "the process of establishing and controlling overt and covert positive consequences of one's own behavior." Holding unrealistically high expectations for oneself and failing to acknowledge one's own successes are possible causes for low frequency of self-reinforcement. The FSRQ was developed to facilitate empirical investigations of the relationship between frequency of self-reinforcement and depression.

Administration

The FSRQ takes 5–10 minutes to complete and 2 minutes to score.

Scoring

Each nondepressed item is given a score of 1 and each depressed item is scored as 0. High scores indicate a favorable attitude toward self-reinforcement and low scores indicate a poor attitude or tendency not to engage in self-reinforcement. Scores range from 0 to 30.

Interpretation

A score of 17 or less indicates a deficit in self-control skills.

Psychometric Properties

Norms. In a test of the FSRQ administered to 300 college undergraduates, the mean score was 17.2 (SD = 2.42).

Reliability. The test–retest reliability of the FSRQ administered to 100 college undergraduates twice over an 8-week period was .92. The Spearman–Brown split-half reliability tested on the same sample was .87.

Validity. The construct validity of the FSRQ was tested by comparing scores on the instrument to the average amount of self-praise behaviors observed while performing an experimental task whereby 300 college undergraduate participants performed 12 analogy tasks and reported whether they experienced any self-satisfaction or self-praise after completing each item. The correlation between the FSRQ and the experimental self-praise task was .69.

The construct validity was assessed a second time on 100 college undergraduates by comparing FSRQ scores to self-praise after performing anagram tasks. The correlation between these tasks was .65.

The factor structure of the FSRQ was tested on a group of 570 college undergraduates. Five factors were identified and characterized as (a) self-evaluation, (b) self reinforcement and self-reward, (c) don't self-praise, (d) be self-critical, and (e) responding emotionally to criticism for males and responding emotionally to self-evaluation for females. Although the factor structure produced five factors for males and females, the factors did not load in the same order for both groups (Wagner, Holden, & Jannarone, 1988).

Because the purpose of the FSRQ is to facilitate the examination of the self-reinforcement–depression relationship, understanding this relationship is important for its validity. One study found that the FSRQ had significant direct, as well as moderating, effects on depression for a group of adults ($N = 366$; Wilkinson, 1997). Another study of 88 nondepressed undergraduates showed a significant interaction between frequency of self-reinforcement and reduction in environmentally controlled reinforcement in predicting depression (Heiby, 1983).

Clinical Utility

High. The FSRQ has been widely studied, as has the self-control theory of depression upon which the instrument is based.

Research Applicability

High. Studies show that the FSRQ is useful in predicting development of depression, especially in college populations.

Source

The FSRQ is reprinted from Heiby (1983) in Appendix B. For more information, contact Elaine Heiby, Ph.D., Department of Psychology, University of Hawaii, 2430 Campus Road, Honolulu, HI 96822.

Cost

None.

Alternate Forms

A Spanish form is available from Jose Garcia Hurtado, Departamento de Psicologia de la Salud, Universidad de Alicante, Campus de San Juan Apdo, 374, 03080, Alicante, Spain. A Japanese interview version as well as an interview version for the elderly is available from Dr. Heiby. A children's version for ages 8–14 years was developed by Joshi-Peters (1991) and information about this version can also be obtained from Dr. Heiby.

GOAL ORIENTATION INVENTORY (GOI)

Original Citation

Dykman, B. M. (1998). Integrating cognitive and motivational factors in depression: Initial tests of a goal-orientation approach. *Journal of Personality and Social Psychology, 74,* 139–159.

Purpose

To assess motivational and cognitive aspects of depression.

Population

Adults age 17 years and older.

Description

The GOI contains 36 items. Respondents rate the degree of agreement with each statement using a 7-point Likert-type scale, where 1 = "strongly disagree" and 7 = "strongly agree." Items are evenly divided between descriptions of validation-seeking (e.g., "My approach to situations is one of always trying to prove my basic worth, competence, or likeability") and growth-seeking (e.g., "Personal growth is more important to me than protecting myself from my mistakes") individuals. Sample items, reprinted with permission of the publisher (© 1998, the American Psychological Association), include the following:

_____ My approach to situations is one of always trying to prove my basic worth, competence, or likeability.

_____ One of the main things I know I'm striving for is to prove that I am good enough.

_____ I feel like I am always testing out whether I "measure-up."

_____ I approach difficult situations welcoming the opportunity to learn from my mistakes.

_____ Personal growth is more important to me than protecting myself from my fears.

_____ I look upon potential problems in life as opportunities for growth rather than as threats to my self-esteem.

Background

The GOI is based on Dykman's goal-orientation model of depression. This model proposes that depression-prone and depression-resistant individuals can be distinguished based on their goal orientation. Validation-seeking individuals are described as continually striving to prove their self-concept. Growth-seeking individuals strive to reach their fullest potential through self-improvement. The interaction of these characteristics is posited as useful in understanding people predisposed to develop depression-related symptoms. Goal-orientation theory suggests that those individuals who score higher in the validation-seeking domain are more likely to exhibit depression than growth-seeking individuals. The theory also suggests that validation-seeking individuals are more likely to view failure as a result of personal inadequacy, abandon difficult tasks, and develop depressive symptoms following a negative life event.

Administration

The GOI can be administered in individual or group formats and requires 12–15 minutes to complete.

Scoring

Separately summing the responses to each subscale and then subtracting the Growth-Seeking subscale from the Validation-Seeking subscale scores the Goal Orientation Inventory. Scores can range from 108 to −108.

Interpretation

Higher scores represent the endorsement of greater validation-seeking thoughts and behaviors.

Psychometric Properties

Norms. The norms for the final 64-item scale were based on 381 undergraduate students.

Reliability. Coefficient alpha estimates for the total inventory and both subscales ranged from .96 to .97. Test–retest reliability over a 10-week period was estimated using 68 undergraduates and resulted in stability estimates ranging from .76 to .82.

Validity. Validity was evaluated using measures of depression, self-actualization, self-esteem, and task-persistence. As expected, Validation-Seeking scores were related to scores on the BDI (p. 29) and inversely related to self-esteem; Growth-Seeking scores were related to task persistence and inversely related to the BDI.

Clinical Utility

Limited. This measure is easily administered and scored. The information would seem particularly useful for clinicians adopting a coping model of depression. However, the lack of extensive norms limits the clinical utility of the inventory.

Research Utility

High. This measure was developed based on sound theoretical reasoning and this is likely to engender considerable heuristic value. Available psychometric data suggest it can be a useful research instrument.

Source

Dykman (1998).

Cost

This instrument can be used without written permission. To obtain additional information contact Benjamin M. Dykman, Department of Psychology, University of Wisconsin, 1202 West Johnson Street, Madison, WI 53706.

Alternative Forms

None.

INTERPERSONAL EVENTS SCHEDULE (IES)

Original Citation

Youngren, M. A., Zeiss, A., & Lewinsohn, P. M. (1975). *Interpersonal Events Schedule.* University of Oregon, Eugene OR (see also Youngren & Lewinsohn, 1980).

Purpose

To measure interpersonal activities and cognitions.

Population

Adults.

Description

The IES has 160 items that relate to activities (e.g., "visiting friends," "helping a stranger," "smiling at someone") and thoughts (e.g., "feeling unpopular at a social event," "knowing someone is sizing me up," "being afraid I will say or do the wrong thing") related to other people. For each item, respondents are requested to indicate the frequency (3-point scale) that it occurred during the past 30 days, as well as the impact (5-point scale ranging from "very uncomfortable or upset" to "very comfortable or good") of the event when it occurred.

The IES has 10 scales based on rational and empirical decisions: Social Activity; Conflict; Cognitions; Give Positive; Give Negative; Receive Positive; Receive Negative; Dysphoria

Related; Positive Mood Related; and Most Discriminating (i.e., those items that best discriminate between depressed and nondepressed individuals; e.g., "being criticized by my spouse," "worrying about seeming foolish to others," "feeling inferior or incompetent socially").

Background

The IES was developed to test the hypothesized relationship between dysfunctional interpersonal behavior and depression (e.g., Lewinsohn, Biglan, & Zeiss, 1976; Weissman & Paykel, 1974).

Administration

Requires about 30 minutes to complete.

Scoring

Scores can be computed for the various scales.

Interpretation

In its present format, no norms exist for comparison, making clinical interpretation difficult. However, it can be used descriptively to develop a finer analysis of a patient's interpersonal difficulties.

Psychometric Properties

Norms.   Not applicable.

Reliability.   Test–retest correlations were computed at 1-month and 3-month intervals. For the 1-month period, correlations ranged between .44 and .83 across scales (average $r = .67$) for frequency scores, and from .49 to .85 (average $r = .66$) for mean impact scores. Similar coefficients were obtained for the 3-month testing.

Validity.   A comparison between depressed and nondepressed adults regarding their responses to the IES indicated strong differences in self-reported frequency and comfort of social situations.

Clinical Utility

Limited due to the absence of norms.

Research Applicability

High. The IES has been used in several investigations addressing interpersonal behavior and depression.

Source

Peter M. Lewinsohn, Ph.D., Oregon Research Institute, 1715 Franklin Blvd., Eugene, OR 97403-1983.

Cost

None.

Alternative Forms

None.

LIFE ATTITUDES SCHEDULE (LAS)

Original Citation

Lewinsohn, P. M., Langhinrichsen-Rohling, J., Langford, R., Rohde, P., Seeley, J. R., & Chapman, J. (1995). The Life Attitudes Schedule: A scale to assess adolescent life-enhancing and life-threatening behaviors. *Suicide and Life-Threatening Behavior*, *25*, 458–474.

Purpose

To assess a broad array of suicidal and life-threatening behaviors.

Population

Adolescents and adults 13 years and older.

Description

There are three different forms of the LAS (Forms A, B, C), each of which contains 96 true/false questions that require the respondent to indicate whether a given statement (e.g., "I relax on a regular basis," "I went to a cemetery," "I dreamed that I was dead") was true of him/her during the past week. In addition, 19 questions are included for validity purposes. The LAS measures four separate content categories (death-related, health-related, injury-related, self-related) which are hypothesized to encompass the entire domain of life-threatening and life-enhancing behaviors. Each category contains an equal number of items that assess relevant thoughts, actions, and feelings. In this manner, the LAS is viewed as being able to measure an individual's degree of suicide-proneness, depression, and certain aspects of life enhancement.

Background

The LAS was originally developed with high school students to identify problem behaviors in adolescents that lead to increased risk for potential difficulties, such as depression. It has since been expanded to include adults. The theoretical underpinnings involve the belief that a single domain of behaviors exists (i.e., "suicide-proneness") to which all life-enhancing and life-threatening behaviors belong. These behaviors fall along a continuum of positive to negative thoughts, actions, and feelings.

Administration

The LAS requires about 30 minutes to complete.

Scoring

The LAS can be scored for the four content areas, as well as an overall score. Higher scores indicate higher levels of suicide behavior.

Interpretation

Normative profiles exist for comparison.

Psychometric Properties

Norms.   Four groups of norms exist to convert raw scores into standardized scores: female adolescents (ages 13–18 years), male adolescents (ages 13–18 years), female adults (ages 19–60 years), and male adults (ages 19–60 years).

Reliability.   Test–retest correlations for the LAS total averaged .83 across the three forms. Such reliability estimates ranged from .59 to .90 across behaviors (thoughts, feelings, actions), and from .66 to .88 across the four content areas.

Validity.   The LAS was found to correlate .43, .59, and .59 with the CES-D scale (p. 39) across the three forms, and .57, .65, and .55 with the Beck Hopelessness Scale (p. 175) across the three forms.

Clinical Utility

High. The LAS can provide for details regarding a patient's suicidal and life-threatening behaviors. In addition to the LAS, Lewinsohn and his colleagues developed the LAIS (Life Attitudes Interview Schedule) for clinicians to use as a semistructured interview to parallel the format of the LAS with specific focus on suicide behavior.

Research Applicability

High, especially as a confirmatory factor analyses has supported the hypothesized structure of the LAS.

Source

Peter M. Lewinsohn, Ph.D., Oregon Research Institute, 1715 Franklin Blvd., Eugene, OR 97403-1983. The LAS is currently under development by Multi-Health Systems, 908 Niagara Falls Blvd., North Tonawanda, NY 14120-2060. Phone: 800-456-3003.

Cost

None.

Alternative Forms

A 24-item short form is available.

PLEASANT EVENTS SCHEDULE (PES)

Original Citations

MacPhillamy, D. J., & Lewinsohn, P. M. (1976). *Manual for the Pleasant Events Schedule*. University of Oregon, Eugene, OR.

MacPhillamy, D. J., & Lewinsohn, P. M. (1982). The Pleasant Events Schedule: Studies on reliability, validity, and scale intercorrelation. *Journal of Consulting and Clinical Psychology*, *50*, 363-380.

Purpose

To assess the frequency and subjective enjoyability of pleasurable or reinforcing events.

Population

Adults.

Description

The PES contains 320 items that describe potentially reinforcing events or activities. Respondents are requested to rate these items twice, once using a 3-point scale of frequency over the past 30 days, and a second time using a 3-point scale of subjective enjoyability. Because the PES is used to help identify potential reinforcers, the respondent is asked to provide a rating of enjoyability regardless of whether he or she actually engaged in the event in the past 30 days.

Various scales have been developed. One scale was derived rationally and provides for a social (e.g., "having a frank and open conversation") versus nonsocial (e.g., "driving skillfully") distinction. Other scales were derived via a principal components analysis (e.g., masculine versus feminine role-related activities, introverted versus extraverted activities).

Background

A major behavioral theory of depression espoused by Lewinsohn and his colleagues (e.g., Lewinsohn, 1974; Lewinsohn, Youngren, & Grosscup, 1979) focused on the role of response-contingent positive reinforcement in the etiopathogenesis of depression. More specifically, a low rate of response-contingent reinforcement in major life areas and/or a high rate of aversive experiences can lead to a reduction of effective behavior and to the experience of dysphoria. This low rate of positive reinforcement can be caused by one of three factors: (a) behavioral skill deficits leading to an inability to obtain such reinforcement, (b) changes in one's environment (e.g., death of a family member), and (c) an increase in an individual's sensitivity to negative events. The PES has been used in various research studies to support these hypotheses. For example, Lewinsohn and Libet (1972) found an association between the rate of positive reinforcement and the intensity of depression.

Administration

The PES takes about 1 hour to complete.

Scoring

The PES was originally designed to be mechanically read (i.e., optical scanner), scored, and fed directly into a computer. Hand scoring can follow the directions in the manual regarding each scale.

Interpretation

Norms exist for comparison by age and gender.

Psychometric Properties

Norms.   The normative group consists of 464 adults.

Reliability.   Test-retest reliability was assessed with three separate samples across three time periods (1, 2, and 3 months) between testings. Correlations between baseline and 1 month across the seven major PES scales ranged from .69 to .88.

Validity.   Concurrent validity was examined by comparing the self-ratings with those of trained observers and found to be significant. Predictive validity was measured by having respondents monitor their daily activities for 1 month after completing the PES. Correlations for two different data sets were .57 and .62. A variety of studies were conducted to assess the construct validity of the PES. For example, the PES was found to discriminate significantly between depressed individuals and both normal and psychiatric control subjects.

Clinical Utility

High. The PES can easily be used to develop a list of potential reinforcers for a given patient.

Research Applicability

High. The PES has been used in a multitude of studies supporting a behavioral model of depression.

Source

The PES is reprinted from MacPhillamy and Lewinsohn (1980) in Appendix B. For additional information, contact Peter M. Lewinsohn, Ph.D., Oregon Research Institute, 1715 Franklin Blvd., Eugene, OR 97403-1983.

Cost

None.

Alternative Forms

The PES was modified for use with a group of adolescents and children in a study by Clarke, Lewinsohn, and Alexander (1985), as well as for use with the elderly (Teri & Lewinsohn, 1982).

PLEASANT EVENTS SCHEDULE-AD (PES-AD)

Original Citation

Logsdon, R. G., & Teri, L. (1997). The Pleasant Events Schedule-AD: Psychometric properties of long and short forms and an investigation of its association to depression and cognition in Alzheimer's disease patients. *The Gerontologist*, *37*, 40–45.

Purpose

To identify pleasant events for people with Alzheimer's disease.

Population

People with Alzheimer's disease.

Description

The PES-AD is a caregiver-completed questionnaire that is available in both a long (53 item) and a short (20 item) form. Both versions contain lists of activities (e.g., being outside, shopping, buying things). Each activity is followed by a 3-point frequency scale ranging from "not at all" to "7 or more times" and a 3-point enjoyment scale ranging from "not at all" to "a great deal." The caregiver is instructed to rate each item based on how frequently the patient has engaged in each activity, as well as how much he or she seemed to enjoy the activity during the past month.

Background

Following behavioral conceptualizations hypothesizing that low rates of response-contingent positive reinforcement contribute to the etiology and maintenance of depression (Lewinsohn & Graf, 1973), the PES-AD was developed to assess the rate of pleasant events (i.e., positive reinforcers) experienced by people suffering from Alzheimer's disease. When developing the PES-AD, the developers took into account the likelihood that positive activities would decrease as cognitive abilities declined, thereby increasing the risk of developing depression. The PES-AD was based on the PES (Lewinsohn & Talkington, 1979) and the PES-Elderly (Teri & Lewinsohn, 1982).

Administration

The PES-AD takes approximately 15 minutes to complete.

Scoring

The PES-AD produces an overall activity frequency rating and an overall enjoyment rating by summing the ratings for each item. In addition, an estimate of frequency of enjoyable activity can be obtained by calculating the cross-product between the two ratings.

Interpretation

Higher scores indicate higher frequency or greater enjoyment of activities.

Psychometric Properties

Norms.   Means and standard deviations for a group of 42 outpatients with Alzheimer's disease are reported in Logsdon and Teri (1997).

Reliability.   Using the sample described above, coefficient alphas ranged from .86 to .95 for the long form and from .76 to .94 for the short form, whereas split-half reliabilities ranged from .78 to .95 for the long form and from .74 to .94 for the short form.

Validity.   Estimates of the concurrent validity of the PES-AD indicate that the frequency × enjoyment cross-product, or frequency of engaging in activity that one enjoys, was most predictive of depression. This calculation was significantly negatively correlated with the HRSD (p. 58) for both the long form and the short form ($-.41$). The correlation between the two versions of the PES-AD was .95.

Clinical Utility

High. The PES-AD proves to be a useful instrument for evaluating depression in a population where reliable and valid assessments are especially difficult. The individual activity ratings provide potential areas to target for intervention.

Research Applicability

Limited. The PES-AD was used in a treatment study on depression in Alzheimer's patients (Teri, Logsdon, Uomoto, & McCurry, 1997). Further investigations utilizing this instrument are needed.

Source

Rebecca G. Logsdon, Ph.D., Department of Psychiatry and Behavioral Sciences, Division of Gerontology and Geriatrics, University of Washington School of Medicine, 1959 NE Pacific St., Box 356560, Seattle, WA 98195-6560.

Cost

None if used in academic settings.

Alternative Forms

A 20-item short-form is available.

POSITIVE AUTOMATIC THOUGHTS QUESTIONNAIRE (ATQ-P)

Original Citation

Ingram, R. E., & Wisnicki, K. S. (1988). Assessment of positive automatic cognitions. *Journal of Consulting and Clinical Psychology*, *56*, 898–902.

Purpose

To assess the frequency of positive self-statements.

Population

Adults and adolescents.

Description

The ATQ-P is a 30-item self-report measure. Each item consists of a single positive statement (e.g., "I'm fun to be with," "There is no problem that is hopeless"). Items are rated on a 5-point scale of frequency, ranging from "never" to "all the time," with instructions emphasizing the rate or frequency with which statements occur, rather than a person's belief in a given statement.

Background

The ATQ-P was developed in response to the Automatic Thoughts Questionnaire (ATQ; p. 172), which assesses frequency of negative self-statements. The ATQ is a well established measure of negative cognitions in depression, but theorists have suggested that positive cognitions may also be important to assess, and that deficits in these may be implicated in depression, just as excessive negative cognitions are (Ingram, Kendall, Siegle, Guarino, & McLaughlin, 1995). The ATQ-P was initially developed on an adult population, but a later study (Jolly & Wiesner, 1996) supported its use with adolescents as well.

Administration

The ATQ-P may be completed in either individual or group self-report administration, requiring 5–10 minutes to complete.

Scoring

ATQ-P scores are obtained by summing all responses, for a range of total scores of 30–150.

Interpretation

Cutoff scores are not available, but scores can be compared with norms for depressed, subclinically depressed, and nondepressed groups; norms are available by individual item scores (Ingram & Wisnicki, 1988) and by total scores (Ingram et al., 1995).

Psychometric Properties

Initial psychometric properties for the ATQ-P were developed in a sample of 480 undergraduate students (197 male, 283 female). Subjects were classified as depressed or nondepressed based on scores on the Beck Depression Inventory (BDI; p. 29). A number of other studies have also examined the psychometric properties of the ATQ-P; these are summarized in some detail in Ingram et al. (1995).

Norms.   The mean score on the ATQ-P across subjects was 103.31. To compare means across levels of depression, groups were formed of depressed, mildly depressed, and nondepressed subjects. Subjects were classified as depressed if they had a BDI score >20, were in treatment for depression, and had a family history of mental health treatment ($N = 16$). A random selection of 24 subjects with BDI scores >12, but with no personal or family treatment history, was classified as mildly depressed, and a random selection of 24 subjects with BDI scores <9 and no personal or family treatment history was classified as nondepressed. Within this subsample, the mean scores were 83.08 ($SD = 15.78$) for the depressed group, 95.96 ($SD = 18.63$) for the mildly depressed group, and 107.15 ($SD = 18.55$) for the nondepressed group.

Reliability.   Split-half reliability for the ATQ-P was .95. Item-total correlations ranged from .42 to .75, with a coefficient alpha of .94, suggesting excellent internal consistency. Temporal stability was supported in a test–retest reliability study by Baldree, Ingram, and Saccuzzo (1991), with a correlation of .80 for two administrations 1 month apart.

Validity.   ATQ-P scores were significantly different between depressed (BDI $\geq$ 10) and nondepressed (BDI < 10) subjects in the initial study. In the subsample described above, ATQ-P scores also differed based on relative levels of depression, further supporting its validity. Factor analyses yielded four orthogonal factors: Positive Daily Functioning, Positive Self-Examination, Others' Evaluations of the Self, and Positive Future Expectations. The authors note that these factors seem to be the positive counterparts of Beck's negative triad (A. T. Beck, 1967), which considerable research has supported as being related to depression. ATQ-P scores were also correlated with several standardized measures of psychopathology, including the BDI, State-Trait Anxiety Inventory-Trait Form (STAI-T; Spielberger, Gorsuch, & Lushene, 1970), and Social Avoidance and Distress Scale (SADS; Watson & Friend, 1969). These correlations were $-.33$, $-.37$, and $-.32$ respectively, all statistically significant.

Clinical Utility

High. The ATQ-P is brief and easy to complete. Whereas most clinical measures focus on negative symptoms, thoughts, and states, the ATQ-P allows for positive cognitions to be assessed as well, which may provide useful information to the clinician while also pleasing clients by its focus on healthy, rather than unhealthy, aspects.

Research Applicability

High. The assessment of cognition has been an important part of depression research, and the assessment of positive, as well as negative, cognitions is supported by a number of theories of depression. The authors particularly emphasize its utility within the States of Mind theory (Schwartz & Garamoni, 1989).

Source

Rick E. Ingram, Ph.D., 6363 Alvarado Court, #103, San Diego State University, San Diego, CA 92120 (items are listed in Ingram & Wisnicki, 1988).

Cost

None.

Alternate Forms

None.

PROBLEM-SOLVING INVENTORY (PSI)

Original Citation

Heppner, P. P., & Petersen, C. H. (1982). The development and implications of a personal problem-solving inventory. *Journal of Counseling Psychology*, *29*, 66–75.

Purpose

To assess individuals' perceptions about how they react to and solve personal problems.

Population

Adults.

Description

The PSI is a 35-item self-report questionnaire. Each item presents a statement reflecting a possible attitude or behavior that a person may experience when facing a personal problem (e.g., "When a solution to a problem was unsuccessful, I did not examine why it didn't work"). Respondents are instructed to indicate the extent to which each statement reflects their own problem-solving approach along a 6-point Likert-type scale ranging from 1 ("Strongly Agree") to 6 ("Strongly Disagree"). The PSI measures three problem-solving factors: problem-solving confidence, approach-avoidance style, and personal control.

Background

Heppner and Petersen developed the PSI to provide a method of assessing personal problem-solving approaches. Although scientific information about the value of problem solving was present in the literature, few studies applied this information to counseling settings. The authors believed that the PSI would promote idiographic assessment of problem-solving skills, measurement of change in personal problem-solving skills after counseling, and systematic application of problem-solving interventions in counseling settings and research evaluating the effects of such interventions. Following the development of the PSI, numerous studies have demonstrated the relationships between problem solving and depression (A. M. Nezu & Ronan, 1985, 1988) and problem solving and suicide ideation or suicide risk (Schotte & Clum, 1982, 1987).

Administration

The PSI takes approximately 10–15 minutes to complete.

Scoring

A total score, as well as scores for each of the three factors, can be obtained simply by summing the scores for each individual item. Eleven items compose the problem-solving confidence factor, 16 items compose the approach-avoidance style factor, and 5 items compose the personal control factor. Seventeen items of the PSI are reverse-scored (e.g., a response of 6 would receive a score of 1). Three items are filler items and their scores are not considered in the interpretation.

Interpretation

High scores indicate poor self-confidence, avoiding problems, and having poor personal control, while low scores indicate the reverse.

Psychometric Properties

Norms.   Normative data for the total PSI as well as each subscale are contained in Heppner (1982).

Reliability.   The internal consistency of the total PSI was (alpha) = .90 for a group of 150 college undergraduates. Test–retest reliability estimates for 31 college undergraduates tested at 2-week intervals were .89 for the total scale, .84 for the problem-solving confidence scale, .88 for the approach–avoidance style scale, and .83 for the personal control scale.

Validity.   With regard to concurrent, as well as construct, validity, the PSI correlated with personal ratings of problem-solving skills using 150 college undergraduates. Scores were also compared to ratings of personal satisfaction with problem-solving skills in the same sample and again produced significant correlations. Conversely, the PSI did not correlate significantly with measures of intelligence or social desirability.

The PSI has also been found to be sensitive to the effects of training in problem-solving skills among clinically depressed adults (A. M. Nezu, 1986b; A. M. Nezu & Perri, 1989).

Clinical Utility

High. The PSI was specifically developed to be used in clinical settings, and research has supported its clinical utility.

Research Application

High. The PSI is sensitive to change and has good psychometric properties.

Source

Consulting Psychologists Press, 3803 East Bayshore Road, P.O. Box 10096, Palo Alto, CA 94303. Phone: 800-624-1765.

Cost

$33.25 for item booklet, scoring key, and manual.

Alternative Forms

A Turkish version of the PSI is described in Sahin, Sahin, and Heppner (1993).

REASONS FOR LIVING INVENTORY (RFL)

Original Citation

Linehan, M. M., Goodstein, J. L., Nielsen, S. L., & Chiles, J. A. (1983). Reasons for staying alive when you are thinking of killing yourself: The Reasons for Living Inventory. *Journal of Consulting and Clinical Psychology, 51,* 276–286.

Purpose

To evaluate a variety of beliefs that people hold as reasons not to commit suicide if suicidal thoughts occur.

Population

The RFL was developed based on a population of adults sampled from the general community and was further refined using samples of psychiatric inpatients. Psychometric properties of the RFL were also examined for normal and juvenile adolescents.

Description

The RFL is a 48-item self-report questionnaire. Each item contains a statement that may be considered a reason for not committing suicide (e.g., "I believe killing myself would not really accomplish or solve anything"). Respondents are requested to rate the importance of each statement as a reason for living on a 6-point scale ranging from 1 = "not at all important" to 6 = "extremely important." The RFL contains six subscales: Survival and Coping Beliefs, Responsibility to Family, Child-Related Concerns, Fear of Suicide, Fear of Social Disapproval, and Moral Objections.

Background

Contrary to other self-report inventories that evaluate maladaptive thoughts or behaviors that increase risk for suicidal behavior, the RFL was designed to evaluate adaptive beliefs that prevent individuals from committing suicide. The investigators hypothesized that peoples' belief systems facilitate their will to live and their desire not to commit suicide. Therefore, these belief systems are different for people who attempt suicide or parasuicide than they are for people who are not suicidal. Models provided by Frankl (1959), who evaluated the belief systems or survivors of Nazi concentration camps, provided some of the early framework for their hypotheses. The items of the RFL were developed by sampling a large and diverse subject pool who generated 343 reaasons for living. Content and factor analyses eventually narrowed the list to 48 items.

Administration

The RFL takes approximately 15 minutes to complete.

Scoring

A score for each subscale is derived by summing the score of each item and dividing by the number of items in the subscale. Scores range from 1 to 6 for each subscale.

Interpretation

Higher scores indicate stronger reasons for living.

Psychometric Properties

Norms. Mean scores on the RFL subscales are reported for samples of 197 Seattle shoppers and for 175 psychiatric inpatients divided into three groups: (a) those without suicidal behavior, (b) those with current suicidal ideation, and (c) those with current parasuicide (Linehan et al., 1983). In addition, means and standard deviations for a sample of 175 students enrolled in an introductory psychology class are reported by Osman, Gregg, Osman, and Jones (1992), and means are reported for a sample of 407 college students by Osman et al. (1993).

Reliability. Internal consistency estimates using Cronbach's alpha are moderately high, with scores ranging from .72 to .89 in one study (Linehan et al., 1983).

Validity. Various analyses support the validity of the RFL for differentiating suicidal from nonsuicidal individuals in the general population as well as psychiatric inpatients (Lineham et al., 1983).

Several factor analyses also support the factorial validity of the RFL. A principal-component factor analyses used to design the original RFL identified six factors (Linehan et al., 1983) and was supported by an exploratory principal-components factor analysis conducted by Osman et al. (1993). Another factor analysis identified a five-factor solution that folded the Fear of Social Disapproval and Fear of Suicide items into one scale, but retained the other four scales delineated in the original analyses (Osman et al., 1992).

Significant correlations were found between subscales of the RFL and subscales of the Suicidal Behaviors Questionnaire (Linehan & Nielsen, 1981) and the Suicide Probability Scale (p. 258; Cull & Gill, 1982) to support its concurrent validity.

Clinical Utility

High. Because research demonstrates that suicide ideators lack certain beliefs that maintain their will to live, the RFL may be a useful instrument for clinical applications, although data are limited concerning this issue at this time.

Research Applicability

High. Factor analyses have been replicated and continue to support the factorial validity of this instrument. In addition, studies demonstrate its significant relationship with other measures of suicidal behavior and psychopathology (Osman et al., 1993).

Source

The items of the RFL can be viewed in Linehan et al. (1983) or can be obtained from Marsha M. Linehan, Ph.D., Department of Psychology, NI-25, University of Washington, Seattle, WA 98195.

Cost

None.

Alternative Forms

A 12-item Brief Reasons for Living Inventory is available to evaluate reasons for living among prison inmates (Ivanoff, Jang, Smyth, & Linehan, 1994), and a College Student Reasons for Living Inventory is also available (Westefeld, Badura, Hiel, & Scheel, 1996).

REVISED GRIEF EXPERIENCE INVENTORY (RGEI)

Original Citation

Lev, E., Munro, B. H., & McCorkle, R. (1993). A shortened version of an instrument measuring bereavement. *International Journal of Nursing Studies*, *30*, 213–226.

Purpose

To assess the experience of grief and bereavement.

Population

Adults.

Description

The RGEI is a 22-item self-report measure. Each item is rated on a 6-point Likert-type scale in which the level of agreement with each statement is indicated (1 = "slight agreement" to 6 = "slight disagreement"). The RGEI has four scales: Depression, Physical Distress, Existential Concerns, and Tension and Guilt.

Background

The original Grief Experience Inventory (GEI; Sanders, Mauger, & Strong, 1979) consisted of 135 items that were rated on a dichotomous yes/no scale. The GEI was developed using a Q-Sort based on interviews of individuals in bereavement, and included several validity scales (e.g., social desirability) as well as nine bereavement scales (despair, anger/hostility, guilt, social isolation, loss of control, rumination, depersonalization, somatization, and death anxiety). The RGEI was developed to provide a briefer measure than the GEI. Items selected for the RGEI were chosen first based on Parkes' (1972) theory of grief and on the professional experiences of the first author, and then included if the item-total correlations were satisfactory. The RGEI differs from the GEI in its scoring system as well: The dichotomous ratings were replaced with a 6-point scale to allow for a greater range of responding.

Administration

The RGEI can be completed in approximately 10 minutes.

Scoring

The RGEI is scored by recoding the scores and then summing them for a total score. Higher scores indicate greater levels of grief. Scores for the four subscales are obtained by following the same procedure for the items within that scale. These are as follows: Existential Concerns (items 5, 11, 14, 15, 20, 21), Depression (7, 8, 9, 13, 16, 17), Guilt (1, 2, 4), Physical Distress (3, 6, 10, 12, 18, 19, 22).

Interpretation

No cutoff scores were provided. However, scores may be compared with norms listed below. Additional norms, broken down by various demographic categories (i.e., gender, marital history), are included in the reference article as well.

Psychometric Properties

Psychometric properties for the RGEI are based on 418 responses to a mailing of 1,116 questionnaires via hospice agencies. Of the 418 respondents, the mean age was 58.1 years, and

78% were female. The majority (88%) were White, with 6% African American and 5% from other ethnic backgrounds.

Norms.   The mean score on the RGEI was 75.5 ($SD = 25.7$), with scores ranging from 22 to 132. The mean scores for the subscales were as follows: Depression (6 items), 23.0 ($SD = 7.0$); Physical Distress (7 items), 22.5 ($SD = 9.3$); Existential Concerns (6 items), 20.1 ($SD = 8.5$); and Tension and Guilt (3 items), 10.0 ($SD = 4.6$). Separate norms are also available based on relationship to the deceased, use of medication, and other demographic variables.

Reliability.   The overall alpha was estimated to be .93. Alphas for the four subscales were .80, .83, .87, and .72 for Depression, Physical Distress, Existential Concerns, and Tension and Guilt, respectively. No data were provided on stability over time.

Validity.   The RGEI was not validated against other standardized measures. Factor analyses of the measure support theoretical conceptualizations of grief as detailed by Lev et al. (1993), thus supporting its construct validity.

Clinical Utility

High. The RGEI is easy to administer and score, and provides a quick check for the clinician regarding both the level and type of clients' bereavement and grief.

Research Applicability

High. Although additional psychometric data are needed, the RGEI provides a useful measure of grief that is not burdensome in terms of time or effort. As there are not many such measures, research in this area is likely to benefit from the use of the RGEI, and thus will also provide the needed data on its validity.

Source

The RGEI is reprinted in Appendix B. For additional information, contact Elise Lev, Ph.D., College of Nursing, Rutgers University, 180 University Avenue, Newark, NJ 07102.

Cost

None.

Alternate Forms

None.

SELF-CONTROL QUESTIONNAIRE FOR DEPRESSION

Original Citation

Anderson, C. B., Metha, P. D., Rehm, L. P., Wagner, A. L., Delaune, K., & Cook, H. (1998). *The Revised Self-Control Questionnaire: Psychometric properties and relation to depression*. Paper presented at the 42nd Annual Convention of the Southwestern Psychological Association, Houston, TX.

Purpose

To measure self-control-related behaviors and thoughts that covary with depression.

Population

Adults.

Description

The Self-Control Questionnaire for Depression is a 47-item self-report measure. Items reflect common deficits in self-control that are hypothesized to contribute to the development of depression (Rehm, 1977). The self-control model of depression suggests that depression is the result of deficits in six areas of self-control: attributional style, focus on immediate consequences, self-monitoring, self-punishment, self-reinforcement, and standard setting. Items are rated using a 5-point Likert-type format.

A modified version of the directions, as well as five sample items, are listed below, with permission of the authors.

> Please read each of the following statements and indicate just how characteristic or descriptive of you the statement is by using the code given below:
> 1 = Very true of me
> 2 = Rather true of me
> 3 = Somewhat true of me
> 4 = Rather untrue of me
> 5 = Very untrue of me
> _____ I have a hard time dismissing the negative thoughts about myself.
> _____ Even though I know that doing something now will produce the most productive results for me in the long run, I tend not to do it.
> _____ When things go wrong it is usually because of something I did.
> _____ I don't feel good about something I've done, unless someone else approves of it.
> _____ When I accomplish something, I reward myself with a pleasant activity.

Background

The Self-Control Questionnaire (Rehm et al., 1981) was initially developed to evaluate the effectiveness of a self-control therapy program that was based on Rehm's self-control model of depression. The construction, standardization, and validation of the Self-Control Questionnaire involved 101 clinically depressed community volunteers, a control sample, and pregnant women. The Self-Control Questionnaire for Depression is an expanded and revised version of the Self-Control Questionnaire.

Administration

The Self-Control Questionnaire for Depression requires about 15 minutes to complete and can be administered in individual or group formats.

Scoring

The Self-Control Questionnaire for Depression is scored by hand. Twenty-seven items reflect negative, depressive attitudes and are reverse-scored. The total score is the sum of all items, allowing for a range of scores from 47 to 235. Scores can be calculated for eight separate subscales.

Interpretation

The Self-Control Questionnaire for Depression was conceptualized as a continuous measure. Therefore, cutoff scores are not available. Higher scores indicate the endorsement of less effective self-control strategies.

Psychometric Properties

Norms.   Normative data have not yet been published.

Reliability.   Coefficient alpha estimates for the original Self-Control Questionnaire ranged from .82 to .88. Five-week test–retest reliability revealed a test–retest correlation of .86. Reliability data for the Self-Control Questionnaire for Depression have not yet been published.

Validity.   Validity data for the Self-Control Questionnaire for Depression are based on a sample of 257 college students with a mean age of 25 ($SD = 6$). Confirmatory factor analysis was used to analyze the measure and generally supported three latent factors: Goal Orientation, Negativity, and Self-Reinforcement. Correlations between these latent factors and a latent factor derived from the Beck Depression Inventory subscales (p. 29) were $-.64$ (Goal Orientation), $-.72$ (Negativity), and $-.28$ (Self-Reinforcement). Additional structural analyses supported the existence of eight subscales: attribution of negative events (three items), attribution of positive events (four items), consequences of behavior (six items), external standards (six items), goal setting (seven items), monitoring and control of mood (eight items), self-punishment (six items), and self-reinforcement (seven items).

Clinical Utility

Limited. The Self-Control Questionnaire for Depression is brief and easily administered. The measure is conceptualized as a continuous measure of self-control skills related to depression. The measure provides a potentially useful means of quantifying self-reported self-control behaviors and thoughts. Unfortunately, the lack of norms and cutoff scores for various pathological groups limits the clinical utility.

Research Utility

High. The Self-Control Questionnaire has been used successfully as an outcome measure and it seems likely that the Self-Control Questionnaire for Depression will function similarly. The Self-Control Questionnaire for Depression can be administered in an individual or group format. The available psychometric data for the Self-Control Questionnaire for Depression suggest it possesses considerable construct validity.

Source

Anderson et al. (1998).

Cost

For additional information and permission to use, contact Lynn P. Rehm, Department of Psychology, University of Houston, Houston, TX 77204-5341. Phone: 713-743-8606; e-mail: lprehm@uhupvml.uh.edu.

Alternative Forms

None available.

SELF-CONTROL SCHEDULE

Original Citation

Rosenbaum, M. (1980). A schedule for assessing self-control behaviors: Preliminary findings. *Behavior Therapy*, *11*, 109–121.

Purpose

To assess the tendency toward applying self-control methods for resolving behavior problems.

Population

Adults.

Description

The SCS is a 36-item self-report measure designed to quantify skills used for coping with problems. Items are worded in the present tense to elicit currently used strategies (e.g., "When I am feeling depressed I try to think about pleasant events," "When I plan to work, I remove all the things that are not relevant to my work"). Twelve items refer to the use of cognitions to control emotional and physiological sensations, 11 items refer to the use of problem-solving strategies, 4 items relate to the respondent's perceived ability to delay immediate gratification, and 9 items assess general expectations for self-efficacy. Items are rated using a 6-point Likert-type format, ranging from -3 ("very uncharacteristic of me") to $+3$ ("very characteristic of me").

Background

The SCS was developed initially in the Hebrew language. Means and standard deviations obtained with an English version completed by American students were similar to those obtained using a Hebrew version completed by Israeli students. The construction, standardization, and validation process involved over 600 subjects. Simons, Lustman, Wetzel, and Murphy (1985) found SCS scores were the single best predictor of success in cognitive therapy of depression.

As noted in Chapter 2, the construct of self-control holds a predominant role in various cognitive-behavioral models of depression (Lewinsohn et al., 1987; A. M. Nezu et al., 1989; Rehm, 1977). As such, the SCS provides for the ability to assess an important variable that may serve as a crucial target problem area in treatment for a given patient.

Administration

The SCS requires between 5 and 10 minutes to complete.

Scoring

Item scores range from -3 to $+3$; there are 10 reverse-scored items. The total score is obtained by summing the item scores, allowing for a range of scores from -108 to $+108$.

Interpretation

Higher scores indicate the endorsement of more varied or effective self-control strategies or both.

Psychometric Properties

Norms. Norms and psychometric properties are based on six samples: four samples of undergraduate students from universities in Israel ($N = 529$), one sample of American undergraduates ($N = 111$), and one sample of nonstudent Israeli men who were randomly chosen from a group who were required to pass a psychological and physical examination prior to renewing their driving licenses ($N = 105$). Means and standard deviations for these samples are contained in Rosenbaum (1980).

Reliability. With regard to internal consistency, coefficient alpha estimates for the six samples ranged from .78 to .86. Four-week test–retest reliability revealed the SCS to be fairly stable over time, $r = .86$.

Validity. The SCS was inversely related ($r = -.40$) to the Rotter Locus of Control Scale (Rotter, 1966). This suggests that the more subjects reported using self-control methods, the more they endorsed an internal locus of control. Subjects who reported greater application of the self-control methods tapped by the SCS also were less likely to hold irrational beliefs ($-.48$) as measured by the Irrational Beliefs Test (Jones, 1969). The SCS was significantly related to the G Factor, and unrelated to other factors, of the 16 Personality Factor Questionnaire (Cattell, Eber, & Tatsuoka, 1970). The G Factor was assumed by Cattell et al. (1970) to measure self-control as a personality pattern and these findings add discriminate validity. High scores on the SCS were also related to coping with laboratory pain (Rosenbaum, 1980), clinical pain (Courey, Feuerstein, & Bush, 1982), and seasickness (Rosenbaum & Rolnick, 1983). Finally, the SCS was also related to self-control of nail biting (Frankel & Merbaum, 1982).

Clinical Utility

High. The SCS is a fairly brief and easily administered inventory and provides a useful means of quantifying self-reported strategies that clients employ when confronted by problems.

Research Utility

High. The available psychometric data suggest it possesses many desirable characteristics, and it has been used successfully in a number of research studies.

Source

The SCS is reprinted in Appendix B.

Cost

Not available.

Alternative Forms

The SCS was originally developed in the Hebrew language.

SELF-ESTEEM WORKSHEET

Original Citation

Overholser, J. C. (1993). Idiographic, quantitative assessment of self-esteem. *Personality and Individual Differences, 14*, 639–646.

Purpose

To measure self-esteem.

Population

Adults.

Description

The Self-Esteem Worksheet is completed through the collaborative effort of a professional and the participant. The worksheet contains a flow-chart format comprised of several boxes with the words "area," "importance," and "success" written inside each box. For each box, the participant is instructed to (a) identify an area relevant to his or her self-esteem (e.g., occupation, friendships), (b) rate on a scale from 0 to 100 how important this area is to him or her, and (c) rate on a scale from 0 to 100 his or her perception of personal success in this area. Participants may use as few as 3 boxes and as many as 15.

Background

Designed to provide a quantitative, yet idiographic assessment of self-esteem, the Self-Esteem Worksheet was developed in response to the belief that self-esteem has different meanings for different people and is influenced by different areas of a person's life rather than a global dimension (Hammen & Goodman-Brown, 1990; Safran, Segal, Hill, & Whiffin, 1990; Wylie, 1989; Griffin, Chassin, & Young, 1981). Overholser believed that existing instruments for self-esteem, which provided general statements of self-esteem, were biased by the developers' values of self-esteem and did not capture the individual nature of this construct or how it varies from person to person. He predicted that the Self-Esteem Worksheet would be related to negative affect, as are other self-esteem instruments.

Administration

The time line for administering the Self-Esteem Worksheet varies from person to person. The instructions provide questions which may facilitate completion (e.g., "What things about you really play a role in how you feel about yourself?"). Choosing specific (e.g., "my sense of humor") rather than general (e.g., "my personality") areas is recommended. Professionals are advised to facilitate completion of the worksheet by helping participants identify all areas related to their self-esteem until they can agree that if they were doing well in all of the areas identified, their self-esteem would be as high as it could possibly be.

Scoring

Multiply each importance rating by its respective success rating. Then, sum the products of each box and divide by 100. Scores range from 0 to 100.

Interpretation

Higher scores indicate higher self-esteem.

Psychometric Properties

Norms. Norms are reported for a group of 323 college undergraduates in Overholser (1993). It should be noted that mean scores were significantly different for males and females, where males placed greater emphasis on task-related areas and females placed greater emphasis on social relationships and personal qualities.

Reliability. The test–retest reliability for a group of 323 college undergraduates was .61 when measured after a 10-week interval.

Validity. The Self-Esteem Worksheet correlated positively and significantly with three other measures of self esteem. It also correlated negatively and significantly with the BDI (p. 29; $r = -.25$) and the UCLA Loneliness Scale (Russell, Peplau, and Cutrona, 1980; $r -.33$).

Clinical Utility

High. The Self-Esteem Worksheet allows for assessment of change in self-esteem over time while also examining the areas that each individual believes are important to his or her own self-esteem.

Research Applicability

High. The quantitative aspects of the Self-Esteem Worksheet allow for comparisons within as well as between individuals or groups.

Source

James C. Overholser, Ph.D., Department of Psychology, Case Western Reserve University, 10900 Euclid Avenue, Cleveland, OH 44106-7123.

Cost

None.

Alternative Forms

None.

SOCIAL ADJUSTMENT SCALE (SAS)

Original Citation

Paykel, E. S., Weissman, M., Prusoff, B. A., & Tonks, C. M. (1971). Dimensions of social adjustment in depressed women. *Journal of Nervous and Mental Disease, 152,* 158–172.

Purpose

To assess the dimensions of social and interpersonal functioning and adjustment.

Population

Adults.

Description

The SAS is a 48-item semistructured interview designed to obtain ratings on a variety of behaviors and feelings related to several different aspects of social functioning and adjustment. Of these 48 items, 42 address specific issues related to the following social roles: work, social and leisure activities, relationships with extended family, intimate relationships, and parenthood. The remaining 6 items involve more global judgments of social adjustment. Items are scored according to defined anchor points; the 42 specific items are rated on a 5-point scale of descending social adjustment, whereas the 6 global items are rated on similarly designed 7-point scales. The order of items, as well as required initial questions, is fixed; however, interviewers are instructed to ask whatever supplementary questions seem necessary. The time period assessed by this measure is the 2 months prior to the interview. Two sample items are reprinted below, with the permission of the author, Myrna Weissman. The first item is from the category of "social and leisure," whereas the second item is from the category "parent."

FRICTION:

"How have you been getting along with friends in the past month? Have they gotten on your nerves or made you angry? Did you tell them or hold the feelings in?

Rate: Overt behavior due to friction, withdrawal. Do not rate inner feeling. Include friends/social acquaintances.

    1 = smooth relationships, no visible annoyance
    2 = not provocative but overt difficulty with sensitive situations
    3 = rather uneasy, tense relationships or one major incident
    4 = moderate friction or friction with many
    5 = many furious clashes or avoided by others

LACK OF INVOLVEMENT:

"What kinds of things have you been doing with your children in the past month? Let's start with —(name)—"

Rate: Rate each child separately and average ratings. Rate activities both at home and school (age dependent). Do not rate feelings, rate behavior.

    1 = active involvement with kids' lives
    2 = good interest, knows kids' lives well
    3 = moderate interest
    4 = little interest
    5 = disinterest, totally uninvolved

Background

Social functioning is frequently disrupted in depressed patients, and in fact such disruption plays a role in a number of theories of depression (see Chapter 3). The SAS was developed to assess in detail the different dimensions of social functioning and adjustment, as well as the interrelationships of these dimensions. This was in response to the observation that most other measures of social functioning focused on global judgments of adjustment, or simply summed scales assessing different components to obtain a unitary measure of social functioning. Othogonal factor-analytically derived dimensions that cut across the roles outlined above (e.g., work, social/leisure) were also delineated, with items loading above .45 included in each factor. These included Work Performance, Interpersonal Friction, Inhibited Communication, Submissive Dependency, Family Attachment, and Anxious Rumination.

The SAS was derived by modification of the Structured and Scaled Interview to Assess Maladjustment (SSIAM; Gurland, Yorkston, Stone, Frank, & Fleiss, 1972), a structured interview which assesses various aspects of social maladjustment as related to work, social, family, marriage, and sex roles.

Administration

The interview takes between 45 minutes and 1.5 hours to administer. Training may be required to ensure reliability with previous data, but advanced professional training is not required.

Scoring

Scores within each dimension are summed, then divided by the number of items included within that dimension, so that each dimension score falls within a range of 1–5. Higher scores reflect poorer social adjustment.

Interpretation

Interpretation guidelines are incorporated within the descriptions of the global role ratings. A rating of 1 indicates excellent status and represents the ideal norm for social adjustment. A score of 2 is representative of mild impairment, and more closely approximates an average rating for the general population. Scores of 3, 4, or 5 reflect increasingly impaired social functioning/adjustment.

Psychometric Properties

Psychometric properties are based on a sample of 40 depressed adult females participating in a trial of maintenance antidepressant medication and individual psychotherapy and 40 adult females from the general population (selected via city directory for living on a parallel street to one of the depressed patients). Groups as a whole were matched on social class, marital status, and race/ethnicity.

Norms.   Psychometric studies indicated that the role categories yielded variable scores, possibly due to the heterogeneity of the items contained within each role category. The factor dimensions explained 57% of the total variance, and were suggested for use as a more sensitive measure of discriminating social functioning. Mean factor scores and standard deviations were thus calculated for the depressed and control groups and are contained in Paykel et al. (1971).

Reliability.   Interrater reliability was established using the trained interviewers and a separate sample of depressed patients from the standardization study. The two interviewers agreed with each other to within 1 point in 86% of ratings, with a mean Pearson correlation between them of .80. With respect to internal consistency, item-to-group correlations within both the social-role groupings and qualitative categories of behavioral, feeling, and global qualities were only moderate. It was for this reason that the factor analysis was conducted.

Validity.   The factor dimensions of the SAS successfully discriminated between the depressed and control groups, with the depressed group more impaired than the control group. When SAS scores were compared with symptom ratings of depression using the Hamilton Rating Scale for Depression (p. 196), the two were not correlated (Paykel, Weissman, & Prusoff, 1978) when administered in the midst of a depressive episode, although a moderate relationship between these was found upon remission from the episode.

Clinical Utility

High. The SAS provides a semistructured method for assessing a variety of aspects of social functioning, which may be implicated in both depression and its treatment.

Research Applicability

High. As quality of life and cost-effectiveness are increasingly emphasized as issues in treatment outcome, there will be an even greater need for measures assessing the range of aspects of social functioning included within the SAS.

Source

Myrna M. Weisman, Ph.D., College of Physicians and Surgeons of Columbia University, Box 14, 722 West 168th Street, New York, NY 10032.

Cost

None.

Alternate Forms

The SAS is also available in a 54-item self-report version.

SOCIAL PROBLEM-SOLVING INVENTORY-REVISED (SPSI-R)

Original Citation

D'Zurilla, T. J., Nezu, A. M., & Maydeu-Olivares, A. (in press). *Social Problem-Solving Inventory-Revised (SPSI-R): Test manual*. North Tonawanda, NY: Multi-Health Systems.

Purpose

To measure various social problem-solving skills and abilities.

Population

Adults.

Description

The SPSI-R is a 52-item self-report measure that requests respondents to rate the degree to which each item best characterizes their feelings, actions, and behavior regarding the way in which they respond to problems in everyday living. The 5-point scale ranges from 0 ("not at all true of me") to 4 ("extremely true of me"). Based on a series of factor analyses, the following five scales were derived: Positive Problem Orientation (e.g., "Whenever I have a problem, I believe it can be solved"); Negative Problem Orientation (e.g., "Difficult problems make me very upset"); Rational Problem-Solving Skills (e.g., "When solving problems, I approach them from as many different angles as possible," "When I have a decision to make, I weigh the consequences of each option and compare them to each other"); Impulsivity/Carelessness Style (e.g., "When solving problems, I act on the first idea that occurs to me"); and Avoidance Style (e.g., "When faced with problems, I go to someone else for help in solving them").

Background

Social problem solving is the process by which people attempt to resolve problems they experience in everyday living. Studies have consistently identified a significant relationship between problem-solving skills and distress, particularly depression (A. M. Nezu, 1987). Further, problem solving has been found to be a significant mediator of the deleterious effects of stressful life events with specific regard to depression (e.g., A. M. Nezu & Ronan, 1985). As such, a problem-solving model of depression has identified problem-solving deficits as a key vulnerability factor for depression under conditions of significant stress (A. M. Nezu et al., 1989).

The SPSI-R is a revision of the original 70-item SPSI (D'Zurilla & Nezu, 1990), which was based on the model of problem solving initially developed by D'Zurilla & Goldfried (1971). This model highlights two general, but partially independent, processes: (a) problem orientation (a motivational process involving the operation of a set of relatively stable cognitive-emotional schemas, both constructive and dysfunctional, that reflect the generalized thoughts and feelings of a person regarding problems in living as well as his or her own ability to resolve them); and (b) problem-solving proper (those rational problem-solving skills used to help a person discover effective coping responses in reaction to stressful problems). Such skills include defining problems, generating potential ideas for solutions, making decisions, carrying out the solution, and verifying the solution outcome.

Administration

The SPSI-R requires about 15–20 minutes to complete.

Scoring

Scores can be generated for each of the five scales as well as for the total score. Higher total scores indicate more effective problem-solving ability.

Interpretation

Normative data exist for comparison purposes.

Psychometric Properties

Norms.   Means and standard deviations for several "normal" individuals (e.g., high school students, college students, middle-ages adults, elderly adults, caregivers of Alzheimer patients, and nursing students) and "distressed" or psychiatric patients (psychiatric adult patients, psychiatric adolescent patients, distressed adult cancer patients, and depressed outpatients) are contained in the manual for comparison purposes.

Reliability.   Internal consistency estimates across four different samples for the five scales range between .69 and .95, with a mean of .86. The test–retest correlations for a group of college students regarding a 3-week period for the five scales ranged from .72 to .88. With regard to a sample of nursing students, the stability correlations ranged from .68 to .91.

Validity. The SPSI-R is characterized by strong structural, concurrent, predictive, convergent, and discriminant validity. For example, the SPSI-R has been found to be significantly correlated with a variety of measures of distress (e.g., SCL-90, p. 117; State-Trait Anxiety Inventory [Spielberger, 1983]; BDI, p. 29; BHS, p. 175; SPS, p. 258; RADS, p. 152). It is also strongly correlated with a measure of problem-solving appraisal (PSI; p. 230).

Clinical Utility

High. The SPSI-R can provide for a profile of an individual's strengths and weaknesses in problem solving.

Research Applicability

High. The SPSI-R has been used in multiple research investigations and has been found to be sensitive to the effects of training in problem-solving skills (A. M. Nezu et al., 1998).

Source

Multi-Health Systems, 908 Niagara Falls Blvd., North Tonawanda, NY 14120-2060. Phone: 800-456-3003.

Cost

Contact publisher, cost not yet determined.

Alternative Forms

Spanish version available. Sadowski, Moore, and Kelly (1994) also adapted the original SPSI for an adolescent population.

SOCIAL RESOURCEFULNESS SCALE (SRS)

Original Citations

Rapp, S. R., Shumaker, S. A., Schmidt, S., McFarlane, M., & Naughton, M. *The Social Resourcefulness Scale: Development and preliminary validation.* Unpublished manuscript.
Rapp, S. R., Shumaker, S. A., Schmidt, S., Naughton, M., & Anderson, R. (1998). Social resourcefulness: Its relationship to social support and well-being among caregivers of dementia victims. *Aging and Mental Health, 2,* 40–48.

Purpose

To measure the frequency of help-seeking behaviors.

Population

Adults aged 18 years or older. This instrument is targeted for populations in need of help from others.

Description

The SRS is a 20-item self-report questionnaire. It begins with the question, "When you need help, how often do you ...," and is followed by 20 items that complete the sentence (e.g., "tell someone how their help makes you feel?"). Each sentence completion represents a help-seeking behavior. Respondents rate each item on a 5-point scale according to how frequently they engage in each behavior. Responses range from "Always do it" to "Never do it."

Background

Research has supported the relationship between social support and emotional distress, as well as the relationship between help-seeking behaviors or social resourcefulness and actual receipt of support or help from others. The SRS was developed to assess quantitatively the degree to which individuals actively pursue social support through their thoughts and actions.

Administration

The SRS takes approximately 5 minutes to complete.

Scoring

The total score is obtained by adding the scores of the individual items. Scores range from 20 to 100.

Interpretation

High scores indicate less frequent help-seeking behavior, whereas low scores indicate greater social resourcefulness.

Psychometric Properties

Norms. Since the SRS can be used for any number of populations, it is important to consider the norms relevant for each population. Means and standard deviations are reported for a group of 65 caregivers of people with dementia in Rapp et al. (1998).

Reliability.   The test–retest reliability of the SRS was .79 for the same group of 65 caregivers noted above. The internal consistency as measured by Cronbach's alpha was .85.

Validity.   With regard to construct validity, the SRS was compared to other measures of social support and well-being in the same 65 caregivers. Significant correlations were found with social support ($r = .43$), social network size ($r = .31$), quality of life ($r = .37$), and health status ($r = .26$), whereas the SRS was not correlated with social desirability or negative affect. In a pilot test of the SRS in a sample of 137 undergraduates, the SRS was significantly negatively correlated with depression.

Clinical Utility

Limited. The SRS is a promising new instrument. It is expected that future studies will support its usefulness in assessment of help-seeking behaviors as either outcome variables or mediator/moderator variables among various populations.

Research Applicability

Limited. The initial evaluations of the SRS support its research applicability. Continued investigations are needed especially to evaluate its sensitivity to change.

Source

The SRS is reprinted in Appendix B. For additional information, contact Stephen R. Rapp, Ph.D., Department of Psychiatry and Behavioral Medicine, Wake Forest University School of Medicine, Medical Center Boulevard, Winston-Salem, NC 27157-1087.

Cost

None.

Alternative Forms

None.

SOCIOTROPY AUTONOMY SCALE (SAS)

Original Citation

Bieling, P. J., Beck, A T., & Brown, G. K. (in press). The Sociotropy Autonomy Scale: Structure and implications. *Cognitive Therapy and Research*.

Purpose

To measure two aspects of personality, sociotropy and autonomy, which are hypothesized to be related to a vulnerability toward depression.

Population

Adults in psychiatric settings. Although the authors hope that the SAS will be applicable to other samples, its reliability and validity have not been replicated adequately in non-psychiatric samples thus far.

Description

Two 30-item scales, the Sociotropy scale and the Autonomy scale, comprise this 60-item self-report questionnaire. Each item presents a statement (e.g., "It is more important that I know I've done a good job than having others know it") for which respondents are requested to indicate how often each statement describes them. Responses are indicated on a 5-point percentage scale ranging from 0% to 100%.

According to the most recent faactor analysis of the SAS (Bieling et al., in press), each scale of this instrument contains two factors. The Sociotropy scale contains the factors Preference for Affiliation, and Excessive Fear of Others' Appraisal. The Autonomy scale contains the factors Independent Goal Attainment and Desire for Control.

Background

A. T. Beck (1983, 1987) hypothesized that two personality factors, sociotropy and autonomy, increase people's vulnerability toward depression in the event of certain types of negative life experiences. Sociotropy refers to a desire for strong interpersonal relationships, whereas autonomy refers to a preference for independence. Beck's cognitive model hypothesizes that these characteristics increase vulnerability toward depression when life events threaten the feasibility of achieving or maintaining one's preferences. The SAS was designed to measure sociotropy and autonomy in order to promote research on these constructs, as well as investigations on the cognitive model of depression.

The 60 items of the SAS, derived from patients' self-reports and clinicians' materials, were narrowed from an original pool of 109 items through factor-analytic procedures. Inconsistent results led to numerous further investigations of the instrument's factor structure and psychometric properties.

Administration

The SAS takes approximately 15 minutes to complete.

Scoring

Scores are obtained by summing the item scores for each subscale, where 0% = 0, 25% = 1, 50% = 2, 75% = 3, and 100% = 4. Scores for each factor can be computed in a similar manner.

Interpretation

Higher scores on the Sociotropy scale indicate a greater tendency to value positive social interaction. Higher scores on the Autonomy scale indicate a greater tendency to value independence and activities related to personal independence.

Psychometric Properties

The psychometric properties of the revised SAS were tested in a sample of 2,067 adult psychiatric outpatients (Bieling et al., in press).

Norms.   Means and standard deviations of the Sociotropy and Autonomy subscales are available for some diagnostic groups (e.g., dysthymic disorder) and can be obtained from the authors.

Reliability.   With regard to internal consistency, coefficient alphas were .90 for the Sociotropy scale and .83 for the Autonomy scale (A. T. Beck, Epstein, Harrison, & Emery, 1983). Alpha reliabilities for the factors within the two subscales were also adequate.

Validity.   Several factor analyses have been conducted to validate the factor structure of the SAS. Most recently, a series of exploratory and confirmatory factor analyses supported a two-factor structure for both the Sociotropy and Autonomy subscales of the SAS (Bieling et al., in press).
Both factors of the Sociotropy scale were positively correlated with various measures of psychopathology, demonstrating this scale's validity as an instrument to measure a depression-related construct. The factors of the Autonomy scale were also correlated, but in different directions. The desire for control/fear of loss of control was positively related to psychopathology, whereas the independent goal attainment subscale was negatively related to psychopathology (Bieling et al., in press).

Clinical Utility

High. The SAS provides a method of understanding personality characteristics and individual preferences that may increase certain individuals' risk for depression under certain circumstances. The information obtained by the SAS can help clinicians understand individual depressive experiences within the frame of a diathesis-stress model.

Research Applicability

High. The most recent factor analysis of the SAS provides further support for the research applicability of this instrument, and further clarification for the construct validity of the subscales. However, additional analyses in clinical and nonclinical samples are needed.

Source

The 60-item version of the SAS is reprinted in the Appendix.

Cost

None.

Alternative Forms

A revised SAS (Clark, Steer, Beck, & Ross, 1995) is available. This is a 59-item version that divides the SAS along three subscales (Sociotropy, Solitude, and Independence).

SUICIDAL IDEATION QUESTIONNAIRE (SIQ)

Original Citation

Reynolds, W. M. (1987). *Suicide Ideation Questionnaire: Professional manual.* Odessa, FL: Psychological Assessment Resources.

Purpose

To assess suicidal ideation in clinic and school settings.

Population

Adolescents and young adults (grades 7–12).

Description

There are two forms of the Suicide Ideation Questionnaire for adolescents: the Suicide Ideation Questionnaire-JR (junior high school version, grades 7–9) and the Suicide Ideation Questionnaire (high school version, grades 10–12). The junior high school version contains 15 items, whereas the high school version contains 30 items. Both versions require individuals to rate self-referent statements using a 7-point frequency scale that ranges from 6 ("almost every day") to 0 ("I have never had this thought"). Items reflect a range of thoughts varying from morbid ideation and wishes that one had never been born to detailed thoughts of killing oneself. Respondents are requested to use the past month as the frame of reference when estimating frequency. Sample items are reprinted below with the permission of the publisher (© 1987, the Psychological Assessment Resources).

> I thought it would be better if I were not alive.
> I thought about telling people that I plan to kill myself.
> I thought that killing myself would solve my problems.
> I thought about having a bad accident.
> I wondered if I had the nerve to kill myself.

Background

These versions of the SIQ were developed by Reynolds (1987) to provide an initial screening measure of the current seriousness of suicidal thoughts in adolescents.

Administration

The SIQ requires approximately 5–10 minutes to complete and can be administered in an individual or a group setting.

Scoring

A total score results from summing over the item scores. Items are scored in a pathology direction; high scores indicate more suicidal thoughts.

Interpretation

According to Reynolds (1987), adolescents scoring at or above 41 on the SIQ, or at or above 31 on the SIQ-JR, should be referred for a suicide risk evaluation.

Psychometric Properties

Norms. Initial information was based on a sample of 2,180 adolescents from one high school (grades 10–12; $N = 890$) and two junior high schools (grades 7–9; $N = 1,290$) located in an urban/suburban community in the midwestern United States. The normative sample was equally distributed across gender. Additional samples totaling 4,000 adolescents and young adults from regular education, special education, and clinical settings were collected. The manual provides detailed descriptive information, as well as tables for converting raw scores to percentile ranks.

Reliability.   Coefficient alpha estimates for the total sample are around .94 for the SIQ-JR and .97 for the SIQ. Four week test–retest reliability for the SIQ was estimated using high school students from the midwest ($N = 801$). The resulting stability coefficient was .72.

Validity.   Content validity was examined using item-total scale correlations. Item-total correlation coefficients ranged from .70 to .90 for the SIQ, and from .46 to .86 for the SIQ-JR. Items appear to sample adequately the dimension of suicidal ideation in adolescents. Item content with specified suicidal cognition on both versions was examined and reflected descriptive components of suicidal ideation. Construct validity was examined in the form of correlations between the SIQ and related constructs. Overall, the correlation coefficients provide support for the validity of the SIQ and the SIQ-JR. Specifically, the SIQ was found to correlate .58 with the RADS (p. 152), .70 with the BDI (p. 29), and .47 with the BHS (p. 175). The SIQ-JR was found to correlate .55 with the RADS, .65 with the BDI, and .65 with the CDI (p. 127).

Factor analyses of both the SIQ and the SIQ-JR were conducted using the normative sample. For both questionnaires, the majority of items loaded on the first unrotated factor, and a three-factor solution was selected. The first factor represented components of suicidal ideation specific to wishes and plans of suicide. The second factor contained items related to the response and aspects of others. Finally, the third factor consisted of items related to morbid ideation.

Clinical Utility

High. These versions of the SIQ are brief and easily administered. They provide a useful self-report measure to screen for the frequency and severity of symptoms related to adolescent suicide.

Research Utility

High. These versions of the SIQ are easily administered and the manual provides clear guidelines for group administration. In addition, they have been found to be useful in previous research studies.

Source

Psychological Assessment Resources, Inc., P.O. Box 998, Odessa, FL 33556. Phone: 800-331-TEST.

Cost

$99 for SIQ Introductory Kit (includes manual, 25 each of the SIQ and SIQ-JR hand-scorable answer sheets, and scoring keys for each).

Alternative Forms

Junior high school, high school, and adult versions are available.

SUICIDE PROBABILITY SCALE (SPS)

Original Citation

Cull, J. G., & Gill, W. S. (1988). *Suicide Probability Scale (SPS) manual.* Los Angeles: Western Psychological Services.

Purpose

To assess suicide risk.

Population

Adolescents and adults 14 years and older.

Description

The SPS is a 36-item self-report measure that requests respondents to rate the frequency of their subjective experience (e.g., "I worry about money") and past behaviors (e.g., "When I get mad, I throw things") along a 4-point scale ranging from "none or little of the time" to "most or all of the time." Assessment of suicide risk is reflected in three summary scores: a total weighted score; a normalized *T*-score, and a Suicide Probability Score that can be adjusted to the base rates of differing clinical populations (e.g., normal individuals, psychiatric inpatients, suicide attempters). In addition, the SPS provides for four clinical subscales based on theoretical and factor-analytic choices: Hopelessness; Suicide Ideation; Negative Self-Evaluation; and Hostility. Additional items, reprinted with the permission of the publisher (© 1982 by Western Psychological Services), include the following: "Others feel hostile toward me," "I plan for the future very carefully," "I feel I can't be happy no matter where I am."

Background

The SPS was developed based a review of various theories and research proposed to explain or predict suicide.

Administration

The SPS requires about 5–10 minutes to complete.

Scoring

Scoring can be completed by hand or through a computer administration procedure. Raw weighted scores can be converted into *T*-scores and a probability score. The higher the score, the higher the level of assessed risk for suicide. Scores also exist for each of the four subscales.

Interpretation

The authors point out that the SPS should be part of an overall assessment approach to the prediction of suicide. Clinical interpretation of the SPS can be based on individual items, subscale scores, and the summary scores. For each total weighted score, there are different categories of probability scores against which to better understand how an individual's score relates to his/her "normative group." More specifically, the test interpreter is able to choose among three categories providing a context within which to understand a group's level of presumptive risk. The "high-risk" group category would be used to classify individuals in settings such as psychiatric inpatient facilities or suicide prevention centers. The "intermediate-risk" category involves a general outpatient clinic population or psychiatric inpatients who do not present any clinical signs of suicide ideation or depression. The "low-risk" group is intended for use with the general population.

Psychometric Properties

Norms.   Norms for each of the clinical subscales and the total score exist for three groups (normal individuals, suicide attempters, psychiatric inpatients).

Reliability.   The internal consistency for the total scale has been estimated to be alpha = .93. In one sample ($N = 80$), test–retest reliability for a period of 3 weeks was found to be .92. In a second study ($N = 478$), the stability correlation over 10 days was .94.

Validity.   A series of studies indicated that the SPS total score, as well as the four clinical subscales, were able to significantly discriminate among groups of normal individuals, psychiatric inpatients, and suicide attempters. Further studies found the SPS to have high levels of classification accuracy (i.e., SPS scores accurately predicted which group a given individual belonged to among these three groups). In one study, the classification accuracies were as follows: 75.4% for psychiatric patients; 94.3% for normal individuals; and 83.9% for suicide attempters.

Clinical Utility

High. The existence of three groups of norms provides for increased accuracy and clinical sophistication.

Research Applicability

High. The SPS has been used in several investigations of suicide risk prediction.

Source

Western Psychological Services, 12031 Wilshire Boulevard, Los Angeles, CA 90025-1251. Phone: 800-648-8857.

Cost

$80 for a manual, 25 test forms, and 25 profile forms.

Alternative Forms

Not available.

UNPLEASANT EVENTS SCHEDULE (UES)

Original Citation

Lewinsohn, P. M., Mermelstein, R., Alexander, C., & MacPhillamy, D. (1983). The Unpleasant Events Schedule: A scale for the measurement of aversive events. *Journal of Clinical Psychology*, *41*, 483–498.

Purpose

To measure the rate of occurrence and experienced aversiveness of stressful events.

Population

Adolescents and adults 12 years and older.

Description

The UES is a 320-item self-report inventory addressing the frequency and subjective aversiveness of various events and activities. In many ways, the UES can be viewed as a measure of stressful life events. Respondents are requested to rate each item twice, once using a 3-point scale of frequency of occurrence over the past 30 days, and a second time using a 3-point scale of subjective unpleasantness.

Various scales are possible to compute based on the UES. These scales were developed rationally, empirically, or via a factor analysis. Nine such scales are recommended for research and clinical purposes due to their psychometric soundness and independence. These scales are labeled: All Items; Major versus Minor Stressors (e.g., "death of my spouse"), Self versus Other (e.g., "having a relative or friend living in unsatisfactory surroundings"), Controllable versus Uncontrollable (e.g., "being hungry or thirsty"), Life Changes (e.g., "retiring or being retired from work"), Death Related (e.g., "attending funerals"), Legal (e.g., "being arrested or detained by legal authorities"), Sexual-Marital-Friendship (e.g., "asking someone for a date"), and Most Discriminating (i.e., items most discriminating between depressed and nondepressed individuals; e.g., "working at something I don't enjoy").

Background

A major behavioral theory of depression as espoused by Lewinsohn and his colleagues (e.g., Lewinsohn, 1974; Lewinsohn et al., 1979) focused on the role of response-contingent positive reinforcement in the etiopathogenesis of depression. More specifically, a low rate of response-contingent reinforcement in major life areas and/or a high rate of aversive experiences can lead to a reduction of effective behavior and to the experience of dysphoria. This low rate of positive reinforcement can be caused by one of three factors: (a) behavioral skill deficits leading to an inability to obtain such reinforcement, (b) changes in one's environment (e.g., death of a family member), and (c) an increase in an individual's sensitivity to negative events. The UES has been used in various research studies to support these hypotheses. For example, Lewinsohn found strong support for the hypothesized association between aversive events and depressed mood (e.g., Lewinsohn & Talkington, 1979).

Administration

The UES takes about 1 hour to complete.

Scoring

The UES was originally designed to be mechanically read (i.e., optical scanner), converted, scored, and fed directly into a computer. Hand scoring can follow the directions in the manual regarding each scale.

Interpretation

Norms exist for comparison by age.

Psychometric Properties

Norms.   The normative group consists of over 1,186 individuals, mostly adults (e.g., approximately 0.1% are < 16 years old).

Reliability.   Certain scales (e.g., Sexual-Marital scale) were found to be characterized by acceptable levels of test–retest reliability (e.g., .60–.80), whereas stability estimates for other scales, due to the infrequency of such events (e.g., Legal scale) were low as expected. Internal consistency, as measured by coefficient alpha, across scales ranged between .76 and .93, where the overall scale was .98.

Validity. The UES was found to correlate .37 with the CES-D (p. 39). It was also found to provide a significant increase in the discrimination of depressed and nondepressed individuals beyond that provided by measures based on the experience of pleasant activities.

Clinical Utility

High. It can be used to identify specific actual or potential areas of distress and discomfort, as well as a measure of stressful life events.

Research Applicability

High. The UES has been used in a variety of studies supporting a behavioral model of depression.

Source

The UES is reprinted in Appendix B. For additional information, contact Peter M. Lewinsohn, Ph.D., Oregon Research Institute, 1715 Franklin Blvd., Eugene, OR 97403-1983.

Cost

None.

Alternative Forms

A 53-item short form version of the UES is available, as well as a version for use with the elderly (Teri & Lewinsohn, 1982).

WAYS OF COPING SCALE (WOC)

Original Citation

Folkman, S., & Lazarus, R. S. (1988). *Manual for the Ways of Coping Questionnaire*. Palo Alto, CA: Mind Garden, Inc.

Purpose

To assess coping processes used in dealing with stressful situations.

Population

Adults.

Description

The Ways of Coping Questionnaire is a 66-item self-report measure of coping processes. Each item is rated on a 4-point scale, based on how often that type of coping strategy is used, with 0 indicating "it is not used or doesn't apply" and 3 indicating "it is used a great deal." The items form eight factors: Confrontive Coping, Distancing, Self-Controlling, Seeking Social Support, Accepting Responsibility, Escape-Avoidance, Planful Problem-Solving, and Positive Reappraisal. Sample items are reprinted below with the permission of the publisher (© 1988 by Mind Garden, Inc.):

> I turned to work or another activity to take my mind off things.
> I stood my ground and fought for what I wanted.
> I took it out on other people.
> I wished that I could change what had happened or how I felt.
> I reminded myself how much worse things could be.

Background

Substantial research in the area of stress points to the significant relationship between stressors and depressive reactions, i.e., the experience of a stressful negative life event, chronic stressors, or a traumatic event can lead to depression (A. M. Nezu & Ronan, 1985). In addition, researchers and clinicians have also identified various mediators of this stressor–depression relationship, a primary one being coping resources and skills (Cronkite & Moos, 1995). Coping, then, may be an area of interest for clinicians and researchers alike when working with depressed individuals.

Early versions of the WOC used a checklist of items to which respondents noted yes or no to indicate whether they used that particular strategy to cope with one specific stressful event, which was described prior to completion of the checklist. These items consisted of both problem-focused and emotion-focused coping strategies (Folkman & Lazarus, 1980). Due to several problems with this limited classification system, the WOC was revised to incorporate a broader range of coping processes; several datasets were factor-analyzed to yield the items currently included in the WOC.

Administration

When self-administered, the WOC takes approximately 10 minutes to complete. The WOC has also been used as a self-report measure following an interview in which a specific stressful event is described; this method would obviously take additional time. A study comparing WOC responses with and without interviews showed no differences in problem-focused coping reported, but greater amounts of emotion-focused coping were reported in the interview condition (Folkman, 1979).

Scoring

Two scoring systems are available for the WOC. In the most commonly used method, the scores of each item comprising a scale are summed to provide the score for that scale. A second system uses relative scoring, in which average scale scores (i.e., the sum of a scale divided by the number of items in that scale) are calculated for each scale, and the relative scale score is calculated by dividing the average item score for a specific scale by the sum of the average item scores for the eight total scales, thus controlling for unequal numbers of items per scale.

Interpretation

No interpretation guidelines are provided; however, norms for both the eight scales as well as the 66 individual items are provided in the manual.

Psychometric Properties

Psychometric properties for the WOC were established in a sample of 75 married couples, in which the wife and husband were interviewed separately. Each couple was White, with at least one child in the home, and was middle-class or upper-middle-class. All subjects completed an interview and the WOC on five separate monthly occasions, yielding a total of 750 WOC observations.

Norms.   Means for the WOC scales were as follows: Confrontive Coping, six items, 3.94 ($SD = 2.09$); Distancing, six items, 3.05 ($SD = 1.78$); Self-Controlling, seven items, 5.77 ($SD = 2.87$); Seeking Social Support, six items, 5.40 ($SD = 2.40$); Accepting Responsibility, four items, 1.87 ($SD = 1.44$); Escape-Avoidance, eight items, 3.18 ($SD = 2.48$); Planful Problem-Solving, six items, 7.25 ($SD = 2.34$); and Positive Reappraisal, seven items, 3.48 ($SD = 2.96$).

Reliability.   The authors noted that test–retest reliability estimates were not calculated due to the variable nature of coping processes. Internal consistencies were moderate, with Cronbach's alpha ranging from .61 (Distancing) to .79 (Positive Reappraisal).

Validity.   The WOC was not validated against other standardized measures. However, the authors note that their studies using the WOC support its construct validity in that their findings matched their theoretical predictions (i.e., which types of coping processes would be used at which points in stressful situations).

Clinical Utility

High. The WOC is relatively easy to administer and can be examined rapidly as an assessment of coping processes employed by clients.

Research Applicability

High. There is a great need for additional psychometric data on the WOC, especially in more heterogeneous samples. Despite this, the WOC has, in its various forms over the years, been one of the most widely used measures of coping in research studies. Thus, there is a large database that can serve as a comparison for new research.

Source

Mind Garden, Inc., 1690 Woodside Rd., Suite 202, Redwood City, CA 94061. Phone: 650-261-3500. Website: www.mindgarden.com.

Cost

A Sampler Set, including the manual, questionnaire/answer sheet, and scoring directions, is available for $25.

Alternate Forms

The WOC is available in several other languages, including Dutch, Hebrew, Spanish, French, and German.

WAYS OF RESPONDING (WOR)

Original Citation

Barber, J. P., & DeRubeis, R. J. (1992). The Ways of Responding: A scale to assess compensatory skills taught in cognitive therapy. *Behavioral Assessment*, *14*, 93–115.

Purpose

To measure compensatory skills in persons with depression.

Population

Adults.

Description

The WOR is an eight-item, self-reported, open-ended, thought-listing questionnaire. Each item presents a vignette describing a particular situation (e.g., difficulty applying for a job) followed by a depressotypic thought (e.g., "Will I ever get a job? There just doesn't seem to be any point in applying.") Respondents are instructed to rate (0–100) how vividly they are able to imagine themselves in the situation, describe the mood they experience while imagining the situation, rate (0–100) the intensity of the mood, rate (0–100) how well they can imagine having the depressotypic thought, describe any further thoughts, describe the action they would take next, and rerate (0–100) the intensity of the mood after they have written down their thoughts and actions.

Background

The WOR was designed to measure the compensatory skills model of change in cognitive therapy. Compensatory skills have been defined as "a set of skills that [people] can use to curtail negative thinking both during the acute episode and while in remission following the episode. These skills include metacognitive (Hollon & Kriss, 1984) and planning or problem-solving skills" (Barber and DeRubeis, 1989). This model purports that cognitive therapy actually provides skills for coping with negative thoughts that individuals produce *in reaction to* stressful situations, which is different than other models of change, which hypothesize that cognitive therapy reduces the tendency for individuals to produce negative thoughts. The specific compensatory skills that have been identified are metacognitive skills and problem-solving skills. When designing the WOR, the authors sought to provide a measure that would present a challenge or stressor to participants, assess compensatory skills in reaction to a particular stressor as close to the time it occurs as possible, guide participants to respond with how they would react, rather than how they *should* react, assess the quality of coping as well as the coping style, and provide some control over the type of stressor to which participants respond (Hollon and Kriss, 1984).

Administration

The WOR takes approximately 20–30 minutes to complete.

Scoring

Scoring the WOR is somewhat detailed and may take as long as its administration. A detailed description for scoring the WOR is provided in Barber and DeRubeis (1992). Scoring consists in categorizing each thought response, finding the total number of positive, negative, and neutral responses, and producing a total (WOR-Total) score representing the difference between the number of positive and negative responses. In addition, raters evaluate the Overall Quality of Responding (WOR-Qal) on a 7-point scale. Rater training is required, and weekly meetings to discuss scoring problems were conducted for the development of the WOR in order to prevent scoring drift.

Interpretation

Higher WOR-Total scores reflect higher levels of compensatory skills. The WOR-Qal score represents the rater's judgment of how well the participant's response will improve mood and meet personal needs.

Psychometric Properties

The psychometric properties of the WOR were tested in two samples. Sample 1 consisted of 43 college undergraduates. Sample 2 consisted of 50 patients diagnosed with unipolar major depression without psychotic features.

Norms. Means and standard deviations for Sample 2 are provided in Barber and DeRubeis (1992).

Reliability. In Sample 1, interrater reliability coefficients for the WOR-Qal score were .79 and .89 for two alternate forms of the WOR. Reliability coefficients for the subscales ranged from .94 to .97. In Sample 2, intraclass correlations ranged from .91 to .97.

Alternate form reliability coefficients in Sample 1 ranged from .60 to .76, and stability coefficients ranged from .45 to .72 with a 12-week lapse between administration.

The internal consistency was measured in both samples. Alpha coefficients in Sample 1 ranged from .58 to .81. Alpha coefficients for alternate forms administered in Sample 2 ranged from .74 to .86.

Validity. With regard to concurrent validity, the WOR-Qual and WOR-Total were compared to the BDI (pp. 29), the Ways of Coping Scale (p. 262), the Self Control Schedule (SCS; p. 240), and a measure of well-being, in Sample 1. Significant Pearson correlation coefficients were found between the WOR-Qual and the well-being measure ($r = .42$) as well as between the WOR-Total and that measure ($r = .36$). After Bonferroni corrections, the SCS correlated significantly with the WOR-Qual ($r = .46$) and the WOR-Total ($r = .32$).

In Sample 2, the WOR-Qual and WOR-Total were compared to the BDI (p. 29), the Cognition Checklist-Depression (CCL-D; Beck, Brown, Steer, Eidelson, & Riskind, 1987), the ASQ (p. 169), and the SCS (p. 262). Using Pearson correlation coefficients, the WOR-Qual correlated significantly with the CCL-D ($r = -.51$) and the ASQ ($r = .58$), whereas the WOR-Total correlated significantly with the BDI ($r = -.32$), the CCL-D ($r = -.52$), the ASQ ($r = .50$) and the SCS ($r = .42$).

The construct validity of the WOR was supported by the significant, but moderate correlation between both WOR scores and the ASQ, and the moderate correlation between the WOR and CCL-D, as well as between the ASQ and the CCL-D in Sample 2.

Further assessment of the validity of the WOR was measured by evaluating the relationship between compensatory skills used in response to negative thoughts and immediate mood change. A mood change index was derived from the responses, and correlated significantly with the WOR-Total (partial $r = .47$) and the WOR-Qual (partial $r = .36$) in Sample 1, as well as in Sample 2 (partial $r = -.30$, partial $r = -.38$, respectively).

Clinical Utility

Limited. The WOR's ability to measure mediators of change in cognitive therapy is promising. Although its utility in clinical settings has not yet been demonstrated, promising new results can be expected from clinical trials currently being conducted in Seattle, Nashville, and Philadelphia.

Research Applicability

Limited. Although its research applicability has been examined more extensively than its clinical utility, more research is needed. The WOR will be useful for studying mediators of change and outcome in cognitive therapy as well as relapse prevention.

Source

Jacques Barber, Ph.D., Department of Psychiatry, University of Pennsylvania Health System, 3600 Market Street, 7th Floor, Philadelphia, PA 19104-2648.

Cost

None.

Alternative Forms

Two alternate forms of the WOR, as well as male and female versions of the instrument, are available from the author.

Appendix A
Quick-View Guides

Table I. Assessment of Depression and Depressive Symptoms Among Adults (Chapter 4)

Name of instrument	Target population	Type of measure	Measurement focus	Time to complete (minutes)	Norms available?	Fee involved?	Alternate forms
Beck Depression Inventory-II	Adults and adolescents 13+	Self-report	Depressive symptoms	5–10	Yes	Yes	Spanish
Brief Psychiatric Rating Scale	Adults	Clinician rating	Psychiatric symptoms	10–40	No	Yes	Various European languages
Brief Symptom Inventory	Adults and adolescents	Self-report	Psychiatric symptoms	10	Yes	Yes	14 other languages
Carroll Depression Scales-Revised	Adults	Self-report	Depressive symptoms	5–10	Yes	Yes	None
Center for Epidemiological Studies Depression Scale	Adults	Self-report	Depressive symptoms	10	Yes	No	Spanish and other languages
Depression Anxiety Stress Scales	Adults and adolescents	Self-report	Depression, anxiety, and stress symptoms	10–20	Yes	Yes	Short form
Depression questionnaire	Adults	Self-report	Depressive symptoms	20	Yes	No	Italian
Depression 30 Scale	Adults	Self-report	Depressive symptoms	10	Yes	Yes	Spanish and other languages
Diagnostic Interview Schedule	Adults	Structured interview	Diagnose DSM-IV disorders	90–120	No	Yes	Various languages and child version
Diagnostic Inventory for Depression	Adults	Self-report	Diagnose DSM-IV Major Depressive Disorder	25	No	No	None
Hamilton Depression Inventory	Adults	Self-report	Depressive symptoms	10–15	Yes	Yes	Short form
Hamilton Rating Scale for Depression	Adults	Clinician rating	Depressive symptoms	30	No	No	Differing lengths
Hopelessness Depressive Symptoms Questionnaire	Adults	Self-report	Hopelessness, depression	10	Yes	Yes	None
Hospital Anxiety and Depression Scale	Medical outpatients (16–65)	Self-report	Anxiety and depressive symptoms	10	Yes	No	Spanish and other languages
Inventory of Depressive Symptomatology	Adults	Self-report and clinician rating	Depressive symptoms	30–45	Yes	No	Italian
IPAT Depression Scale	Adults and adolescents 16+	Self-report	Depressive symptoms	10–20	Yes	Yes	None
Manual for the Diagnosis of Major Depression	Adults	Clinician rating	Depression diagnosis	20–30	No	No	None

Instrument	Population	Format	Focus	Time			Other forms/languages
MMPI-D Scale	Adults	Self-report	Psychiatric symptoms	12	Yes	Yes	Spanish and other languages
Montgomery-Asberg Depression Rating Scale	Adults	Clinincian rating	Depressive symptoms	5	Yes	No	None
MOS 8-Item Depression Screener	Adults	Self-report	Screen for MDD and dysthymia	5	No	No	None
Multiple Affect Adjective Checklist-Revised	Adults and adolescents	Self-report	Various emotions	5–10	Yes	Yes	None
Multiscore Depression Inventory for Adolescents and Adults	Adults and adolescents 13+	Self-report	Depressive symptoms	20–25	Yes	Yes	Short form
Newcastle Scales	Adults	Clinician rating	Differentiate endogenous and reactive depression	10–30	No	No	None
Positive and Negative Affect Scales	Adults	Self-report	Positive and negative affect	5	Yes	Yes	None
Primary Care Evaluation of Mental Disorders	Adults	Clinician rating	Differential diagnosis including depression	5–10	No	No	None
Profile of Mood States	Adults	Self-report	Mood states	3–5	Yes	Yes	Short form
Raskin Three-Area Scale	Adults	Clinician rating	Depressive symptoms	30	N/A	No	None
Revised HRSD-Clinical Rating Form	Adults	Clinician rating	Depression diagnosis	5–10	Yes	Yes	None
Revised HRSD-Self-Report Problem Inventory	Adults	Self-report	Depression diagnosis	10–20	Yes	Yes	None
Reynolds Depression Screening Inventory	Adults	Self-report	Depressive symptoms	5–10	Yes	Yes	None
Rimon's Brief Depression Scale	Adults	Clinician Rating	Depressive symptoms	15–30	Yes	No	None
Schedule for Affective Disorders and Schizophrenia	Adults	Structured interview	Differential diagnosis	90–120	No	Yes	Different versions exist to capture varying periods of time
State-Trait Depression Adjective Check Lists	Adults and adolescents, 14–89	Self-report	Depressive mood	3	Yes	Yes	Alternative equivalent forms
Structured Clinical Interview for DSM-IV Axis I Disorders	Adults	Semistructured interview	DSM-IV Axis I disorders	45–90	No	Yes	Research version
Symptom Checklist-90-Revised	Adults and adolescents	Self-report	Psychiatric symptoms	30	Yes	Yes	Spanish and other languages
Zung Self-Rating Depression Scale	Adults	Self-report	Depressive symptoms	5	Yes	No	Various languages

Table II. Measures of Depression: Special Populations (Chapter 5)

Name of instrument	Target population	Type of measure	Measurement focus	Time to complete (minutes)	Norms available?	Fee involved?	Alternate forms
Calgary Depression Scale for Schizophrenia	Adults with schizophrenia	Clinician rating	Depressive symptoms	30	Yes	No	Spanish and other languages
Children's Depression Inventory	Children and adolescents 7–17	Self-report	Depressive symptoms	10–15	Yes	Yes	Short form; Spanish and other languages
Children's Depression Rating Scale-Revised	Children 6–12	Semistructured interview	Depression	20–30	Yes	Yes	None
Cornell Scale for Depression in Dementia	Patients with dementia	Clinician rating	Depressive symptoms	30	Yes	No	German, French, Chinese
Depression Rating Scale	Elderly in nursing homes	Caregiver rating	Depressed affect	15	No	No	None
Geriatric Depression Scale	Adults 65+	Self-report	Depressive symptoms	30	Yes	No	Spanish and other languages
Kiddie-SADS-PL	Children 6–17	Structured interview	Depression diagnosis	35–45	No	No	None
Medical-Based Emotional Distress Scale	Adults with physical disabilities	Clinician rating	Emotional reactions	45	Yes	No	None
Multiscore Depression Inventory for Children	Children 8–17	Self-report	Depressive symptoms	15–20	Yes	Yes	None
Postpartum Depression Interview Schedule	Postpartum women	Semistructured interview	Depression	30	Yes	No	None
Psychopathology Inventory for Mentally Retarded Adults	Adults with mental retardation	Clinician rating	Clinical disorders, including affective disorder	30–45	No	No	Self-report version
Reynolds Adolescent Depression Scale	Adolescents 13–18	Self-report	Depressive symptoms	5–10	Yes	Yes	None
Reynolds Child Depression Scale	Children 8–12	Self-report	Depressive symptoms	10	Yes	Yes	None
Visual Analog Mood Scales	Adults with verbal or cognitive difficulties	Self-report	Depressive and anxiety symptoms	5	Yes	Yes	None
Youth Depression Adjective Checklist	Children and adolescents 11–17	Self-report	Dysphoric mood	5–10	Yes	No	State and trait versions; Spanish version.

Table III. Measures of Depression-Related Constructs (Chapter 6)

Name of instrument	Target population	Type of measure	Purpose	Time to complete (minutes)	Norms available?	Fee involved?	Alternate forms
Actigraphy	Children, adolescents, adults	Physiological measure	Activity and movement	—	No	Yes	None
Anticipatory Cognitions Questionnaire	Adults	Self-report	Negative anticipatory thoughts	20	No	No	French and German
Attributional Style Questionnaire	Adults	Self-report	Causal ascriptions	15	Yes	No	Children; other languages
Automatic Thoughts Questionnaire-Revised	Adults	Self-report	Negative and positive automatic thoughts	5–10	Yes	No	None
Beck Hopelessness Scale	Adults and adolescents	Self-report	Negative beliefs about the future	5–10	Yes	Yes	Spanish
Beck Scale for Suicide Ideation	Adults and adolescents 17+	Self-report	Suicidal ideation	5–10	Yes	Yes	Spanish
Children's Attributional Style Questionnaire-Revised	Children and adolescents 8–18	Self-report	Attributional style	10–15	Yes	No	None
Cognitive Bias Questionnaire	Adults	Self-report	Cognitive distortions	15	Yes	No	None
Cognitive Error Questionnaire	Adults	Self-report	Cognitive distortions	15	Yes	No	Lower-back-pain patients
Cognitive Events Schedule	Adults	Self-report	Beck's cognitive triad	30	No	No	Short form
Cognitive Triad Inventory	Adults	Self-report	Beck's cognitive triad	10	Yes	No	None
Coping Inventory for Stressful Situations	Adults and adolescents 13+	Self-report	Coping resources	10	Yes	Yes	Spanish
Coping Resources Inventory	Adults and adolescents 14–83	Self-report	Coping resources	10	Yes	Yes	None
Coping Resources Inventory	Adults	Self-report	Coping styles	15	Yes	Yes	Youth version
Depression Beliefs Questionnaire-Version I	Adults and adolescents	Self-report	Beliefs about the causes of depression	10–15	No	No	None
Depression Check Questionnaire	Adults	Observer ratings	Nonverbal depressive behavior	15	Yes	No	None

(continued)

Table III. (*Continued*)

Name of instrument	Target population	Type of measure	Purpose	Time to complete (minutes)	Norms available?	Fee involved?	Alternate forms
Depression Proneness Rating Scale	Adults	Self-report	Depression-proneness	10	Yes	No	None
Depressive Personality Disorder Inventory	Adults	Self-report	Thoughts related to depressive personality disorder	15–20	Yes	No	None
Divorce Dysfunctional Attitudes Scale	Adults	Self-report	Dysfunctional attitudes related to divorce	30	Yes	No	Short form
Dysfunctional Attitude Scale	Adults	Self-report	Maladaptive thinking patterns	10–15	Yes	Yes	Various languages
Frequency of Self-Reinforcement Questionnaire	Adults and adolescents	Self-report	Self-reinforcement	5–10	Yes	No	Spanish, Japanese, and children's forms
Goal Orientation Inventory	Adults 17+	Self-report	Motivational and cognitive aspects of depression	12–15	Yes	No	None
Interpersonal Events Schedule	Adults	Self-report	Interpersonal activities and cognitions	30	No	No	None
Life Attitudes Schedule	Adults and adolescents 13+	Self-report	Suicidal and life-threatening behaviors	30	Yes	Yes	Short form
Pleasant Events Schedule	Adults	Self-report	Pleasurable activities and events	60	Yes	No	Child form
Pleasant Events Schedule-AD	Adults with Alzheimer's disease	Caregiver rating	Pleasurable activities and events	15	Yes	No	Short form

Instrument	Population	Format	Construct	Time (min)			Versions
Positive Automatic Thoughts Questionnaire	Adults and adolescents	Self-report	Positive self-statements	5–10	Yes	No	None
Problem-Solving Inventory	Adults	Self-report	Self-appraised problem-solving ability	10–15	Yes	Yes	Turkish version
Reasons for Living Inventory	Adults	Self-report	Reasons not to commit suicide	15	Yes	No	Brief version for inmates; college student version
Revised Grief Experience Inventory	Adults	Self-report	Feelings of grief and bereavement	10	Yes	No	None
Self-Control Questionnaire for Depression	Adults	Self-report	Self-control behaviors and thoughts	5–10	No	No	None
Self-Control Schedule	Adults	Self-report	Self-control behaviors	5–10	Yes	No	Hebrew version
Self-Esteem Worksheet	Adults	Self-report	Self-esteem	Variable	Yes	No	None
Social Adjustment Scale	Adults	Semistructured interview	Social adjustment and functioning	45–60	Yes	No	Self-report version
Social Problem-Solving Inventory-Revised	Adults	Self-report	Social problem-solving skills and abilities	15–20	Yes	Yes	Short-form; Spanish version; adolescent version
Social Resourcefulness Scale	Adults	Self-report	Help-seeking behaviors	5	Yes	No	None
Sociotropy-Autonomy Scale	Adults	Self-report	Depression-related personality characteristics	15	Yes	No	None
Suicide Ideation Scale	Adolescents (grades 7–12)	Self-report	Suicidal ideation	5–10	Yes	Yes	Junior high, high school, and adult versions
Suicide Probability Score	Adults and adolescents 14+	Self-report	Suicidal risk	5–10	Yes	Yes	None
Unpleasant Events Schedule	Adults and adolescents 12+	Self-report	Stressful events	60	Yes	No	Short form
Ways of Coping Scale	Adults	Self-report	Coping processes	10	Yes	Yes	Several languages
Ways of Responding	Adults	Self-report	Compensatory skills	20–30	Yes	No	Equivalent forms

Appendix B
Reprinted Measures

Automatic Thoughts Questionnaire-Revised

Reprinted with permission from the author (Kendall, P.C., et al., 1989).

Instructions

Listed below are a variety of thoughts that pop into people's heads. Please read each thought and indicate how frequently, if at all, the thought occurred to you over the last week. Please read each item carefully and circle the appropriate answers in the following fashion 0 = "not at all," 1 = "sometimes," 2 = "moderately often," 3 = "often," and 4 = "all the time."

Responses   Thoughts

0 1 2 3 4   1. I feel like I'm up against the world.

0 1 2 3 4   2. I'm no good.

0 1 2 3 4   3. I'm proud of myself.

0 1 2 3 4   4. Why can't I ever succeed?

Remember, each sentence that you read is a thought that you may have had often, less frequently, or not at all. Tell us how often over the last week you have had each of the thoughts.

0 1 2 3 4   5. No one understands me.

0 1 2 3 4   6. I've let people down.

0 1 2 3 4   7. I feel fine.

0 1 2 3 4   8. I don't think I can go on.

0 1 2 3 4   9. I wish I were a better person.

0 1 2 3 4   10. No matter what happens, I know I'll make it.

0 1 2 3 4   11. I'm so weak.

0 1 2 3 4   12. My life's not going the way I want it to.

0 1 2 3 4   13. I can accomplish anything.

0 1 2 3 4   14. I'm so disappointed in myself.

0 1 2 3 4   15. Nothing feels good anymore.

0 1 2 3 4   16. I feel good.

0 1 2 3 4   17. I can't stand this anymore.

0 1 2 3 4   18. I can't get started.
0 1 2 3 4   19. What's wrong with me?
0 1 2 3 4   20. I'm warm and comfortable.
0 1 2 3 4   21. I wish I were somewhere else.
0 1 2 3 4   22. I can't get things together.
0 1 2 3 4   23. I hate myself.
0 1 2 3 4   24. I feel confident I can do anything I set my mind to.

Remember, each sentence that you read is a <u>thought</u> that you may have had often, less frequently, or not at all. Tell us how often <u>over</u> the last week you have had each of the thoughts.

0 1 2 3 4   25. I'm worthless.
0 1 2 3 4   26. Wish I could just disappear.
0 1 2 3 4   27. What's the matter with me?
0 1 2 3 4   28. I feel very happy.
0 1 2 3 4   29. I'm a loser.
0 1 2 3 4   30. My life is a mess.
0 1 2 3 4   31. I'm a failure.
0 1 2 3 4   32. This is super!
0 1 2 3 4   33. I'll never make it.
0 1 2 3 4   34. I feel so helpless.
0 1 2 3 4   35. Something has to change.
0 1 2 3 4   36. There must be something wrong with me.
0 1 2 3 4   37. I'm luckier than most people.
0 1 2 3 4   38. My future is bleak.
0 1 2 3 4   39. It's just not worth it.
0 1 2 3 4   40. I can't finish anything.

Center for Epidemiological Studies Depression Scale

Circle the number for each statement which best describes how often you felt or behaved this way—DURING THE PAST WEEK.

	Rarely or None of the Time (Less than 1 Day)	Some or a Little of the Time (1–2 Days)	Occasionally or a Moderate Amount of Time (3–4 Days)	Most or All of the Time (5–7 Days)
DURING THE PAST WEEK:				
1. I was bothered by things that usually don't bother me	0	1	2	3
2. I did not feel like eating; my appetite was poor	0	1	2	3
3. I felt that I could not shake off the blues even with help from my family or friends	0	1	2	3
4. I felt that I was just as good as other people	0	1	2	3
5. I had trouble keeping my mind on what I was doing	0	1	2	3
6. I felt depressed	0	1	2	3
7. I felt that everything I did was an effort	0	1	2	3
8. I felt hopeful about the future	0	1	2	3
9. I thought my life had been a failure	0	1	2	3
10. I felt fearful	0	1	2	3
11. My sleep was restless	0	1	2	3
12. I was happy	0	1	2	3
13. I talked less than usual	0	1	2	3
14. I felt lonely	0	1	2	3
15. People were unfriendly	0	1	2	3
16. I enjoyed life	0	1	2	3
17. I had crying spells	0	1	2	3
18. I felt sad	0	1	2	3
19. I felt that people disliked me	0	1	2	3
20. I could not get "going"	0	1	2	3

Cognitive Triad Inventory

©1986 E. E. Beckham, W. R. Leber, J. T. Watkins, J. Boyer, & J. Cook

This inventory lists different ideas that people sometimes have. For each of these ideas, show how much you agree with it by circling the answer which best describes your opinion. Be sure to <u>choose only one answer for each idea.</u> Answer the ideas for what you are thinking RIGHT NOW.

EXAMPLE:

TA = TOTALLY AGREE	SD = SLIGHTLY DISAGREE
MA = MOSTLY AGREE	MD = MOSTLY DISAGREE
SA = SLIGHTLY AGREE	TD = TOTALLY DISAGREE
N = NEUTRAL	

1. Life has its ups and downs.   TA MA (SA) N SD MD TD

In the example above, the circle at "SA" indicates that this statement agrees somewhat with the ideas held by the person completing this inventory.

NOW TURN THE PAGE AND BEGIN

Answering Codes: Circle the answer which best describes your opinion. <u>Choose only one answer for each idea.</u> Answer the items for what you are feeling RIGHT NOW.

TA = TOTALLY AGREE	SD = SLIGHTLY DISAGREE
MA = MOSTLY AGREE	MD = MOSTLY DISAGREE
SA = SLIGHTLY AGREE	TD = TOTALLY DISAGREE
N = NEUTRAL	

ANSWER THE ITEMS FOR WHAT YOU ARE THINKING RIGHT NOW.

1. I have many talents and skills.   TA MA SA N SD MD TD
2. My job (housework, school work, daily duties) is unpleasant.   TA MA SA N SD MD TD
3. Most people are friendly and helpful.   TA MA SA N SD MD TD
4. Nothing is likely to work out for me.   TA MA SA N SD MD TD
5. I am a failure.   TA MA SA N SD MD TD
6. I like to think about the good things that lie ahead for me.   TA MA SA N SD MD TD
7. I do my work (job, schoolwork, housework) adequately.   TA MA SA N SD MD TD
8. The people I know help me when I need it.   TA MA SA N SD MD TD
9. I expect that things will be going very well for me a few years from now.   TA MA SA N SD MD TD
10. I have messed up almost all the important relationships I have ever had.   TA MA SA N SD MD TD
11. The future holds a lot of excitement for me.   TA MA SA N SD MD TD
12. My daily activities are fun and rewarding.   TA MA SA N SD MD TD
13. I can't do anything right.   TA MA SA N SD MD TD
14. People like me.   TA MA SA N SD MD TD

15. There is nothing left in my life to look forward to.   TA MA SA N SD MD TD
16. My current problems or concerns will always be there in one way or another.   TA MA SA N SD MD TD
17. I am as adequate as other people I know.   TA MA SA N SD MD TD
18. The world is a very hostile place.   TA MA SA N SD MD TD
19. There is no reason for me to be hopeful about my future.   TA MA SA N SD MD TD
20. The important people in my life are helpful and supportive.   TA MA SA N SD MD TD
21. I hate myself.   TA MA SA N SD MD TD
22. I will overcome my problems.   TA MA SA N SD MD TD
23. Bad things happen to me a lot.   TA MA SA N SD MD TD
24. I have a spouse or friend who is warm and supportive.   TA MA SA N SD MD TD
25. I can do a lot of things well.   TA MA SA N SD MD TD
26. My future is simply too awful to think about.   TA MA SA N SD MD TD
27. My family doesn't care what happens to me.   TA MA SA N SD MD TD
28. Things will work out well for me in the future.   TA MA SA N SD MD TD
29. I am guilty of a great many things.   TA MA SA N SD MD TD
30. No matter what I do, others make it difficult for me to get what I need.   TA MA SA N SD MD TD
31. I am a worthwhile human being.   TA MA SA N SD MD TD
32. There is nothing to look forward to in the years ahead.   TA MA SA N SD MD TD
33. I like myself.   TA MA SA N SD MD TD
34. I am faced with many difficulties.   TA MA SA N SD MD TD
35. I have serious flaws   TA MA SA N SD MD TD
36. I expect to be content and satisfied as the years go by.

Cornell Scale for Depression in Dementia

Reprinted by permission of Elsevier Science, copyright 1988, by The Society of Biological Psychiatry.

Scoring System

a = unable to evaluate
0 = absent
1 = mild or intermittent
2 = severe

Ratings should be based on symptoms and signs occurring during the week prior to interview. No score should be given if symptoms result from physical disability or illness.

A. Mood-Related Signs

1. Anxiety	a	0	1	2
anxious expression, ruminations, worrying				
2. Sadness	a	0	1	2
sad expression, sad voice, tearfulness				
3. Lack of reactivity to pleasant events	a	0	1	2
4. Irritability	a	0	1	2
easily annoyed, short tempered				

B. Behavioral Disturbance

5. Agitation	a	0	1	2
restlessness, hand wringing, hair pulling				
6. Retardation	a	0	1	2
slow movements, slow speech, slow reactions				
7. Multiple physical complaints	a	0	1	2
(score 0 if GI symptoms only)				
8. Loss of interest	a	0	1	2
less involved in usual activities				
(score only if change occurred acutely, i.e., in less than 1 month)				

C. Physical Signs

9. Appetite loss	a	0	1	2
eating less than normal				
10. Weight loss	a	0	1	2
(score 2 if greater than 5 lb in 1 month)				
11. Lack of energy				
fatigues easily, unable to sustain activities				
(score only if change occurred acutely, i.e., in less than 1 month)				

D. Cyclic Functions

12. Diurnal variation of mood	a	0	1	2
symptoms worse in the morning				
13. Difficulty falling asleep	a	0	1	2
later than usual for this individual				

APPENDIX

14. Multiple awakenings during sleep	a	0	1	2
15. Early morning awakening earlier than usual for this individual	a	0	1	2

E. Ideational Disturbance

16. Suicide feels life is not worth living, has suicidal wishes or makes suicide attempt	a	0	1	2
17. Poor self-esteem self-blame, self-depreciation, feelings of failure	a	0	1	2
18. Pessimism anticipation of the worst	a	0	1	2
19. Mood-congruent delusions delusions of poverty, illness, or loss	a	0	1	2

Depression Anxiety Stress Scales

Please read each statement and circle a number 0, 1, 2, or 3 which indicates how much the statement applied to you *over the past week*. There are no right or wrong answers. Do not spend too much time on any statement.

The rating scale is as follows:
0   Did not apply to me at all
1   Applied to me to some degree, or some of the time
2   Applied to me to a considerable degree, or a good part of time
3   Applied to me very much, or most of the time

1	I found myself getting upset by quite trivial things	0	1	2	3
2	I was aware of dryness of my mouth	0	1	2	3
3	I couldn't seem to experience any positive feeling at all	0	1	2	3
4	I experienced breathing difficulty (e.g., excessively rapid breathing, breathlessness in the absence of physical exertion)	0	1	2	3
5	I just couldn't seem to get going	0	1	2	3
6	I tended to over-react to situations	0	1	2	3
7	I had a feeling of shakiness (e.g., legs going to give way)	0	1	2	3
8	I found it difficult to relax	0	1	2	3
9	I found myself in situations that made me so anxious I was relieved when they ended	0	1	2	3
10	I felt that I had nothing to look forward to	0	1	2	3
11	I found myself getting upset rather easily	0	1	2	3
12	I felt that I was using a lot of nervous energy	0	1	2	3
13	I felt sad and depressed	0	1	2	3
14	I found myself getting impatient when I was delayed in any way (e.g., lifts, traffic lights, being kept waiting)	0	1	2	3
15	I had a feeling of faintness	0	1	2	3
16	I felt that I had lost interest in just about everything	0	1	2	3
17	I felt I wasn't worth much as a person	0	1	2	3
18	I felt that I was rather touchy	0	1	2	3
19	I perspired noticeably (e.g,. hands sweaty) in the absence of high temperatures or physical exertion	0	1	2	3
20	I felt scared without any good reason	0	1	2	3
21	I felt that life wasn't worthwhile	0	1	2	3
22	I found it hard to wind down	0	1	2	3
23	I had difficulty in swallowing	0	1	2	3
24	I couldn't seem to get any enjoyment out of the things I did	0	1	2	3
25	I was aware of the action of my heart in the absence of physical exertion (e.g., sense of heart rate increase, heart missing a beat)	0	1	2	3
26	I felt down-hearted and blue	0	1	2	3
27	I found that I was very irritable	0	1	2	3
28	I felt I was close to panic	0	1	2	3
29	I found it hard to calm down after something upset me	0	1	2	3
30	I feared that I would be "thrown" by some trivial but unfamiliar task	0	1	2	3

31 I was unable to become enthusiastic about anything   0   1   2   3

32 I found it difficult to tolerate interruptions to what I was doing   0   1   2   3

33 I was in a state of nervous tension   0   1   2   3

34 I felt I was pretty worthless   0   1   2   3

35 I was intolerant of anything that kept me from getting on with
what I was doing   0   1   2   3

36 I felt terrified   0   1   2   3

37 I could see nothing in the future to be hopeful about   0   1   2   3

38 I felt that life was meaningless   0   1   2   3

39 I found myself getting agitated   0   1   2   3

40 I was worried about situations in which I might panic and make a
fool of myself   0   1   2   3

41 I experienced trembling (e.g., in the hands)   0   1   2   3

42 I found it difficult to work up the initiative to do things   0   1   2   3

Depression Check Questionnaire

[Reprinted with permission of the authors (Tan, J. C. and Stoppard, J. M., 1994)]

Instructions: Please rate your OVERALL impression of the person you have just interacted with:

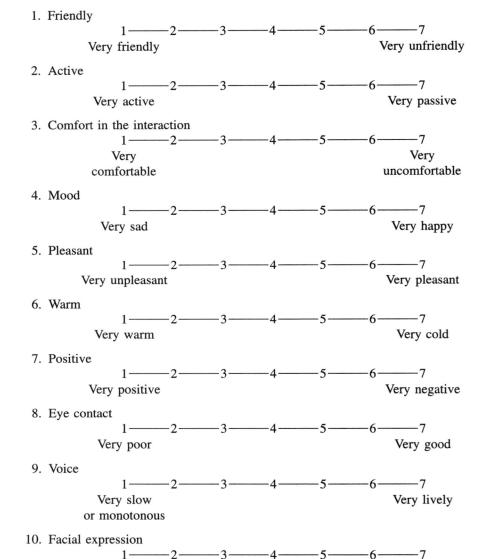

1. Friendly

    1———2———3———4———5———6———7

    Very friendly   Very unfriendly

2. Active

    1———2———3———4———5———6———7

    Very active   Very passive

3. Comfort in the interaction

    1———2———3———4———5———6———7

    Very   Very
    comfortable   uncomfortable

4. Mood

    1———2———3———4———5———6———7

    Very sad   Very happy

5. Pleasant

    1———2———3———4———5———6———7

    Very unpleasant   Very pleasant

6. Warm

    1———2———3———4———5———6———7

    Very warm   Very cold

7. Positive

    1———2———3———4———5———6———7

    Very positive   Very negative

8. Eye contact

    1———2———3———4———5———6———7

    Very poor   Very good

9. Voice

    1———2———3———4———5———6———7

    Very slow   Very lively
    or monotonous

10. Facial expression

    1———2———3———4———5———6———7

    Very pleasant   Very unpleasant

11. Smiling

    1———2———3———4———5———6———7

    Frowning   Smiling fully
    or tearful   or laughing

12. Head posture

1———2———3———4———5———6———7

Head up   Head hung

13. Shoulder posture

1———2———3———4———5———6———7

Shoulder   Shoulder erect
slumped

Depression Proneness Rating Scale

[Reprinted with permission of the author, Robert Zemore (Zemore, R. et al., 1990)]

INSTRUCTIONS: This questionnaire is concerned with your feelings and attitudes over the past two years. Answer each question by circling the appropriate number on the scale below that question. For example, the first question asks how often you become depressed. If, during the past two years, you were depressed about as often as most people, then circle the 5. On the other hand, if you were depressed more often than most people, but not extremely often, then circle one of the numbers between 5 and 9, etc. Sometimes it is very difficult to know how one's feelings compare with the feelings of others. Just do the best you can. Remember, you are being asked to summarize your feelings and attitudes over the past **two years**, not just the past two days. Try to avoid being overly influenced by your present mood.

1. Compared to others, how often did you get depressed?

   1 ___ 2 ___ 3 ___ 4 ___ 5 ___ 6 ___ 7 ___ 8 ___ 9
   Much   About   Much
   less often   the same   more often

2. Compared to others, how long did your depression last?

   1 ___ 2 ___ 3 ___ 4 ___ 5 ___ 6 ___ 7 ___ 8 ___ 9
   Much   About   Much
   shorter   the same   longer

3. Compared to others, how deeply depressed did you become?

   1 ___ 2 ___ 3 ___ 4 ___ 5 ___ 6 ___ 7 ___ 8 ___ 9
   Much   About   Much
   less deeply   the same   more deeply

4. Compared to others, how often did you feel discouraged about the future?

   1 ___ 2 ___ 3 ___ 4 ___ 5 ___ 6 ___ 7 ___ 8 ___ 9
   Much   About   Much
   less often   the same   more often

5. Compared to others, how often did you feel distant or isolated from people?

   1 ___ 2 ___ 3 ___ 4 ___ 5 ___ 6 ___ 7 ___ 8 ___ 9
   Much   About   Much
   less often   the same   more often

6. Compared to others, how often did you see yourself as a failure?

   1 ___ 2 ___ 3 ___ 4 ___ 5 ___ 6 ___ 7 ___ 8 ___ 9
   Much   About   Much
   less often   the same   more often

7. Compared to others, how often did you feel guilty or unworthy?

   1 ___ 2 ___ 3 ___ 4 ___ 5 ___ 6 ___ 7 ___ 8 ___ 9
   Much   About   Much
   less often   the same   more often

8. Compared to others, how often did you have difficulty concentrating or making a decision?

    1 —— 2 —— 3 —— 4 —— 5 —— 6 —— 7 —— 8 —— 9
    Much   About   Much
    less often   the same   more often

9. Compared to others, how often did you feel tired and lacking energy?

    1 —— 2 —— 3 —— 4 —— 5 —— 6 —— 7 —— 8 —— 9
    Much   About   Much
    less often   the same   more often

10. Compared to others, how often did you feel disappointed in yourself?

    1 —— 2 —— 3 —— 4 —— 5 —— 6 —— 7 —— 8 —— 9
    Much   About   Much
    less often   the same   more often

11. Compared to others, how often did you feel sad or blue?

    1 —— 2 —— 3 —— 4 —— 5 —— 6 —— 7 —— 8 —— 9
    Much   About   Much
    less often   the same   more often

12. Compared to others, how often did you think seriously about suicide?

    1 —— 2 —— 3 —— 4 —— 5 —— 6 —— 7 —— 8 —— 9
    Much   About   Much
    less often   the same   more often

13. Compared to others, how often did you suffer from lack of appetite?

    1 —— 2 —— 3 —— 4 —— 5 —— 6 —— 7 —— 8 —— 9
    Much   About   Much
    less often   the same   more often

Depression Rating Scale

1. How frequently does the participant seem sad or depressed? (Notice: sad face, slumped body, and voice, crying, or verbalizations of sadness. Do not include agitation, physical complaints, sleep, or appetite problems.)
   1. Never
   2. Less than once a week, but still occurring
   3. Once or twice a week
   4. Several times a week
   5. Once or twice a day
   6. Several times a day
   7. A few times an hour

2. How severe is the participant's depression when it occurs?
   1. Never occurs
   2. Very mild
   3. Mild
   4. Moderate
   5. Moderate to severe
   6. Severe
   7. Extreme

3. Rate the participant's ability to communicate
   1. Always clear and retains information
   2. Can indicate needs and understand information, though manifests some decline in level of expression or comprehension.
   3. Can indicate needs. Can understand simple verbal directions. Can deal with simple information.
   4. Understands simple verbal and non-verbal information but does not indicate needs.
   5. Requires much assistance or coaching to communicate.
   6. Cannot understand simple verbal or non-verbal information but retains some expressive ability.
   7. No effective contact.

4. How frequently does the participant engage in social activities (with residents, family, visitors, etc.)?
   1. Never
   2. Less than once a week, but still occurring
   3. Once or twice a week
   4. Several times a week
   5. Once or twice a day
   6. Several times a day
   7. A few times an hour

5. What is the quality of the social interactions the participant engages in?
   1. Always very negative, abusive, or angry
   2. Frequently negative
   3. Sometimes negative (more frequently than positive)

4. Usually indifferent or about equally positive and negative
5. Sometimes positive
6. Frequently positive
7. Always positive, very warm

6. How frequently does the participant participate in activities (e.g., music, occupational therapy) or read, write, take a walk, or engage in any other activity which is meaningful for his/her level of functioning?
   1. Never
   2. Less than once a week, but still occurring
   3. Once or twice a week
   4. Several times a week
   5. Once or twice a day
   6. Several times a day
   7. A few times an hour

Divorce Dysfunctional Attitudes Scale

This questionnaire lists some of the things that people might think about the subject of divorce. For each one, circle the letters which best fits whether you agree or disagree with the statement. Use these abbreviations for your answers

SA = Strongly Agree; A = Agree; U = Unsure; D = Disagree; SD = Strongly Disagree

Getting divorced means that ...

SA A U D SD   1. It is difficult to be happy if you're not married.
SA A U D SD   2. You can socialize and have fun without being in a couple.
SA A U D SD   3. People will generally think less of you.
SA A U D SD   4. People will wonder if there is something wrong with you.
SA A U D SD   5. You will always be lonely.
SA A U D SD   6. You just didn't try hard enough in the marriage.
SA A U D SD   7. You wanted too much and didn't compromise.
SA A U D SD   8. You were selfish.
SA A U D SD   9. You lack character.
SA A U D SD   10. You won't stick with anyone else either.
SA A U D SD   11. You've failed as a person.
SA A U D SD   12. Love does not really mean anything.
SA A U D SD   13. People can't be trusted in close relationships.
SA A U D SD   14. People who say they love you don't really mean it.
SA A U D SD   15. If a person says he/she loves you and will stay with you, it doesn't mean anything.
SA A U D SD   16. You're just going to keep repeating the same types of relationships and problems.
SA A U D SD   17. You're not able to choose a good partner.
SA A U D SD   18. Others think you're "damaged goods."
SA A U D SD   19. You can't be happy until you get remarried.
SA A U D SD   20. You're codependent.
SA A U D SD   21. You'll have damaged children.
SA A U D SD   22. You don't care about your children.
SA A U D SD   23. Your children will have good marriages when they are adults.
SA A U D SD   24. Your children will always have psychological problems.
SA A U D SD   25. You won't be able to provide adequate discipline for your children.
SA A U D SD   26. Your children will not grow up normally without a same-sex parent in the home.
SA A U D SD   27. Your children will always resent you for the divorce.
SA A U D SD   28. It's ruined your life.
SA A U D SD   29. You will probably never be happy.
SA A U D SD   30. If your friends stay in touch with your ex-spouse, they are siding against you.
SA A U D SD   31. You will always be drawn to people who aren't good for you.
SA A U D SD   32. You had the courage to do what you needed to do.
SA A U D SD   33. You care too much about your kids to have them grow up in an unhappy home.

SA A U D SD   34. You'll just get used in romantic relationships.
SA A U D SD   35. You've lost your chance to be loved.
SA A U D SD   36. You can't keep a stable, mature relationship.
SA A U D SD   37. You can't count on people to be there for the long haul.
SA A U D SD   38. You failed in a very important task in life.
SA A U D SD   39. With such an example, your children won't have healthy families themselves.

Frequency of Self-Reinforcement Questionnaire

[Reprinted with permission of the author and publisher (© 1983, the American Psychological Association)]

Below are a number of statements concerning beliefs or attitudes people have. Indicate whether the statements are characteristic and descriptive of you by circling T if the statement is somewhat or *very true* for yourself. Circle F if the statement is somewhat or *very false* for yourself. Please be as honest as possible. Your answers are completely anonymous.

1. When I fail at something, generally I am still able to feel good about myself.   T   F
2. I can stick to a tiresome task that I need to complete for a long time without someone encouraging me.   T   F
3. I don't often think positive thoughts about myself.   T   F
4. When I do something right, I take time to enjoy the feeling.   T   F
5. I have such high standards for what I demand of myself that I rarely meet those standards.   T   F
6. I seem to blame myself when things go wrong and am very critical of myself.   T   F
7. There are pleasurable activities which I enjoy doing alone at my leisure.   T   F
8. I usually get upset when I make mistakes because I rarely learn from them.   T   F
9. My feelings of self-confidence and self-esteem fluctuate a great deal.   T   F
10. When I succeed at small things, I become encouraged to go on.   T   F
11. Unless I do something absolutely perfectly, it gives me little satisfaction.   T   F
12. I get myself through hard things mostly by planning to enjoy myself afterwards.   T   F
13. When I make mistakes, I take time to criticize myself.   T   F
14. I encourage myself to improve by feeling good about myself or giving myself something special whenever I make some progress.   T   F
15. If I didn't criticize myself frequently, I would continue to do things poorly forever.   T   F
16. I think talking about what you've done right is being too boastful.   T   F
17. I find I feel better and do better when I silently praise myself for even small achievements.   T   F
18. I can keep trying at something when I stop to think of what I've accomplished.   T   F
19. The way I keep up my confidence is by acknowledging any success I have.   T   F
20. The way I achieve my goals is by rewarding myself every step along the way.   T   F
21. Praising yourself is being selfish and egotistical.   T   F
22. When someone criticizes me, my self-confidence is shattered.   T   F
23. I criticize myself more frequently than others criticize me.   T   F
24. I have a lot of worthwhile qualities.   T   F
25. I silently praise myself even when others do not praise me.   T   F
26. Any activity can provide some pleasure regardless of how it comes out.   T   F
27. If I don't do the best possible job, I think less of myself.   T   F
28. I should be upset if I make a mistake.   T   F
29. My happiness depends more on myself than it does on other people.   T   F
30. People who talk about their own better points are just bragging.   T   F

Geriatric Depression Scale

Reprinted with permission of Elsevier Science, © 1983.

Administration. These items may be administered in written format, but oral presentation is preferred for medical patients. If written format is used, the answer sheet must have printed YES/NO after each question, and the subject is instructed to circle the better response. If administered orally, the examiner may have to repeat the question in order to get a response that is more clearly a "yes" or "no."

1. Are you basically satisfied with your life?	YES	NO
2. Have you dropped many of your activities and interests?	YES	NO
3. Do you feel that your life is empty?	YES	NO
4. Do you often get bored?	YES	NO
5. Are you hopeful about the future?	YES	NO
6. Are you bothered by thoughts you can't get out of your head?	YES	NO
7. Are you in good spirits most of the time?	YES	NO
8. Are you afraid that something bad is going to happen to you?	YES	NO
9. Do you feel happy most of the time?	YES	NO
10. Do you often feel helpless?	YES	NO
11. Do you often get restless and fidgety?	YES	NO
12. Do you prefer to stay at home, rather than going out and doing new things?	YES	NO
13. Do you frequently worry about the future?	YES	NO
14. Do you feel you have more problems with memory than most?	YES	NO
15. Do you think it is wonderful to be alive now?	YES	NO
16. Do you often feel downhearted and blue?	YES	NO
17. Do you feel pretty worthless the way you are now?	YES	NO
18. Do you worry a lot about the past?	YES	NO
19. Do you find life very exciting?	YES	NO
20. Is it hard for you to get started on new projects?	YES	NO
21. Do you feel full of energy?	YES	NO
22. Do you feel that your situation is hopeless?	YES	NO
23. Do you think that most people are better off then you are?	YES	NO
24. Do you frequently get upset over little things?	YES	NO
25. Do you frequently feel like crying?	YES	NO
26. Do you have trouble concentrating?	YES	NO
27. Do you enjoy getting up in the morning?	YES	NO
28. Do you prefer to avoid social gatherings?	YES	NO
29. Is it easy for you to make decisions?	YES	NO
30. Is your mind as clear as it used to be?	YES	NO

Hamilton Rating Scale for Depression

Reprinted with permission from John Waterhouse and the British Psychological Society.

Instructions: For each item, select the number that corresponds to the statement that best characterizes the patient.

1. **DEPRESSED MOOD** (Sadness, hopeless, helpless, worthless)
   0   Absent
   1   These feeling states indicated only on questioning
   2   These feeling states spontaneously reported verbally
   3   Communicates feeling states non-verbally—i.e., through facial expression, posture, voice, and tendency to weep
   4   Patient reports VIRTUALLY ONLY these feeling states in his spontaneous verbal and nonverbal communication

2. **FEELINGS OF GUILT**
   0   Absent
   1   Self reproach, feels he has let people down
   2   Ideas of guilt or rumination over past errors or sinful deeds
   3   Present illness is a punishment. Delusions of guilt
   4   Hears accusatory or denunciatory voices and/or experiences threatening visual hallucinations

3. **SUICIDE**
   0   Absent
   1   Feels life is not worth living
   2   Wishes he were dead or any thoughts of possible death to self
   3   Suicidal ideas or gestures
   4   Attempts at suicide (any serious attempt rates 4)

4. **INSOMNIA EARLY**
   0   No difficulty falling asleep
   1   Complains of occasional difficulty falling asleep—i.e., more than ½ hour
   2   Complains of nightly difficulty falling asleep

5. **INSOMNIA MIDDLE**
   0   No difficulty
   1   Patient complains of being restless and disturbed during the night
   2   Waking during the night—any getting out of bed rates 2 (except for purposes of voiding)

6. **INSOMNIA LATE**
   0   No difficulty
   1   Waking in early hours of the morning but goes back to sleep
   2   Unable to fall asleep again if he gets out of bed

7. **WORK AND ACTIVITIES**
   0   No difficulty
   1   Thoughts and feelings of incapacity, fatigue or weakness related to activities, work or hobbies
   2   Loss of interest in activity, hobbies, or work—either directly reported by patient, or indirect in listlessness, indecision and vacillation (feels he has to push self to work or activities)

3 Decrease in actual time spent in activities or decrease in productivity
4 Stopped working because of present illness

8. **RETARDATION: PSYCHOMOTOR** (Slowness of thought and speech; impaired ability to concentrate; decreased motor activity)
   0 Normal speech and thought
   1 Slight retardation at interview
   2 Obvious retardation at interview
   3 Interview difficult
   4 Complete stupor

9. **AGITATION**
   0 None
   1 Fidgetiness
   2 Playing with hands, hair, etc.
   3 Moving about, can't sit still
   4 Hand wringing, nail biting, hair-pulling, biting of lips

10. **ANXIETY (PSYCHOLOGICAL)**
    0 No difficulty
    1 Subjective tension and irritability
    2 Worrying about minor matters
    3 Apprehensive attitude apparent in face or speech
    4 Fears expressed without questioning

11. **ANXIETY SOMATIC:** Physiological concomitants of anxiety (i.e., effects of autonomic overactivity, "butterflies," indigestion, stomach cramps, belching, diarrhea, palpitations, hyperventilation, paresthesia, sweating, flushing, tremor, headache, urinary frequency). Avoid asking about possible medication side effects (i.e., dry mouth, constipation)
    0 Absent
    1 Mild
    2 Moderate
    3 Severe
    4 Incapacitating

12. **SOMATIC SYMPTOMS (GASTROINTESTINAL)**
    0 None
    1 Loss of appetite but eating without encouragement from others. Food intake about normal
    2 Difficulty eating without urging from others. Marked reduction of appetite and food intake

13. **SOMATIC SYMPTOMS GENERAL**
    0 None
    1 Heaviness in limbs, back or head. Backaches, headache, muscle aches. Loss of energy or fatigability
    2 Any clear-cut symptom rates 2

14. **GENITAL SYMPTOMS** (Symptoms such as: loss of libido; impaired sexual performance; menstrual disturbances)
    0 Absent
    1 Mild
    2 Severe

15. **HYPOCHONDRIASIS**
    0   Not present
    1   Self-absorption (bodily)
    2   Preoccupation with health
    3   Frequent complaints, requests for help, etc.
    4   Hypochondriacal delusions

16. **LOSS OF WEIGHT**
    A. When rating by history:
       0   No weight loss
       1   Probably weight loss associated with present illness
       2   Definite (according to patient) weight loss
       3   Not assessed
    B. On weekly ratings by ward psychiatrist, when actual weight changes are measured
       0   Less than 1 lb weight loss in a week
       1   Greater than 1 lb weight loss in a week
       2   Greater than 2 lb weight loss in a week

17. **INSIGHT**
    0   Acknowledges being depressed and ill
    1   Acknowledges illness but attributes cause to bad food, climate, overwork, virus, need for rest, etc.
    2   Denies being ill at all

18. **DIURNAL VARIATION**
    A. Note whether symptoms are worse in morning or evening. If NO diurnal variation, mark none
       0   No variation
       1   Worse in A.M.
       2   Worse in P.M.
    B. When present, mark the severity of the variation. Mark "None" if NO variation
       0   None
       1   Mild
       2   Severe

19. **DEPERSONALIZATION AND DEREALIZATION** (Such as: feelings of unreality; nihilistic ideas)
    0   Absent
    1   Mild
    2   Moderate
    3   Severe
    4   Incapacitating

20. **PARANOID SYMPTOMS**
    0   None
    1   Suspicious
    2   Ideas of reference
    3   Delusions of reference and persecution

21. **OBSESSIONAL AND COMPULSIVE SYMPTOMS**
    0   Absent
    1   Mild
    2   Severe

Total score _____

Hopeless Depression Symptom Questionnaire

Instructions: On this questionnaire are groups of statements. Please read all of the statements in a given group. Then pick out the one in each group which describes you best for the past TWO WEEKS. If several statements in the group seem to apply equally well, choose the higher number. Do not choose more than one number for a given group of statements. BE SURE TO READ ALL OF THE STATEMENTS IN EACH GROUP BEFORE MAKING YOUR CHOICE

1.
0 = I have not stopped trying to get what I want.
1 = I have stopped trying to get what I want in some situations.
2 = I have stopped trying to get what I want in most situations.
3 = I have stopped trying to get what I want in all situations.

2.
0 = I am not passive when it comes to getting what I want these days.
1 = In some situations I'm passive when it comes to getting what I want these days.
2 = In most situations I'm passive when it comes to getting what I want these days.
3 = In all situations I'm passive when it comes to getting what I want these days.

3.
0 = I have not given up trying to accomplish what's important to me.
1 = I have given up trying to accomplish some things that are important to me.
2 = I have given up trying to accomplish most things that are important to me.
3 = I have given up trying to accomplish all things that are important to me.

4.
0 = My motivation to get things done is as good as usual.
1 = In some situations my motivation to get things done is lower than usual.
2 = In most situations my motivation to get things done is lower than usual.
3 = In all situations my motivation to get things done is lower than usual.

5.
0 = I need little or no support from other people.
1 = I need some support from other people.
2 = I need a lot of support from other people.
3 = I need total support from other people.

6.
0 = I don't rely on other people to do things for me.
1 = Sometimes I rely on other people to do things for me.
2 = Most of the time I rely on other people to do things for me.
3 = All of the time I rely on other people to do things for me.

7.
0 = These days I am not overly dependent on other people.
1 = Sometimes these days I am overly dependent on other people.
2 = Most of the time these days I am overly dependent on other people.
3 = These days I am always overly dependent on other people.

8.
0 = I am not a burden to other people.
1 = I am a burden to other people sometimes.
2 = I am a burden to other people most of the time.

3 = I am a burden to other people all of the time.

9.

0 = I am not doing things in "slow motion" these days.

1 = Sometimes I do things in "slow motion" these days.

2 = Most of the time I do things in "slow motion" these days.

3 = I always do things in "slow motion" these days.

10.

0 = I do not walk around like a zombie these days.

1 = Sometimes I walk around like a zombie these days.

2 = Most of the time I walk around like a zombie these days.

3 = I always walk around like a zombie these days.

11.

0 = My speech is not slowed down.

1 = My speech is somewhat slowed down.

2 = My speech is very slowed down.

3 = My speech is extremely slowed down.

12.

0 = My thoughts are not slowed down.

1 = My thoughts are somewhat slowed down.

2 = My thoughts are very slowed down.

3 = My thoughts are extremely slowed down.

13.

0 = My energy is not lower than usual.

1 = My energy is somewhat lower than usual.

2 = My energy is much lower than usual.

3 = My energy is extremely lower than usual.

14.

0 = I can get things done as well as usual.

1 = In some situations I can't get things done as well as usual.

2 = In most situations I can't get things done as well as usual.

3 = In all situations I can't get things done as well as usual.

15.

0 = I have as much energy as usual.

1 = In some situations I have less energy than usual.

2 = In most situations I have less energy than usual.

3 = In all situations I have less energy than usual.

16.

0 = I do not get tired out more easily than usual.

1 = In some situations I get tired out more easily than usual.

2 = In most situations I get tired out more easily than usual.

3 = In all situations I get tired out more easily than usual.

17.

0 = I enjoy things as much as usual.

1 = In some situations I don't enjoy things as much as usual.

2 = In most situations I don't enjoy things as much as usual.

3 = In all situations I don't enjoy things as much as usual.

18.

0 = When doing things I normally enjoy (e.g., work; being with people) I have as much fun as usual.

1 = When doing things I normally enjoy (e.g., work; being with people) I have somewhat less fun than usual.

2 = When doing things I normally enjoy (e.g., work; being with people) I have much less fun than usual.

3 = When doing things I normally enjoy (e.g., work; being with people) I don't have fun at all anymore.

19.

0 = When it comes to the things in life that count, I am as interested as usual.

1 = When it comes to the things in life that count, I am somewhat less interested than usual.

2 = When it comes to the things in life that count, I am much less interested than usual.

3 = When it comes to the things in life that count, I don't have any interest at all anymore.

20.

0 = I enjoy sex as much as usual.

1 = I enjoy sex somewhat less than usual.

2 = I enjoy sex much less than usual.

3 = I do not enjoy sex at all anymore.

21.

0 = I do not have trouble falling asleep.

1 = It takes me somewhat longer to fall asleep than usual (i.e., up to one hour longer).

2 = It takes me much longer to fall asleep than usual (i.e., up to 2 hours longer).

3 = It takes me substantially longer to fall asleep than usual (i.e., more than 2 hours longer).

22.

0 = I do not have trouble sleeping through the night.

1 = Sometimes I have trouble sleeping through the night.

2 = Most of the time I have trouble sleeping through the night.

3 = I always have trouble sleeping through the night.

23.

0 = I do not wake up early in the morning and have trouble falling back to sleep.

1 = Sometimes I wake up early in the morning and have trouble falling back to sleep.

2 = Most of the time I wake up early in the morning and have trouble falling back to sleep.

3 = I always wake up early in the morning and have trouble falling back to sleep.

24.

0 = I can fall asleep as well as usual.

1 = Sometimes I have trouble falling asleep.

2 = Most of the time I have trouble falling asleep.

3 = I always have trouble falling asleep.

25.

0 = My concentration is as good as usual.

1 = My concentration is somewhat less focused than usual.

2 = My concentration is much less focused than usual.

3 = I can hardly concentrate at all anymore.

26.

0 = I can concentrate as well as usual.

1 = In some situations I cannot concentrate as well as usual.

2 = In most situations I cannot concentrate as well as usual.

3 = In all situations I cannot concentrate as well as usual.

27.

0 = I do not brood about unpleasant events these days.

1 = Sometimes I brood about unpleasant events these days.

2 = Most of the time I brood about unpleasant events these days.

3 = I always brood about unpleasant events these days.

28.

0 = I am not distracted by unpleasant thoughts.

1 = In some situations I am distracted by unpleasant thoughts.

2 = In most situations I am distracted by unpleasant thoughts.

3 = In all situations I am distracted by unpleasant thoughts.

29.

0 = I do not have thoughts of killing myself.

1 = Sometimes I have thoughts of killing myself.

2 = Most of the time I have thoughts of killing myself.

3 = I always have thoughts of killing myself.

30.

0 = I am not having thoughts about suicide.

1 = I am having thoughts about suicide but have not formulated any plans.

2 = I am having thoughts about suicide and am considering possible ways of doing it.

3 = I am having thoughts about suicide and have formulated a definite plan.

31.

0 = I am not having thoughts about suicide.

1 = I am having thoughts about suicide but have these thoughts completely under my control.

2 = I am having thoughts about suicide but have these thoughts somewhat under my control.

3 = I am having thoughts about suicide and have little or no control over these thoughts.

32.

0 = I am not having impulses to kill myself.

1 = In some situations I have impulses to kill myself.

2 = In most situations I have impulses to kill myself.

3 = In all situations I have impulses to kill myself.

Inventory of Depressive Symptomatology (Self-Report)

Reprinted with permission from Elsevier Science, © 1986.

Please circle the one response to each item that best described you for the past seven days.

1. Falling Asleep:
   0   I never take longer than 20 minutes to fall asleep.
   1   I take at least 30 minutes to fall asleep, less than half the time.
   2   I take at least 30 minutes to fall asleep, more than half the time.
   3   I take more than 60 minutes to fall asleep, more than half the time.
2. Sleep During the Night:
   0   I do not wake up at night.
   1   I have a restless, light sleep with a few brief awakenings each night.
   2   I wake up at least once a night, but I go back to sleep easily.
   3   I awaken more than once a night and stay awake for 20 minutes or more, more than half the time.
3. Waking Up Too Early:
   0   Most of the time, I awaken no more than 30 minutes before I need to get up.
   1   More than half the time, I awaken more than 30 minutes before I need to get up.
   2   I almost always awaken at least one hour or so before I need to, but I go back to sleep eventually.
   3   I awaken at least one hour before I need to, and can't go back to sleep.
4. Sleeping Too Much:
   0   I sleep no longer than 7–8 hours/night, without napping during the day.
   1   I sleep no longer than 10 hours in a 24-hour period including naps.
   2   I sleep no longer than 12 hours in a 24-hour period including naps.
   3   I sleep longer than 12 hours in a 24-hour period including naps.
5. Feeling Sad:
   0   I do not feel sad.
   1   I feel sad less than half the time.
   2   I feel sad more than half the time.
   3   I feel sad nearly all of the time.
6. Feeling Irritable:
   0   I do not feel irritable.
   1   I feel irritable less than half the time.
   2   I feel irritable more than half the time.
   3   I feel extremely irritable nearly all of the time.
7. Feeling Anxious or Tense:
   0   I do not feel anxious or tense.
   1   I feel anxious (tense) less than half the time.
   2   I feel anxious (tense) more than half the time.
   3   I feel extremely anxious (tense) nearly all of the time.
8. Response of Your Mood to Good or Desired Events:
   0   My mood brightens to a normal level which lasts for several hours when good events occur.
   1   My mood brightens but I do not feel like my normal self when good events occur.
   2   My mood brightens only somewhat to a rather limited range of desired events.

3. My mood does not brighten at all, even when very good or desired events occur in my life.

9. Mood in Relation to the Time of Day:
   0 There is no regular relationship between my mood and the time of day.
   1 My mood often relates to the time of day because of environmental events (e.g., being alone, working)
   2 In general, my mood is more related to the time of day than to environmental events.
   3 My mood is clearly and predictably better or worse at a particular time each day.
   9A. Is your mood typically worse in the morning, afternoon, or night? (circle one)
   9B. Is your mood variation attributed to the environment? (yes or no) (circle one)

10. The Quality of Your Mood:
   0 The mood (internal feelings) that I experience is very much a normal mood.
   1 My mood is sad, but this sadness is pretty much like the sad mood I would feel if someone close to me died or left.
   2 My mood is sad, but this sadness has a rather different quality to it than the sadness I would feel if someone close to me died or left.
   3 My mood is sad, but this sadness is different from the type of sadness associated with grief or loss.

Please complete either 11 or 12 (not both)

11. Decreased Appetite:
   0 There is no change in my usual appetite.
   1 I eat somewhat less often or lesser amounts of food than usual.
   2 I eat much less than usual and only with personal effort.
   3 I rarely eat within a 24-hour period, and only with extreme personal effort or when others persuade me to eat.

12. Increased Appetite:
   0 There is no change from my usual appetite.
   1 I feel a need to eat more frequently than usual.
   2 I regularly eat more often and/or greater amounts of food than usual.
   3 I feel driven to overeat both at mealtime and between meals.

Please complete either 13 or 14 (not both)

13. Within the Last Two Weeks:
   0 I have not had a change in my weight.
   1 I feel as if I've had a slight weight loss.
   2 I have lost 2 pounds or more.
   3 I have lost 5 pounds or more.

14. Within the Last Two Weeks:
   0 I have not had a change in my weight.
   1 I feel as if I've had a slight weight gain.
   2 I have gained 2 pounds or more.
   3 I have gained 5 pounds or more.

15. Concentration/Decision Making:
   0 There is no change in my usual capacity to concentrate or make decisions.
   1 I occasionally feel indecisive or find that my attention wanders.
   2 Most of the time, I struggle to focus my attention or to make decisions.
   3 I cannot concentrate well enough to read or cannot make even minor decisions.

16. View of Myself:
    0   I see myself as equally worthwhile and deserving as other people.
    1   I am more self-blaming than usual.
    2   I largely believe that I cause problems for others.
    3   I think almost constantly about major and minor defects in myself.
17. View of My Future:
    0   I have an optimistic view of my future.
    1   I am occasionally pessimistic about my future, but for the most part I believe things will get better.
    2   I'm pretty certain that my immediate future (1–2 months) does not hold much promise of good things for me.
    3   I see no hope of anything good happening to me anytime in the future.
18. Thoughts of Death or Suicide:
    0   I do not think of suicide or death.
    1   I feel that life is empty or wonder if it's worth living.
    2   I think of suicide or death several times a week for several minutes.
    3   I think of suicide or death several times a day in some detail, or I have made specific plans for suicide or have actually tried to take my life.
19. General Interest:
    0   There is no change from usual in how interested I am in other people or activities.
    1   I notice that I am less interested in people or activities
    2   I find I have interest in only one or two of my formerly pursued activities.
    3   I have virtually no interest in formerly pursued activities.
20. Energy Level:
    0   There is no change in my usual level of energy.
    1   I get tired more easily than usual.
    2   I have to make a big effort to start or finish my usual daily activities (for example, shopping, homework, cooking or going to work).
    3   I really cannot carry out most of my usual daily activities because I just don't have the energy.
21. Capacity for Pleasure or Enjoyment (excluding sex):
    0   I enjoy pleasurable activities just as much as usual.
    1   I do not feel my usual sense of enjoyment from pleasurable activities.
    2   I rarely get a feeling of pleasure from any activity.
    3   I am unable to get any pleasure or enjoyment from anything.
22. Interest in Sex (Please Rate Interest, not Activity):
    0   I'm just as interested in sex as usual.
    1   My interest in sex is somewhat less than usual or I do not get the same pleasure from sex as I used to.
    2   I have little desire for or rarely derive pleasure from sex.
    3   I have absolutely no interest in or derive no pleasure from sex.
23. Feeling slowed down:
    0   I think, speak, and move at my usual rate of speed.
    1   I find that my thinking is slowed down or my voice sounds dull or flat.
    2   It takes me several seconds to respond to most questions and I'm sure my thinking is slowed.
    3   I am often unable to respond to questions without extreme effort.

24. Feeling restless:
    - 0   I do not feel restless.
    - 1   I'm often fidgety, wring my hands, or need to shift how I am sitting.
    - 2   I have impulses to move about and am quite restless.
    - 3   At times, I am unable to stay seated and need to pace around.
25. Aches and pains:
    - 0   I don't have any feeling of heaviness in my arms or legs and don't have any aches or pains.
    - 1   Sometimes I get headaches or pains in my stomach, back or joints but these pains are only sometimes present and they don't stop me from doing what I need to do.
    - 2   I have these sorts of pains most of the time.
    - 3   These pains are so bad they force me to stop what I am doing.
26. Other bodily symptoms:
    - 0   I don't have any of these symptoms: heart pounding fast, blurred vision, sweating, hot and cold flashes, chest pain, heart turning over in my chest, ringing in my ears, or shaking.
    - 1   I have some of these symptoms but they are mild and are present only sometimes.
    - 2   I have several of these symptoms and they bother me quite a bit.
    - 3   I have several of these symptoms and when they occur I have to stop doing whatever I am doing.
27. Panic/Phobic symptoms:
    - 0   I have no spells of panic or specific fears (phobia) (such as animals or heights).
    - 1   I have mild panic episodes or fears that do not usually change my behavior or stop me from functioning.
    - 2   I have significant panic episodes or fears that force me to change my behavior but do not stop me from functioning.
    - 3   I have panic episodes at least once a week or severe fears that stop me from carrying on my daily activities.
28. Constipation/diarrhea:
    - 0   There is no change in my usual bowel habits.
    - 1   I have intermittent constipation or diarrhea which is mild.
    - 2   I have diarrhea or constipation most of the time but it does not interfere with my day-to-day functioning.
    - 3   I have constipation or diarrhea for which I take medicine or which interferes with my day-to-day activities.
29. Interpersonal Sensitivity:
    - 0   I have not felt easily rejected, slighted, criticized or hurt by others at all.
    - 1   I have occasionally felt rejected, slighted, criticized or hurt by others.
    - 2   I have often felt rejected, slighted, criticized or hurt by others, but these feelings have had only slight effects on my relationships or work.
    - 3   I have often felt rejected, slighted, criticized or hurt by others and these feelings have impaired my relationships and work.
30. Leaden Paralysis/Physical Energy:
    - 0   I have not experienced the physical sensation of feeling weighted down and without physical energy.
    - 1   I have occasionally experienced periods of feeling physically weighted down and without physical energy, but without a negative effect on work, school, or activity level.

2   I feel physically weighted down (without physical energy) more than half the time.
3   I feel physically weighted down (without physical energy) most of the time, several hours per day, several days per week.

Please review this test and write in this space _____ the numbers of the 3 items that were the most difficult to understand.
Which 3 items (questions) were the easiest to understand? _____
Thank you
Range 0–90   Score: _____
©1982, A. John Rush, M.D.   Revised 6/1/88

Medically-Based Emotional Distress Scale

NOTE:	Each interview section begins with a "Skip" question. If the individual reports no problem in that area, the interviewer may skip the rest of the items in that section. However, if the individual reports a problem, or the "equal amounts of both" response, then all questions in that section must be answered.
TIME FRAME:	All questions refer to your feelings during the past week.
SCORING:	As you proceed through this interview, two types of questions are used: FREQUENCY (How Often?) and INTENSITY (How Much?). Use the following rating scales for the different questions.

HOW OFTEN?
0 = Never
1 = Rarely
2 = Sometimes
3 = Frequently
4 = Always

HOW MUCH?
0 = Not at all
1 = A little bit
2 = Somewhat
3 = A fair amount
4 = Very much

DEPRESSED
CHEERFUL
EQUAL

How has your mood been this past week; have you been feeling fairly depressed or fairly cheerful ... or equal amounts of both?

0 1 2 3 4	In the last week, how often have you felt depressed?
0 1 2 3 4	How often have you felt like crying?
0 1 2 3 4	How often have you actually cried?
0 1 2 3 4	How often have you felt sorry for yourself?
0 1 2 3 4	How often have you felt that nothing matters anymore?
0 1 2 3 4	When you have felt very sad, how often did you hold it in and keep your feelings to yourself?
0 1 2 3 4	How often have you felt sad because of your injury?

IRRITABLE
EASY-GOING
BOTH

Lately, would you say you've been feeling irritable or easy-going ... or equal amounts of both?

0 1 2 3 4	In the past week how often have you felt angry/irritable?
0 1 2 3 4	How often have people bothered you just by being around you?
0 1 2 3 4	How often have you felt like a powder keg ready to explode?
0 1 2 3 4	How often do you feel others have better luck than you?
0 1 2 3 4	When you are feeling low, how often do you take it out on other people?
0 1 2 3 4	How often have you felt like yelling or screaming at people?
0 1 2 3 4	How often have you really lost your temper and shouted or snapped at others?
0 1 2 3 4	How often do you get angry with yourself or call yourself names?

ENJOY
EMPTY
DIFFERENT

Are there still some things in your life you really enjoy or has everything seemed empty lately ... or does everything just seem different?

0 1 2 3 4	How often do you feel nothing matters to you anymore?

0 1 2 3 4   When you feel very sad, how often do you try to do some things that you enjoy doing?

Please list one activity you really enjoyed doing before your injury, and that you can still do?

_____

0 1 2 3 4   How often have you done this activity during the last week?
0 1 2 3 4   If you did it now, how much would you enjoy it?
0 1 2 3 4   How much do you enjoy: Having a pleasant chat with a friend
0 1 2 3 4   Watching a good movie on TV
0 1 2 3 4   Getting a compliment from someone
0 1 2 3 4   Giving someone else a compliment
0 1 2 3 4   Winning a small amount in a lottery.

OTHERS
ALONE
BOTH   During this past week, have you enjoyed spending time with other people or did you just want everyone to leave you alone ... or equal amounts of both?

0 1 2 3 4   How often do you feel bettter if you are with other people?
0 1 2 3 4   How often do you discuss your feelings with your friends?
0 1 2 3 4   How much does your mood improve when you're with friends?
0 1 2 3 4   How often do you feel lonely even when you're with others?
0 1 2 3 4   How often do you wish you could avoid other people?
0 1 2 3 4   How often do you feel close to other people?
0 1 2 3 4   How much do you feel isolated from others?
0 1 2 3 4   How often can you feel companionship when you want it?

BETTER
WORSE
NO DIFFERENCE   When you think about your past, does it make you feel better or worse ... or doesn't it make a difference?

0 1 2 3 4   How often do you think about the way things were before your injury?
0 1 2 3 4   How often do you become depressed when you think about your injury?
0 1 2 3 4   How much do you blame yourself for your injury?
0 1 2 3 4   How much do you think you could have avoided what happened?
0 1 2 3 4   How often do you ask yourself "Why did this happen to me?"

PLEASANT
UPSETTING
BOTH   Do you tend to think more about pleasant things or upsetting things ... or equal amounts of both?

0 1 2 3 4   How often can you find something to do to take your mind off your problems?
0 1 2 3 4   How often are you able to just ignore your problems?
0 1 2 3 4   How often do you feel your life has been destroyed?
0 1 2 3 4   How often do you tend to think about your problems over and over again?
0 1 2 3 4   When you feel very sad, how often do you try to focus on the good things you still have in your life?
0 1 2 3 4   How often do you tell yourself you can handle any problems that happen to you?

0 1 2 3 4   How often do you tell yourself you can make the best of your situation?

WORRY   When you think about your future, do you worry about how things
PLAN   will be or do you plan what you'd like to do ... or equal amounts of
BOTH   planning and worrying?

0 1 2 3 4   How often do you tell yourself things will be better in the future?

0 1 2 3 4   How much pleasantness can you see ahead of you?

0 1 2 3 4   How happy do you think you will be in the future?

0 1 2 3 4   How much do you feel life is still worth living?

0 1 2 3 4   How often do you tell yourself life will never be the same again?

0 1 2 3 4   How often do you live one day at a time and try to not think about the future?

0 1 2 3 4   How often do you tell yourself you will still be able to do things you enjoy?

0 1 2 3 4   How much hope do you have for the future?

Pleasant Events Schedule

[Reprinted with permission from the author and publisher (© 1997, the American Psychological Association)]

This schedule is designed to find out about the things you have enjoyed during the past month. The schedule contains a list of events or activities which people sometimes enjoy. You will be asked to go over the list twice, the first time rating each event on how many times it has happened in the past month and the second time rating each event on how pleasant it has been for you. There are no right or wrong answers.

Please rate every event. Work quickly; there are many items and you will not be asked to make fine distinctions on your ratings. The schedule should take about an hour to complete. Please make your ratings on the answer sheets provided. You should find two of them. Use the answer sheet labeled "A" to answer Question A; use the sheet labeled "B" to answer Question B. When you mark the answer sheet, be very careful to completely fill the little box corresponding to your rating. Use only a soft pencil, and erase completely any answers you have changed.

Directions—Question A

On the following pages you will find a list of activities, events, and experiences. HOW OFTEN HAVE THESE EVENTS HAPPENED IN YOUR LIFE IN THE PAST MONTH? Please answer this question by rating each item on the following scale:

0 = This has not happened in the past 30 days.
1 = This has happened *a few times* (1 to 6) in the past 30 days.
2 = This has happened *often* (7 or more) in the past 30 days.

Place your rating for each item on the answer sheet labeled "A." Here is an example:

Item number 1 is "Being in the country." Suppose you have been in the country three times during the past 30 days. Then you would mark a "1" on the answer sheet in the row of boxes for item number 1. On the answer sheet "A" your mark would look like this:

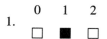

Important: Some items will list *more than one event*; for these items, mark how often you have done *any* of the listed events. For example, item number 12 is "Doing art work (painting, sculpture, drawing, movie-making, etc.)." You should rate item 12 on how often you have done *any* form of art work in the past month.

Since this list contains events that might happen to a wide variety of people, you may find that many of the events have not happened to you in the past 30 days. It is not expected that anyone will have done all of these things in the past one month.

Now turn the page and begin.

1. Being in the country
2. Wearing expensive or formal clothes
3. Making contributions to religious, charitable, or other groups
4. Talking about sports
5. Meeting someone new of the same sex
6. Taking tests when well prepared
7. Going to a rock concert
8. Playing baseball or softball
9. Planning trips or vacations
10. Buying things for myself
11. Being at the beach

12. Doing art work (painting, sculpture, drawing, movie-making, etc.)
13. Rock climbing or mountaineering
14. Reading the Scriptures or other sacred work
15. Playing golf
16. Taking part in military activities
17. Re-arranging or redecorating my room or house
18. Going naked
19. Going to a sports event
20. Reading a "How to Do It" book or article
21. Going to the races (horse, car, boat, etc.)
22. Reading stories, novels, poems, or plays
23. Going to a bar, tavern, club, etc.
24. Going to lectures or hearing speakers
25. Driving skillfully
26. Breathing clean air
27. Thinking up or arranging songs or music
28. Getting drunk
29. Saying something clearly
30. Boating (canoeing, kayaking, motorboating, sailing, etc.)
31. Pleasing my parents
32. Restoring antiques, refinishing furniture, etc.
33. Watching TV
34. Talking to myself
35. Camping
36. Working in politics
37. Working on machines (cars, bikes, motorcycles, tractors, etc.)
38. Thinking about something good in the future
39. Playing cards
40. Completing a difficult task
41. Laughing
42. Solving a problem, puzzle, crossword, etc.
43. Being at weddings, baptisms, confirmations, etc.
44. Criticizing someone
45. Shaving
46. Having lunch with friends or associates
47. Taking powerful drugs
48. Playing tennis
49. Taking a shower
50. Driving long distances
51. Woodworking, carpentry
52. Writing stories, novels, plays or poetry
53. Being with animals
54. Riding in an airplane
55. Exploring (hiking away from known routes, spelunking, etc.)
56. Having a frank and open discussion
57. Singing in a group
58. Thinking about myself or my problems
59. Working on a job
60. Going to a party
61. Going to church functions (socials, classes, bazaars, etc.)
62. Speaking a foreign language
63. Going to service, civic, or social club meetings
64. Going to a business meeting or convention
65. Being in a sporty or expensive car
66. Playing a musical instrument
67. Making snacks
68. Snow skiing
69. Being helped
70. Wearing informal clothes
71. Combing or brushing my hair
72. Acting
73. Taking a nap
74. Being with friends
75. Canning, freezing, making preserves, etc.
76. Driving fast
77. Solving a personal problem
78. Being in a city
79. Taking a bath
80. Singing to myself
81. Making food or crafts to sell or give away
82. Playing pool or billiards
83. Being with my grandchildren
84. Playing chess or checkers
85. Doing craft work (pottery, jewelry, leather, beads, weaving, etc.)
86. Weighing myself
87. Scratching myself
88. Putting on make-up, fixing my hair, etc.
89. Designing or drafting
90. Visiting people who are sick, shut in, or in trouble
91. Cheering, rooting
92. Bowling
93. Being popular at a gathering
94. Watching wild animals
95. Having an original idea
96. Gardening, landscaping, or doing yard work
97. Shoplifting
98. Reading essays or technical, academic, or professional literature
99. Wearing new clothes
100. Dancing
101. Sitting in the sun
102. Riding a motorcycle
103. Just sitting and thinking
104. Social drinking
105. Seeing good things happen to my family or friends
106. Going to a fair, carnival, circus, zoo, or amusement park
107. Talking about philosophy or religion
108. Gambling
109. Planning or organizing something
110. Smoking marijuana
111. Having a drink by myself
112. Listening to the sounds of nature
113. Dating, courting, etc.
114. Having a lively talk
115. Racing in a car, motorcycle, boat, etc.
116. Listening to the radio
117. Having friends come to visit
118. Playing in a sporting competition
119. Introducing people who I think would like each other

120. Giving gifts
121. Going to school or governmental meetings, court sessions, etc.
122. Getting massages or backrubs
123. Getting letters, cards, or notes
124. Watching the sky, clouds, or a storm
125. Going on outings (to the park, a picnic or a barbecue, etc.)
126. Playing basketball
127. Buying something for my family
128. Photography
129. Giving a speech or lecture
130. Reading maps
131. Gathering natural objects (wild foods or fruit, rocks, driftwood, etc.)
132. Working on my finances
133. Wearing clean clothes
134. Making a major purchase or investment (car, appliance, house, stocks, etc.)
135. Helping someone
136. Being in the mountains
137. Getting a job advancement (being promoted, given a raise, or offered a better job, accepted into a better school, etc.)
138. Hearing jokes
139. Winning a bet
140. Talking about my children or grandchildren
141. Meeting someone new of the opposite sex
142. Going to a revival or crusade
143. Talking about my health
144. Seeing beautiful scenery
145. Eating good meals
146. Improving my health (having my teeth fixed, getting new glasses, changing my diet, etc.)
147. Being downtown
148. Wrestling or boxing
149. Hunting or shooting
150. Playing in a musical group
151. Hiking
152. Going to a museum or exhibit
153. Writing papers, essays, articles, reports, memos, etc.
154. Doing a job well
155. Having spare time
156. Fishing
157. Loaning something
158. Being noticed as sexually attractive
159. Pleasing employers, teachers, etc.
160. Counseling someone
161. Going to a health club, sauna bath, etc.
162. Having someone criticize me
163. Learning to do something new
164. Going to a "Drive-in" (Dairy Queen, McDonald's, etc.)
165. Complimenting or praising someone
166. Thinking about people I like
167. Being at a fraternity or sorority
168. Taking revenge on someone
169. Being with my parents
170. Horseback riding
171. Protesting social, political, or environmental conditions
172. Talking on the telephone
173. Having daydreams
174. Kicking leaves, sand, pebbles, etc.
175. Playing lawn sports (badminton, croquet, shuffleboard, horseshoes, etc.)
176. Going to school reunions, alumni meetings, etc.
177. Seeing famous people
178. Going to the movies
179. Kissing
180. Being alone
181. Budgeting my time
182. Cooking meals
183. Being praised by people I admire
184. Outwitting a "superior"
185. Feeling the presence of the Lord in my life
186. Doing a project in my own way
187. Doing "odd jobs" around the house
188. Crying
189. Being told I am needed
190. Being at a family reunion or get-together
191. Giving a party or get-together
192. Washing my hair
193. Coaching someone
194. Going to a restaurant
195. Seeing or smelling a flower or plant
196. Being invited out
197. Receiving honors (civic, military, etc.)
198. Using cologne, perfume, or aftershave
199. Having someone agree with me
200. Reminiscing, talking about old times
201. Getting up early in the morning
202. Having peace and quiet
203. Doing experiments or other scientific work
204. Visiting friends
205. Writing a diary
206. Playing football
207. Being counseled
208. Saying prayers
209. Giving massages or backrubs
210. Hitchhiking
211. Meditating or doing yoga
212. Seeing a fight
213. Doing favors for people
214. Talking to people on the job or in class
215. Being relaxed
216. Being asked for my help or advice
217. Thinking about other people's problems
218. Playing board games (Monopoly, Scrabble, etc.)
219. Sleeping soundly at night
220. Doing heavy outdoor work (cutting or chopping wood, clearing land, farm work, etc.)
221. Reading the newspaper
222. Shocking people, swearing, making obscene gestures, etc.

223. Snowmobiling or dune-buggy riding
224. Being in a body-awareness, sensitivity encounter, therapy, or "rap" group
225. Dreaming at night
226. Playing ping pong
227. Brushing my teeth
228. Swimming
229. Being in a fight
230. Running, jogging, or doing gymnastic, fitness, or field exercises
231. Walking barefoot
232. Playing frisbee or catch
233. Doing housework or laundry; cleaning things
234. Being with my roommate
235. Listening to music
236. Arguing
237. Knitting, crocheting, embroidery, or fancy needle-work
238. Petting, necking
239. Amusing people
240. Talking about sex
241. Going to a barber or beautician
242. Having house guests
243. Being with someone I love
244. Reading magazines
245. Sleeping late
246. Starting a new project
247. Being stubborn
248. Having sexual relations with a partner of the opposite sex
249. Having other sexual satisfactions
250. Going to the library
251. Playing soccer, rugby, hockey, lacrosse, etc.
252. Preparing a new or special food
253. Birdwatching
254. Shopping
255. Watching people
256. Building or watching a fire
257. Winning an argument
258. Selling or trading something
259. Finishing a project or task
260. Confessing or apologizing
261. Repairing things
262. Working with others as a team
263. Bicycling
264. Telling people what to do
265. Being with happy people
266. Playing party games
267. Writing letters, cards, or notes
268. Talking about politics or public affairs
269. Asking for help or advice
270. Going to banquets, luncheons, potlucks, etc.
271. Talking about my hobby or special interest
272. Watching attractive women or men
273. Smiling at people
274. Playing in sand, a stream, the grass, etc.
275. Talking about other people
276. Being with my husband or wife
277. Having people show interest in what I have said
278. Going on field trips, nature walks, etc.
279. Expressing my love to someone
280. Smoking tobacco
281. Caring for houseplants
282. Having coffee, tea, a Coke, etc., with friends
283. Taking a walk
284. Collecting things
285. Playing handball, paddleball, squash, etc.
286. Sewing
287. Suffering for a good cause
288. Remembering a departed friend or loved one, visiting the cemetery
289. Doing things with children
290. Beachcombing
291. Being complimented or told I have done well
292. Being told I am loved
293. Eating snacks
294. Staying up late
295. Having family members or friends do something that makes me proud of them
296. Being with my children
297. Going to auctions, garage sales, etc.
298. Thinking about an interesting question
299. Doing volunteer work; working on community service projects
300. Water skiing, surfing, scuba diving
301. Receiving money
302. Defending or protecting someone; stopping fraud or abuse
303. Hearing a good sermon
304. Picking up a hitchhiker
305. Winning a competition
306. Making a new friend
307. Talking about my job or school
308. Reading cartoons, comic strips, or comic books
309. Borrowing something
310. Traveling with a group
311. Seeing old friends
312. Teaching someone
313. Using my strength
314. Traveling
315. Going to office parties or departmental get-togethers
316. Attending a concert, opera, or ballet
317. Playing with pets
318. Going to a play
319. Looking at the stars or moon
320. Being coached

STOP

If you have just gone through the list for the first time, go to the next page and follow the directions for Question B.

If you have just finished answering Question B you have completed the test.

Directions—Question B

Now please go over the list once again. This time the question is: HOW PLEASANT, ENJOYABLE, OR REWARDING WAS EACH EVENT DURING THE PAST MONTH? Please answer this question by rating each event on the following scale:

0 = This was *not* pleasant. (Use this rating for events which were either neutral or unpleasant.)

1 = This was *somewhat* pleasant. (Use this rating for events which were mildly or moderately pleasant.)

2 = This was *very* pleasant. (Use this rating for events which were strongly or extremely pleasant.)

Important: If an event has happened to you *more than once* in the past month, try to rate roughly how pleasant it was *on the average. If an event has not happened to you during the past month, then rate it according to how much fun you think it would have been.* When an item lists *more than one event*, rate it on the events *you have actually done*. (If you haven't done any of the events in such an item, give it the average rating of the events in that item which you would like to have done.)

Place your rating for each event on the answer sheet labeled "B." Here is an example.:

Event number 1 is "Being in the country." Suppose that each time you were in the country in the past 30 days you enjoyed it a great deal. Then you would rate this event "2" since it was "very pleasant." On answer sheet "B" your mark would look like this:

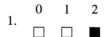

The list of items may have some events which you would not enjoy. The list was made for a wide variety of people, and it is not expected that one person would enjoy them all.

Now go back to the list of events, start with item 1, and go through the entire list rating each event on *roughly how pleasant it was (or would have been) during the past 30 days.* Please be sure that you rate each item and that your marks completely fill the boxes on the answer sheet.

Positive and Negative Affect Scales

Reprinted with permission from the authors and the publisher, © by the American Psychological Association.

This scale consists of a number of words that describe feelings and emotions. Read each item and then mark the appropriate answer in the space next to the word. Indicate to what extent (INSERT APPROPRIATE TIME INSTRUCTIONS HERE). Use the following scale to record your answers.

1	2	3	4	5
very slightly or not at all	a little	moderately	quite a bit	extremely

_____ interested	_____ irritable
_____ distressed	_____ alert
_____ excited	_____ ashamed
_____ upset	_____ inspired
_____ strong	_____ nervous
_____ guilty	_____ determined
_____ scared	_____ attentive
_____ hostile	_____ jittery
_____ enthusiastic	_____ active
_____ proud	_____ afraid

Various time instructions:

Moment	(You feel this way right now, that is, at the present moment)
Today	(You have felt this way today)
Past few days	(You have felt this way during the past few days)
Week	(You have felt this way during the past week)
Past few weeks	(You have felt this way during the past few weeks)
Year	(You have felt this way during the past year)
General	(You generally feel this way, that is, how you feel on the average).

Raskin Three-Area Severity of Depression Scale

Reprinted with permission of author.

Severity of Depression: **To what extent does the individual evidence depression or despondency in verbal report, behavior, and secondary symptoms of depression?**

Cues	Very Much	Consider-ably	Moder-ately	Some-what	Not At All
Verbal Report Says he feels blue; talks of feeling helpless, or worthless; complains of loss of interest; may wish he were dead; reports crying spells	5	4	3	2	1
Behavior Looks sad; cries easily; speaks in a sad voice; appears slowed down; lacking in energy.	5	4	3	2	1
Secondary Symptoms of Depression Insomnia, G.I. complaints; dry mouth; history of recent suicide attempt; lack of appetite; difficulty concentrating or remembering	5	4	3	2	1
TOTAL Add the scale points checked for severity of depression in verbal report, behavior and secondary symptoms of depression					

TOTAL: _____

Revised Grief Experience Inventory

Reprinted with permission of Dr. Elise Lev. Note that permission to reproduce this measure is based on the researcher's willingness to send Dr. Lev a copy of the abstract for their work using the measure.

Below are a series of general statements. You are to indicate how much you agree or disagree with them. Be as honest as possible. Remember, there are no right or wrong answers to these questions.

Read each item and decide quickly how you feel about it; then circle the number of the item that best describes your feelings. Put down your first impressions. Please answer <u>every</u> item.

	Agreement			Disagreement		
	Slight	**moderate**	**strong**	**strong**	**moderate**	**slight**
1. I tend to be more irritable with others since the death of my loved one.	1	2	3	4	5	6
2. I frequently experience angry feelings.	1	2	3	4	5	6
3. My arms and legs feel very heavy.	1	2	3	4	5	6
4. I have feelings of guilt because I was spared and the deceased was taken.	1	2	3	4	5	6
5. I feel lost and helpless.	1	2	3	4	5	6
6. I have had frequent headaches since the death.	1	2	3	4	5	6
7. I cry easily.	1	2	3	4	5	6
8. Concentrating on things is difficult.	1	2	3	4	5	6
9. I feel extremely anxious and unsettled.	1	2	3	4	5	6
10. Sometimes I have a strong desire to scream.	1	2	3	4	5	6
11. Life has lost its meaning for me.	1	2	3	4	5	6
12. I am not feeling healthy.	1	2	3	4	5	6
13. I frequently feel depressed.	1	2	3	4	5	6
14. I have the feeling that I am watching myself go through the motions of living.	1	2	3	4	5	6
15. Life seems empty and barren.	1	2	3	4	5	6
16. I have frequent mood changes.	1	2	3	4	5	6

17. Small problems seem overwhelming.	1	2	3	4	5	6
18. I have lost my appetite.	1	2	3	4	5	6
19. I seem to have lost my energy.	1	2	3	4	5	6
20. I seem to have lost my self-confidence.	1	2	3	4	5	6
21. I am usually unhappy.	1	2	3	4	5	6
22. I am awake most of the night.	1	2	3	4	5	6

Rimon's Brief Depression Scale

[Keltikangas-Järvinen & Rimon, 1987 (reprinted with permission)]

(Note that the testing is carried out by interviewing the patient, not by applying a self-report technique)

1. Have you noticed a recent decrease in your interest in your work and/or hobbies?
   - 0 = no
   - 1 = a little
   - 2 = moderate
   - 3 = severe

2. Has your ability to make decisions and/or to concentrate been impaired lately?
   - 0 = no
   - 1 = a little
   - 2 = moderately
   - 3 = severely

3. Have you recently observed any changes in your appetite and/or in your general physical well-being (for example, abnormal tiredness or headache), or have you experienced unusual pains and/or diminished sexual interest?
   - 0 = no
   - 1 = a little
   - 2 = moderate
   - 3 = severe

4. Have you recently observed any change in your general appearance?
   - 0 = no
   - 1 = a little
   - 2 = moderate
   - 3 = severe

5. Have you recently consumed alcohol more than usual, and/or taken drugs that have affected your nerves, for example pain killers, sleeping pills, or drugs to decrease anxiety?
   - 0 = no
   - 1 = a little
   - 2 = moderately
   - 3 = severely

6. Have you recently blamed yourself for your thoughts or reactions, or had thoughts of not wanting to live?
   - 0 = no
   - 1 = a little
   - 2 = moderate
   - 3 = severe

7. Have you recently been unusually irritable, tense, sensitive or had crying spells?
   - 0 = no
   - 1 = a little
   - 2 = moderate
   - 3 = severe

Self-Control Schedule

[Reprinted with permission from the author and publisher (1980, Association for the Advancement of Behavior Therapy).]

Directions: Indicate how characteristic or descriptive each of the following statements is of you by using the code given below:

+3 very characteristic of me, extremely descriptive
+2 rather characteristic of me, quite descriptive
+1 somewhat characteristic of me, slightly descriptive
−1 somewhat uncharacteristic of me, slightly undescriptive
−2 rather uncharacteristic of me, quite undescriptive
−3 very uncharacteristic of me, extremely nondescriptive

1. When I do a boring job, I think about the less boring parts of the job and the reward that I will receive once I am finished.
2. When I have to do something that is anxiety arousing for me, I try to visualize how I will overcome my anxieties while doing it.
3. Often by changing my way of thinking I am able to change my feelings about almost everything.
4. I often find it difficult to overcome my feelings of nervousness and tension without any outside help.*
5. When I am feeling depressed I try to think about pleasant events.
6. I cannot avoid thinking about mistakes I have made in the past.*
7. When I am faced with a difficult problem, I try to approach its solution in a systematic way.
8. I usually do my duties quicker when somebody is pressuring me.*
9. When I am faced with a difficult decision, I prefer to postpone making a decision even if all the facts are at my disposal.*
10. When I find that I have difficulties in concentrating on my reading, I look for ways to increase my concentration.
11. When I plan to work, I remove all the things that are not relevant to my work.
12. When I try to get rid of a bad habit, I first try to find out all the factors that maintain this habit.
13. When an unpleasant thought is bothering me, I try to think about something pleasant.
14. If I would smoke two packages of cigarettes a day, I probably would need outside help to stop smoking.*
15. When I am in a low mood, I try to act cheerful so my mood will change.
16. If I had the pills with me, I would take a tranquilizer whenever I felt tense and nervous.
17. When I am depressed, I try to keep myself busy with things that I like.
18. I tend to postpone unpleasant duties even if I could perform them immediately.*
19. I need outside help to get rid of some of my bad habits.*
20. When I find it difficult to settle down and do a certain job, I look for ways to help me settle down.
21. Although it makes me feel bad, I cannot avoid thinking about all kinds of possible catastrophes in the future.*

22. First of all I prefer to finish a job that I have to do and then start doing the things I really like.
23. When I feel pain in a certain part of my body, I try not to think about it.
24. My self-esteem increases once I am able to overcome a bad habit.
25. In order to overcome bad feelings that accompany failure, I often tell myself that is it not so catastrophic and that I can do something about it.
26. When I feel that I am too impulsive, I tell myself "stop and think before you do anything."
27. Even when I am terribly angry at somebody, I consider my actions very carefully.
28. Facing the need to make a decision, I usually find out all the possible alternatives instead of deciding quickly and spontaneously.
29. Usually I do first the things I really like to do even if there are more urgent things to do.*
30. When I realize that I cannot help but be late for an important meeting, I tell myself to keep calm.
31. When I feel pain in my body, I try to divert my thoughts from it.
32. I usually plan my work when faced with a number of things to do.
33. When I am short of money, I decide to record all my expenses in order to plan more carefully for the future.
34. If I find it difficult to concentrate on a certain job, I divide the job into smaller segments.
35. Quite often I cannot overcome unpleasant thoughts that bother me.*
36. Once I am hungry and unable to eat, I try to divert my thoughts away from my stomach or try to imagine that I am satisfied.

*Reverse items.

Social Resourcefulness Scale

We are interested in how people take care of their needs, for example, getting advice, asking for money, or having someone run errands for them. For each of the following statements, place a check in the box indicating how often you do each of these things when you need help. Some of the statements may be similar, but it is important that you read and answer each statement. Please remember that there are no right or wrong answers.

When you need help, how often do you ...

	Always do it	Usually do it	Sometimes do it	Rarely do it	Never do it
1. tell someone how their help makes you feel?	☐	☐	☐	☐	☐
2. look for professionals who could help you?	☐	☐	☐	☐	☐
3. remind yourself that everybody needs help?	☐	☐	☐	☐	☐
4. tell yourself that receiving help is not a sign of weakness?	☐	☐	☐	☐	☐
5. tell someone who was **not** very helpful how they could be more helpful?	☐	☐	☐	☐	☐
6. divide your requests for help among friends and family members?	☐	☐	☐	☐	☐
7. try to change what a helper is doing if you think it will serve your needs better?	☐	☐	☐	☐	☐
8. let friends or family members choose which of your needs they want to help with?	☐	☐	☐	☐	☐
9. try to think of as many friends and family members as possible who could help you?	☐	☐	☐	☐	☐
10. tell a helper exactly when, where, and what you want them to do?	☐	☐	☐	☐	☐
11. remind yourself that it is OK to receive help?	☐	☐	☐	☐	☐
12. accept the help you need?	☐	☐	☐	☐	☐
13. try to keep the favors you give and the favors you receive about equal?	☐	☐	☐	☐	☐
14. try to keep track of who has done you favors?	☐	☐	☐	☐	☐
15. remind someone to do something they said they would do for you?	☐	☐	☐	☐	☐

16. suggest a person who is trying to help you how they could help you better? ☐ ☐ ☐ ☐ ☐

17. avoid asking the same people for help over and over? ☐ ☐ ☐ ☐ ☐

18. remind yourself that those who help you now may need your help in the future? ☐ ☐ ☐ ☐ ☐

19. remind yourself that it is OK to ask for help? ☐ ☐ ☐ ☐ ☐

20. look for government, religious, or other charitable organizations that could give you help? ☐ ☐ ☐ ☐ ☐

Sociotropy Autonomy Scale

INSTRUCTIONS
Please indicate what percentages of the time each of the statements below applies to you by using the scale to the left of the items. Choose the percentage that comes closest to how often the item describes you.

0%	25%	50%	75%	100%	
( )	( )	( )	( )	( )	1. I feel I have to be nice to other people.
( )	( )	( )	( )	( )	2. It is important to me to be free and independent.
( )	( )	( )	( )	( )	3. It is more important that I know I've done a good job than having others know it.
( )	( )	( )	( )	( )	4. Being able to share experiences with other people makes them much more enjoyable for me.
( )	( )	( )	( )	( )	5. I am afraid of hurting other people's feelings.
( )	( )	( )	( )	( )	6. It bothers me when people try to direct my behavior or activity.
( )	( )	( )	( )	( )	7. I find it difficult to say "no" to people.
( )	( )	( )	( )	( )	8. I feel bad if I do not have some social plans for the weekend.
( )	( )	( )	( )	( )	9. I prize being a unique individual more than being a member of a group.
( )	( )	( )	( )	( )	10. When I feel sick, I like to be left alone.
( )	( )	( )	( )	( )	11. I am concerned that if people know my faults or weaknesses they would not like me.
( )	( )	( )	( )	( )	12. If I think I am right about something, I feel comfortable expressing myself even if others don't like it.
( )	( )	( )	( )	( )	13. When visiting people, I get fidgety when sitting around talking and would rather get up and do something.
( )	( )	( )	( )	( )	14. It is more important to meet your own objectives on a task than to meet another person's objectives.
( )	( )	( )	( )	( )	15. I do things that are not in my best interest in order to please others.
( )	( )	( )	( )	( )	16. I like to take long walks by myself.
( )	( )	( )	( )	( )	17. I am more concerned that people like me than I am with important achievements.
( )	( )	( )	( )	( )	18. I would be uncomfortable dining out in a restaurant by myself.
( )	( )	( )	( )	( )	19. I don't enjoy what I am doing when I don't feel that someone in my life really cares about me.

0%	25%	50%	75%	100%	
( )	( )	( )	( )	( )	20. I am not influenced by others in what I decide to do.
( )	( )	( )	( )	( )	21. It is very important that I feel free to get up and go wherever I want.
( )	( )	( )	( )	( )	22. I value work accomplishments more than I value making friends.
( )	( )	( )	( )	( )	23. I find it is of importance to be in control of my emotions.
( )	( )	( )	( )	( )	24. I get uncomfortable when I am not sure how I am expected to behave in the presence of other people.
( )	( )	( )	( )	( )	25. I feel more comfortable helping others than receiving help.
( )	( )	( )	( )	( )	26. It would not be much fun for me to travel to a new place all alone.
( )	( )	( )	( )	( )	27. If a friend has not called for a while, I get worried that he or she has forgotten me.
( )	( )	( )	( )	( )	28. It is more important to be active and doing things than having close relations with other people.
( )	( )	( )	( )	( )	29. I get uncomfortable around a person who does not clearly like me.
( )	( )	( )	( )	( )	30. If a goal is important to me, I will pursue it even if it may make other people uncomfortable.
( )	( )	( )	( )	( )	31. I find it difficult to be separated from people I love.
( )	( )	( )	( )	( )	32. When I achieve a goal I get more satisfaction from reaching the goal than from any praise I might get.
( )	( )	( )	( )	( )	33. I censor what I say because I am concerned that the other person may disapprove or disagree.
( )	( )	( )	( )	( )	34. I get lonely when I am home by myself at night.
( )	( )	( )	( )	( )	35. I often find myself thinking about friends or family.
( )	( )	( )	( )	( )	36. I prefer to make my own plans, so I am not controlled by others.
( )	( )	( )	( )	( )	37. I can comfortably be by myself all day without feeling a need to have someone around.
( )	( )	( )	( )	( )	38. If someone criticizes my appearance, I feel I am not attractive to other people.
( )	( )	( )	( )	( )	39. It is more important to get a job done than to worry about people's reactions.
( )	( )	( )	( )	( )	40. I like to spend my free time with others.

0%	25%	50%	75%	100%		
( )	( )	( )	( )	( )	41.	I don't like to answer personal questions because they feel like an invasion of my privacy.
( )	( )	( )	( )	( )	42.	When I have a problem, I like to go off on my own and think it through rather than being influenced by others.
( )	( )	( )	( )	( )	43.	In relationships, people often are too demanding of each other.
( )	( )	( )	( )	( )	44.	I am uneasy when I cannot tell whether or not someone I've met likes me.
( )	( )	( )	( )	( )	45.	I set my own standards and goals for myself rather than accepting those of other people.
( )	( )	( )	( )	( )	46.	I am more apologetic to others than I need to be.
( )	( )	( )	( )	( )	47.	It is important for me to be liked and approved of by others.
( )	( )	( )	( )	( )	48.	I enjoy accomplishing things more than being given credit for them.
( )	( )	( )	( )	( )	49.	Having close bonds with other people makes me feel secure.
( )	( )	( )	( )	( )	50.	When I am with other people, I look for signs whether or not they like being with me.
( )	( )	( )	( )	( )	51.	I like to go off on my own, exploring new places without other people.
( )	( )	( )	( )	( )	52.	If I think somebody may be upset at me, I want to apologize.
( )	( )	( )	( )	( )	53.	I like to be certain that there is somebody close I can contact in case something unpleasant happens to me.
( )	( )	( )	( )	( )	54.	I feel confined when I have to sit through a long meeting.
( )	( )	( )	( )	( )	55.	I don't like people to invade my privacy.
( )	( )	( )	( )	( )	56.	I feel uncomfortable being a nonconformist.
( )	( )	( )	( )	( )	57.	The worst part about being in jail would be not being able to move around freely.
( )	( )	( )	( )	( )	58.	The worst part about growing old is being left alone.
( )	( )	( )	( )	( )	59.	I worry that somebody I love will die.
( )	( )	( )	( )	( )	60.	The possibility of being rejected by others for standing up for my rights would not stop me.

Unpleasant Events Schedule

[Reprinted with permission from the author and publisher (© 1983, American Psychological Association)]

This schedule is designed to find out about the things you have disliked during the past month. The schedule contains a list of events or activities which people sometimes find unpleasant, painful, disturbing, annoying, upsetting, or otherwise aversive. You will be asked to go over the list twice, the first time rating each event on how many times it has happened in the past month and the second time rating each event on how unpleasant it has been for you. There are no right or wrong answers.

Please rate every event. Work quickly; there are many items and you will not be asked to make fine distinctions on your ratings. The schedule should take about an hour to complete. Please make your ratings on the answer sheets provided. You should find two of them. Use the answer sheet labeled "A" to answer Question A; use the sheet labeled "B" to answer Question B. When you mark the answer sheet, be very careful to *completely* fill the little box corresponding to your rating. Use only a soft pencil, and erase completely any answers you have changed.

Directions—Question A

On the following pages you will find a list of activities, events, and experiences. HOW OFTEN HAVE THESE EVENTS HAPPENED IN YOUR LIFE IN THE PAST MONTH? Please answer this question by rating each item on the following scale:

0 = This has not happened in the past 30 days.
1 = This has happened *a few times* (1 to 6) in the past 30 days.
2 = This has happened *often* (7 or more) in the past 30 days.

Place your rating for each item on the answer sheets labeled "A-1" and "A-2." Here is an example:

Item number 1 is "Listening to people complain." If this happened to you three times during the past 30 days, then you would mark a "2" on the answer sheet in the row of boxes for item number 1. On the answer sheet "A" your mark would look like this:

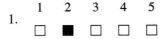

Important: Some items will list *more than one event*; for these items, mark how often you have done *any* of the listed events. For example, item number 12 is "Doing art work (painting, sculpture, drawing, movie-making, etc.)." You should rate item 12 on how often you have done *any* form of art work in the past month.

Since this list contains events that might happen to a wide variety of people, you may find that many of the events have not happened to you in the past 30 days. It is not expected that anyone will have done all of these things in the past one month.

Now turn the page and begin!

1. Listening to people complain.
2. Being talked down to.
3. Being in very hot weather.
4. Having to obtain the assistance of a lawyer.
5. Talking with an unpleasant person (stubborn, unreasonable, aggressive, conceited, etc.).

6. Being alone.
7. Having a relative or friend living in unsatisfactory surroundings.
8. Being hungry or thirsty.
9. Having my belongings stolen.
10. Getting separated or divorced from my spouse.
11. Having someone disagree with me.
12. Change of residence (to different city or area).
13. Being in a situation where I don't know many people.
14. Being asked something I could not, or did not want to answer.
15. Being with sad people.
16. Having family members or friends do something I disapprove of (giving up religious training, dropping out of school, drinking, taking drugs, etc.).
17. Cooking things that don't turn out right (burning toast, too much seasoning, etc.).
18. Being expected to take on more work.
19. Automotive mishaps (car won't start, blowout, etc.).
20. Living in a polluted (dirty, crowded) area.
21. Being with people who don't share my interests.
22. Being awakened when I'm trying to sleep.
23. Being fired or laid off from work.
24. Being dissatisfied with my spouse (living partner, mate).
25. Having to compete against others.
26. Coming home to a messy house.
27. Having someone owe me money or something else that belongs to me.
28. Death of my spouse.
29. Doing heavy outdoor work (cutting or chopping wood, clearing land, putting up fences, farmwork, etc.).
30. Not knowing how much money I have available.
31. Counseling someone.
32. Making household improvements.
33. Attending funerals.
34. Experiencing an abortion, miscarriage, or pregnancy complications.
35. Arguments with spouse (living partner, mate).
36. Finding only 1 of a pair of something (socks, gloves, etc.).
37. Close friend institutionalized (nursing home, mental hospital).
38. Losing property (through repossession, legal settlement, etc.).
39. Having to get up early.
40. Parent or child moves away (to another city or area).
41. Seeing a dead animal.
42. Being with children.
43. Having attention directed toward me at a gathering; being put on the spot.
44. Having a drain plugged or other plumbing problems.
45. Finding I don't have enough money when I need it.

46. Having a project or assignment overdue.
47. Being told what to do.
48. Asking someone for a date.
49. Learning of local, national, or international news (corruptions, government decisions, etc.).
50. Losing or misplacing something (wallet, keys, golf ball, fish on a line, etc.).
51. Having someone forget my name.
52. Working in a job beneath my experience or training.
53. Being with someone I do not trust.
54. Talking in a group.
55. Getting locked out (of a car, house, etc.).
56. Smelling a strong odor (paint, smoke, etc.).
57. Seeing someone cry.
58. 'Realistic' fears (being alone in a strange place, dark street at night, etc.).
59. Having too much to do.
60. Being blamed or accused (of cheating, breaking the law, etc.).
61. Being in a crowded place.
62. Shopping for groceries, clothes, daily necessities.
63. Knowing a close friend or relative is working under adverse conditions.
64. Being away from someone I love for an extended period of time (more than one day).
65. Not being able to find a parking place.
66. Ceasing formal schooling (graduating).
67. Being with my parents.
68. Having someone close to me in trouble with the law.
69. Having a major unexpected expense (hospital bill, home repair, etc.).
70. Not waking up in time to get to work or keep an appointment.
71. Not having a newspaper, magazine, or mail delivered on time.
72. Asking for help or advice.
73. Being refused help (counsel, advice, etc.).
74. Performing poorly in sports.
75. Experiencing childbirth.
76. Having a new person move into my home (childbirth, adoption, grand-parents, etc.).
77. Starting a new job.
78. Seeing children physically or psychologically abused, neglected, or treated unfairly.
79. Having a relative or friend with a mental health problem.
80. Change of residence (within same city or area).
81. Asking to borrow something.
82. Having something break or run poorly (car, appliances, etc.).
83. Knowing that someone I'm close to is disabled or handicapped.
84. Receiving junk mail.
85. Doing housework or laundry; cleaning things.
86. Going through changes at work (promotion, demotion, transfer, reorganization, etc.).

87. Having a minor illness or injury (toothache, allergy attack, cold, flu, hangover, acne breakout, etc.).
88. Realizing that someone I love and I are growing apart.
89. Having something that I own damaged (car wrecked, fire, flood, vandalism, etc.).
90. Learning that I am pregnant or have caused a pregnancy.
91. Paying high prices.
92. Doing something I don't want to in order to please someone else.
93. Being paid attention to or admired by someone I do not like.
94. Breathing foul air.
95. Working on something when I am tired.
96. Learning that an operation (surgery or other major treatment) was not helpful, for someone close to me.
97. Being unable to help someone.
98. Having a mistake I made reported to someone in authority (boss, etc.).
99. Death of an acquaintance (neighbor, co-worker, etc.).
100. Failing at something (a test, a class, etc.).
101. Looking for a job.
102. Working under pressure.
103. Being arrested or detained by authorities.
104. Being kept waiting.
105. Being a victim of a criminal activity (theft, rape, assault, etc.).
106. Lying to someone.
107. Hearing a loud noise.
108. Parents getting divorced or separated.
109. Household chores (washing dishes, mopping the floor, picking up, etc.).
110. Being away from someone I love.
111. Being drunk.
112. Learning that someone would stop at nothing to get ahead.
113. Getting lost, being unable to find a place.
114. Being involved in a law suit.
115. Seeing animals mistreated.
116. Having a friend or relative (including spouse) who is ill or injured.
117. Being the agent of bad news (terminating an employee, evicting someone, telling someone of a death, etc.).
118. Having relatives or friends whose belongings were stolen, damaged or destroyed.
119. Being accused of having committed a crime.
120. Receiving unwanted phone calls (wrong numbers, crank calls, etc.).
121. Disobeying rules or conventions.
122. Having my child get divorced or experience serious marital difficulties.
123. Being interrupted.
124. Paying taxes.
125. Seeing a fight.

126. Disciplining a child.
127. Being forced to do something.
128. Visiting the cemetery, remembering a departed friend or loved one.
129. Quitting my job.
130. Meeting someone who is late.
131. Performing in public.
132. Receiving contradictory information from different sources.
133. Working at something I don't enjoy.
134. Seeing someone I no longer love.
135. Having someone I know drink, smoke, or take drugs.
136. Having my child become romantically involved, engaged or married.
137. Spouse beginning work outside the house.
138. Saying "no."
139. Attending classes or lessons.
140. Being rejected sexually.
141. Driving under adverse conditions (heavy traffic, poor weather, night, etc.).
142. Riding on a bus, train, or subway.
143. Being insulted.
144. Reminding people that they owe me money or something else that belongs to me.
145. Being in very cold weather.
146. Liking someone who does not feel the same way about me.
147. A friend moved away (to another city).
148. Having one of my checks bounce.
149. Being misunderstood or misquoted.
150. Facing financial ruin (bankruptcy, broke, etc.).
151. Writing papers, essays, articles, reports, memos, etc.
152. Being misled, bluffed or tricked.
153. Having insects, rodents, or other unwanted animals where I live or work.
154. Missing an appointment.
155. Encountering a poor driver.
156. Having something fit poorly (clothes, etc.).
157. Retiring or being retired from work.
158. Son or daughter leaving home.
159. Being near unpleasant people (drunk, bigoted, inconsiderate, etc.).
160. Trying to impress someone.

TO ANSWER SHEET NO. 2

1. Shaving.
2. Appearance in court.
3. Leaving a task uncompleted.
4. Encountering the police (being stopped, questioned, searched, etc.).
5. Being stood up for an appointment.
6. Working on something I don't care about.
7. Being on a fixed income.
8. Having family members or friends do something that makes me ashamed of them.
9. Having an application rejected.

10. Losing my job or profession due to legal, health, or financial difficulties.
11. Being found guilty of a major crime (burglary, theft, murder, etc.).
12. Working at a difficult task.
13. Riding in a car with a poor driver.
14. Problems with the mail (not getting yours, getting someone else's).
15. Seeing animals misbehave (make a mess, chase cars, etc.).
16. Being clumsy (dropping, spilling, knocking something over, etc.).
17. Having someone criticize me.
18. Meeting someone who has had a recent death in the family.
19. Being overcharged or receiving inferior merchandise.
20. Being physically uncomfortable (dizzy, constipated, headachy, itchy, cold, having the hiccups, undergoing a rectal exam, etc.).
21. Having relatives or friends with marital problems (divorced, separated, engagement broken, etc.).
22. Political disappointments (person you want not elected, referendum you want voted down, etc.).
23. Being bothered with red tape, administrative hassles, paperwork, etc.
24. Taking an exam (test, license examination, or other evaluation).
25. Losing a friend.
26. Marriage proposal turned down.
27. Lying.
28. Being refused credit (loan, charge card, etc.).
29. Having plans spoiled by poor weather.
30. Being excluded or left out.
31. Not enough money to buy necessities.
32. Being near someone who smells bad.
33. Not having enough money for hobbies, recreation, entertainment.
34. Falling behind in mortgage or loan payments.
35. Having shopping bags rip, a pot boil over, or other minor accidents.
36. Being blamed for doing something wrong.
37. Making a major purchase (car, appliance, house, stocks, etc.).
38. Receiving a check that bounces.
39. Gambling.
40. Having a physical handicap (poor eyesight, hard of hearing, loss of leg, etc.).
41. Having trespassers on my property.
42. Not having enough time to be with people I care about (spouse, close friend, living partner, etc.).
43. Seeing a dead person.
44. Being unable to enroll in a course or training program I would like to take.
45. Losing my girl/boyfriend.
46. Injuring someone else.
47. Having a houseguest.
48. Taking care of a sick person.
49. Working for little reward or pay.

50. Deterioration of living conditions (neighborhood, home run down, etc.)
51. Being socially rejected.
52. Being in dirty or dusty places.
53. Bad weather.
54. Being rushed.
55. Being denied a job benefit.
56. Cooking or preparing meals.
57. Being physically threatened or attacked.
58. Having my finances (tax-return) audited.
59. Accepting money without having earned it (charity, welfare, unemployment, etc.).
60. Having someone I love leave me.
61. Being kept waiting (in lines, for service, etc.).
62. Learning of poor governmental practices (poor decisions, money spent unwisely, abuse of power, etc.).
63. Learning that a friend or relative (including spouse) has just become ill, injured, hospitalized, or in need of an operation.
64. Attending meetings.
65. Having a plant sicken or die.
66. Losing a competition.
67. Being with someone I dislike.
68. Being nagged.
69. Being jealous of someone; envying someone.
70. Having someone I care about fail at something (job, school, etc.) that is important to them.
71. Being in an unfamiliar place.
72. Saying something unclearly.
73. Changing plans suddenly (restaurant closed, store out of desired merchandise, TV shows preempted, etc.).
74. Seeing suffering on the media (terrorism, starvation, war, etc.).
75. Living in a dirty or messy place.
76. Being in a fight.
77. Owing money.
78. Paying for repairs on a machine that still doesn't work.
79. Having my spouse (living partner, mate) dissatisfied with me.
80. Being with my spouse (living partner, mate).
81. Going to the hospital.
82. Hearing gossip.
83. Being treated as inferior.
84. Returning an item to a store.
85. Going to a doctor.
86. Lending money or possessions.
87. Working on my finances (keeping books, preparing tax returns, etc.).
88. Paying a bill.
89. Getting grades or being evaluated.
90. Changing schools.
91. Having someone I know contemplate or attempt suicide.
92. Having my spouse (living partner, mate) be unfaithful.

93. Not getting any mail.
94. Being with my boss.
95. Hearing or seeing swear words.
96. Being late.
97. Giving a speech or lecture.
98. Being dirty.
99. Taking medicines.
100. 'In-law' trouble.
101. Disciplining an animal.
102. Doing school work (studying, writing reports, etc.).
103. Having a friend or relative in financial trouble.
104. Eating a disliked food.
105. Meeting girl/boy friend's parents.
106. Being hounded by creditors (letters, phone calls, etc.).
107. Having people ignore what I have said.
108. Being without privacy.
109. Listening to someone who doesn't stop talking, can't keep to the point, or talks only about one subject.
110. Losing an argument.
111. Displeasing others (parents, employee, teachers, friends, etc.).
112. Doing something embarrassing in the presence of others.
113. Talking with a person in authority (boss, professor, etc.).
114. Learning that my child is having difficulties in school (truancy, misbehavior, poor academic performance, etc.).
115. Poor economic conditions (stock market, low sales, high prices, etc.).
116. Losing a bet.
117. Experiencing a pregnancy.
118. Being put in jail.
119. Being interviewed for a job or school.
120. Hurting myself (falling down stairs, cutting myself, bumping into something).
121. Watching someone in danger.
122. Having my spouse or someone I know experience an abortion, miscarriage, or pregnancy complications.
123. Hearing brags or boasts.
124. Making a mistake (in sports, my job, etc.).
125. Forgetting something (a name or appointment, etc.).
126. Not talking to anyone all day.
127. Having a boring job.
128. Having to leave school (flunk out, expelled, finances, etc.).
129. Knowing you have to take an exam or be evaluated.
130. Evaluating or criticizing someone.
131. Death of a close relative (parent, child).
132. Death of another family member (grandparent, uncle, cousin, in-law, etc.).
133. Breaking up of a fight between others.
134. Learning that someone is angry with me or wants to hurt me.
135. Going to the dentist.
136. Being legally separated from my children.
137. Having my pet sicken and die.
138. Living with a relative or roommate who is in poor physical or mental health.
139. Seeing someone in pain (bleeding, unconscious).
140. Having to cancel a planned vacation.
141. Being betrayed (friend repeating a confidence, etc.).
142. Losing money in a vending machine.
143. Being unemployed.
144. Having things I have lent not returned.
145. Death of a close friend.
146. Talking about a subject I'm not interested in (sports, recipes, etc.).
147. Being exposed to boring conversation.
148. Having a major injury or physical illness (heart trouble, severe burns, etc.).
149. Having someone ask me for money.
150. Having someone not keep their word (bad debt, broken promise, something borrowed not returned, etc.).
151. Not being home to receive an important phone call.
152. Not getting a job advancement (promotion, raise, accepted into a better school, etc.).
153. Being in danger (fire, plane crash, car accident, etc.).
154. Having an operation.
155. Being found guilty of a minior legal violation (traffic ticket, jaywalking, driver's license suspended, etc.).
156. Being in rainy weather.
157. Being unable to call or reach someone when it is important.
158. Seeing someone receive something they haven't earned (food stamps, raise, etc.).
159. Doing a job poorly.
160. Being treated discourteously by a sales or service person.

STOP

If you have just gone through the list for the first time, go to page 10 and follow the directions for Question B.

If you have just finished answering Question B you have completed the test.

Directions—Question B

Now please go over the list once again. This time the question is: HOW UNPLEASANT,

ANNOYING, UPSETTING, OR OTHERWISE AVERSIVE WAS EACH EVENT DURING THE PAST MONTH? Please answer this question by rating each event on the following scale:

0 = This was *not unpleasant.* (Use this rating for events which were either neutral or pleasant.)

1 = This was *somewhat unpleasant.* (Use this rating for events which were mildly or moderately unpleasant.)

2 = This was *very unpleasant.* (Use this rating for events which were strongly or extremely unpleasant.)

Important: If an event has happened to you *more than once* in the past month, try to rate roughly how unpleasant it was *on the average. If an event has not happened to you during the past month, then rate it according to how unpleasant you think it would have been.* When an item lists more than one event, rate it on the events which have actually happened.

Place your rating for each event on the answer sheet labeled "B," starting with "B-1." Here is an example.:

Event number 1 is "Listening to people complain." Suppose that each time you listened to people complain in the past 30 days you disliked it a great deal. Then you would rate this event "3" since it was "very unpleasant." On answer sheet "B" your mark would look like this:

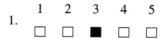

The list of items may have some events which you would not enjoy. The list was made for a wide variety of people, and it is not expected that one person would dislike them all.

Now go back to the list of events, start with item 1, and go through the entire list rating each event on *roughly how pleasant it was (or would have been) during the past 30 days.* Please be sure that you rate each item and that your marks completely fill the boxes on the answer sheet.

Glossary

Sharon L. Foster and Arthur M. Nezu

Concurrent validity
> The extent to which scores on a target measure can be used to predict an individual's score on a measure of performance collected at the same time as the target measure.

Construct validity
> The extent to which scores on a measure enter into relationships in ways predicted by theory or by previous investigations. Examinations of construct validity address the *meaning* of scores on a measure, and are relevant to the issue of whether the instrument assesses what it purports to assess. Construct validity has several specific subtypes; other investigations that speak to construct validity, but do not fall into any of the specific subtypes, are generally called "investigations of construct validity."

Content validity
> Whether the measure appropriately samples or represents the domain being assessed. Substantiation of content validity requires systematic, replicable development of the assessment device, often with formal review by clients or experts to ensure appropriate material is included and excluded.

Convergent validity
> The extent to which scores on the target measure correlate with scores on measures of the same construct.

Criterion-related validity
> The extent to which test scores can be used to predict an individual's performance on some important task or behavior. Examinations of criterion-related validity speak to the utility of scores on a measure rather than to their meaning. Often one ideally would like a perfect match between scores on that target measure and those on the criterion measure. There are two subtypes of criterion-related validity—concurrent validity and predictive validity.

Discriminant validity
> The extent to which scores on a measure are unrelated to scores on measures assessing other, theoretically unrelated constructs.

Discriminative validity

The extent to which scores on a measure distinguish between groups known or suspected to differ on the construct assessed by the target measure.

Internal consistency

A form of reliability indicating the extent to which different item groupings produce consistent scores on a measure, usually measured by (Cronbach's) coefficient alpha or KR-20.

Interrater reliability

The extent to which two individuals who rate (score, or observe) the same person (or stimulus material) score the person (person's behavior, or stimulus material) consistently; usually established by having two independent observers or raters evaluate the same stimulus material at approximately the same time.

Predictive validity

The extent to which scores on a target measure can be used to predict an individual's score on a measure of performance collected some time after the target measure (i.e., in the future).

Sensitivity

The level at which a measure accurately identifies individuals who have a given characteristic in question using a given criterion or cutoff score (e.g., the proportion of people with major depression who are correctly identified as depressed by their score on a given measure of depression).

Specificity

The degree to which a measure accurately identifies people who do *not* have a characteristic that is being measured (e.g., the proportion of people who do *not* have a diagnosis of major depression and who are correctly identified as *not* depressed by their score on a given measure of depression).

Test–retest reliability

The extent to which scores on a measure are consistent over a specified period of time, established by administering the same instrument on two separate occasions.

Treatment sensitivity

Whether the measure is sensitive to changes produced by treatment that have been documented or corroborated by other measures. Note that a measure can have good content and construct validity, but still not be sensitive to treatment effects.

References

Abramson, L. Y., Metalsky, G. I., & Alloy, L.B. (1989). Hopelessness depression: A theory-based subtype of depression. *Psychological Review, 96,* 358–372.

Abramson, L. Y., Seligman, M. E. P., & Teasdale, J. D. (1978). Learned helplessness in humans: Critique and reformulation. *Journal of Abnormal Psychology, 87,* 49–74.

Addington, D., Addington, J., & Atkinson, M. (1996). A psychometric comparison of the Calgary Depression Scale for Schizophrenia and the Hamilton Depression Rating Scale. *Schizophrenia Research, 19,* 205–212.

Addington, D., Addington, J., & Maticka-Tyndale, E. (1993a). Rating depression in schizophrenia: A comparison of a self-report and an observer report scale. *Journal of Nervous and Mental Disease, 181,* 561–565.

Addington, D., Addington, J., & Maticka-Tyndale, E. (1994). Specificity of the Calgary Depression Scale for schizophrenics. *Schizophrenia Research, 11,* 239–244.

Addington, D., Addington, J., Maticka-Tyndale, E., & Joyce, J. (1992). Reliability and validity of a depression rating scale for schizophrenia. *Schizophrenia Research, 6,* 201–208.

Addington, D., Addington, J., & Schissel, B. A. (1990). A depression rating scale for schizophrenics. *Schizophrenia Research, 3,* 247–251.

Aiken, L. S., West, W. G., Sechrest, L., & Reno, R. R. (1990). Graduate school training in statistics, methodology, and measurement in psychology. *American Psychologist, 45,* 721–734.

American Psychiatric Association. (1952). *Diagnostic and statistical manual of mental disorders* (DSM-I; 1st ed.). Washington, DC: Author.

American Psychiatric Association. (1968). *Diagnostic and statistical manual of mental disorders* (DSM-II; 2nd ed.). Washington, DC: Author.

American Psychiatric Association. (1980). *Diagnostic and statistical manual of mental disorders* (DSM-III; 3rd ed.). Washington, DC: Author.

American Psychiatric Association. (1987). *Diagnostic and statistical manual of mental disorders* (DSM-III-R; 3rd ed.-revised). Washington, DC: Author.

American Psychiatric Association. (1994). *Diagnostic and statistical manual of mental disorders* (DSM-IV; 4th ed.). Washington, DC: Author.

American Psychological Association. (1985). *Standards for educational and psychological testing.* American Educational Research Association, American Psychological Association, National Council on Measurement in Education. Washington, DC: American Psychological Association.

Anderson, K. W., & Skidmore, J. R. (1995). Empirical analysis of factors in depressive cognition: The Cognitive Triad Inventory. *Journal of Clinical Psychology, 51,* 603–609.

Antony, M. M., Bieling, P. J., Cox, B. J., Enns, M. W., & Swinson, R. P. (1998). Psychometric properties of the 42-item and 21-item versions of the Depression Anxiety Stress Scales (DASS) in clinical groups and a community sample. *Psychological Assessment, 10,* 176–181.

Archer, R. P. (1992). Review of the Minnesota Multiphasic Personality Inventory-2. In *Mental Measurement Yearbook* (pp. 558–562). Lincoln, NB: Buros Institute of Mental Measurement of the University of Nebraska-Lincoln.

Arean, P. A., Perri, M. G., Nezu, A. M., Schein, R. L., Christopher, F., & Joseph, T. X. (1993). Comparative effectiveness of social problem-solving therapy and reminiscence therapy as treatments for depression in older adults. *Journal of Consulting and Clinical Psychology, 61,* 1003–1010.

Arkes, H. R. (1981). Impediments to accurate clinical judgment and possible ways to minimize their impact. *Journal of Consulting and Clinical Psychology, 49*, 323–330.

Arruda, J. E., Stern, R. A., & Legendre, S. A. (1997). Assessment of mood state in patients undergoing electroconvulsive therapy: The utility of Visual Analog Mood Scales developed for cognitively-impaired patients. *Convulsive Therapy, 12*, 207–212.

Asberg, M., Montgomery, S., Perris, C., Schalling, D., & Sevall, G. (1978). A comprehensive psychopathological rating scale. *Acta Psychiatrica Scandinavica (Supplement), 272*.

Baldree, B. F., Ingram, R. E., & Saccuzzo, D. (1991, August). Cross-validation and social desirability bias in automatic positive cognitions. Paper presented at the Annual Meeting of the American Psychological Association, San Francisco.

Bech, P., Gjerris, A., Andersen, J., Bojholm, S., Krampt, P., Bolwig, T. G., Kastrup, M., Clemmesen, L., & Rafaelsen, O. J. (1983). Melancholia Scale and the Newcastle Scales: Item-combinations and inter-observer reliability. *British Journal of Psychiatry, 143*, 58–63.

Beck, A. T. (1967). *Depression: Clinical, experimental, and theoretical aspects*. New York: Harper & Row.

Beck, A. T. (1976). *Cognitive therapy and the emotional disorders*. New York: Harper & Row.

Beck, A. T. (1983). Cognitive therapy of depression: New perspectives. In P. J. Clayton & J. E. Barrett (Eds.), *Treatment of depression: Old controversies and new approaches* (pp. 265–284). New York: Raven Press.

Beck, A. T. (1987). Cognitive model of depression. *Journal of Cognitive Psychotherapy, 1*, 2–27.

Beck, A. T., Brown, G., Steer, R. A., Eidelson, J. I., & Riskind, J. II. (1987). Differentiating anxiety and depression: A test of the cognitive content-specificity hypothesis. *Journal of Abnormal Psychology, 96*, 179–183.

Beck, A. T., Brown, G., Steer, R. A., & Weissman, A. N. (1991). Factor analysis of the Dysfunctional Attitude Scale in a clinical population. *Psychological Assessment, 3*, 478–483.

Beck, A. T., Epstein, N., Harrison, R. P., & Emery, G. (1983). *Development of the Sociotropy-Autonomy Scale: A measure of personality factors in psychopathology*. Unpublished manuscript, University of Pennsylvania, Philadelphia.

Beck, A. T., Kovacs, M., & Weissman, A. (1975). Hopelessness and suicidal behavior: An overview. *Journal of the American Medical Association, 234*, 1146–1149.

Beck, A. T., Kovacs, M., & Weissman, A. (1979). Assessment of suicidal intention: The Scale for Suicide Ideation. *Journal of Consulting and Clinical Psychology, 47*, 343–352.

Beck, A. T., Rush, A. J., Shaw, B. F., & Emery, G. (1979). *Cognitive therapy of depression*. New York: Guilford Press.

Beck, A. T., & Steer, R. A. (1987). *Manual for the Beck Depression Inventory*. San Antonio, TX: The Psychological Corporation.

Beck, A. T., & Steer, R. A. (1988). *Manual for the Beck Hopelessness Scale*. San Antonio, TX: The Psychological Corporation.

Beck, A. T., & Steer, R. A. (1990). *Manual for the Beck Anxiety Inventory*. San Antonio, TX: The Psychological Corporation.

Beck, A. T., & Steer, R. A. (1991). *Beck Scale for Suicide Ideation*. San Antonio, TX: The Psychological Corporation.

Beck, A. T., Steer, R. A., & Brown, G. K. (1996). *Manual for the BDI-II*. San Antonio, TX: The Psychological Corporation.

Beck, A. T., Steer, R. A., & Garbin, M. G. (1988). Psychometric properties of the Beck Depression Inventory: Twenty-five years of evaluation. *Clinical Psychology Review, 8*, 77–100.

Beck, A. T., Ward, C. H., Mendelson, M., Mock, J., & Erbaugh, J. (1961). An inventory for measuring depression. *Archives of General Psychiatry, 4*, 561–571.

Beck, J. S. (1995). *Cognitive therapy: Basics and beyond*. New York: Guilford Press.

Becker, R. E., & Heimberg, R. G. (1985). Social skills training approaches. In M. Hersen & A. S. Bellack (Eds.), *Handbook of clinical behavior therapy with adults* (pp. 201–226). New York: Plenum Press.

Becker, R. E., Heimberg, R. G., & Bellack, A. S. (1987). *Social skills training treatment for depression*. New York: Pergamon Press.

Beckham, E. E., & Leber, W. R. (1995). *Handbook of depression* (2nd ed.). New York: Guilford Publications.

Bellack, A. S., & Hersen, M. (Eds.) (1988). *Behavioral assessment: A practical handbook*. Boston: Allyn and Bacon.

Bellack, A. S., Hersen, M., & Himmelhoch, J. (1981). Social skills training compared with pharmacotherapy and psychotherapy in the treatment of unipolar depression. *American Journal of Psychiatry, 138*, 1562–1567.

Bellack, A. S., Hersen, M., & Himmelhoch, J. (1983). A comparison of social skills training, pharmacotherapy, and psychotherapy for depression. *Behavior Research and Therapy, 21*, 101–107.

Berndt, D. J. (1981). How valid are the subscales of the Multiscore Depression Inventory? *Journal of Clinical Psychology, 37*, 564–570.

Bertolotti, G., Zotti, A. M., Michielin, P., Vidotto, G., & Sanavio, E. (1990). A computerized approach to cognitive behavioural assessment: An introduction to CBA-2.0 Primary Scales. *Journal of Behavior Therapy and Experimental Psychiatry, 21*, 21–27.

Biggs, J. T., Wylie, L. T., & Ziegler, V. E. (1978). Validity of the Zung Self-Rating Depression Scale. *British Journal of Psychiatry, 132*, 381–385.

Borus, J. F., Howes, M. J., Devins, N. P., Rosenberg, R., & Livingston, W. W. (1988). Primary health care providers' recognition and diagnosis of mental disorders in their patients. *General Hospital Psychiatry, 10*, 317–321.

Bradburn, N. M. (1969). *The structure of psychological well being*. Chicago: Aldine.

Brink, T. L., Yesavage, J. A., Lum, O., Heersema, P. H., Adey, M., & Rose, T. L. (1982). Screening tests for geriatric depression. *Clinical Gerontologist, 1*, 37–43.

Brophy, C. J., Norvell, N. K., & Kiluk, D. J. (1988). An examination of the factor structure and convergent and discriminant validity of the SCL-90-R in an outpatient clinic population. *Journal of Personality Assessment, 52*, 334–340.

Brown, R. A., & Lewinsohn, P. M. (1984). A psychoeducational approach to the treatment of depression: Comparison of group, individual, and minimal contact procedures. *Journal of Consulting and Clinical Psychology, 52*, 774–783.

Brown, T. A., Korotitsch, W., Chorpita, B. F., & Barlow, D. H. (1997). Psychometric properties of the Depression Anxiety Stress Scales (DASS) in clinical samples. *Behaviour Research and Therapy, 35*, 79–89.

Campbell, S. B., & Cohn, J. F. (1991). Prevalence and correlates of postpartum depression in first-time mothers. *Journal of Abnormal Psychology, 100*, 594–599.

Carney, M. W., & Sheffield, B. F. (1972). Depression and the Newcastle Scales: The relationship to Hamilton's Scale. *British Journal of Psychiatry, 121*, 35–40.

Carroll, B. J., Fielding, J. M., & Blashki, T. G. (1973). Depression rating scales: A critical review. *Archives of General Psychiatry, 28*, 361–366.

Carroll, B. J., Feinberg, M., Smouse, P. E., Rawson, S. G., & Greden, J. F. (1981). The Carroll Rating Scale for Depression: I. Development, reliability, and validation. *British Journal of Psychiatry, 138*, 194–200.

Carroll, B. J., Feinberg, M., Smouse, P. E., & Rawson, S. G. (1981). The Carroll Rating Scale for Depression: III. Comparison with other rating instruments. *British Journal of Psychiatry, 138*, 205–209.

Cattell, R. B., Eber, H. W., & Tatsuoka, M. M. (1970). *Handbook for the 16PF*. Champaign, IL: Institute for Personality and Ability Testing.

Chambers, W., Puig-Antich, J., Hirsch, M., Paez, P., Ambrosini, P., Tabrizi, M. A., & Davies, M. (1985). The assessment of affective disorders in children and adolescents by semi-structured interview: Test retest reliability of the Schedule for Affective Disorders and Schizophrenia for School-Age Children, Present Episode version. *Archives of General Psychiatry, 42*, 696–702.

Chang, C. H. (1996). Finding two dimensions in MMPI-2 depression. *Structural Equation Modeling, 3*, 41–49.

Choquette, K. A. (1994). Assessing depression in alcoholics with the BDI, SCL-90-R, and DIS criteria. *Journal of Substance Abuse, 6*, 295–304.

Clark, A., & Friedman, M. J. (1983). Factor structure and discriminant validity of the SCL-90 in a veteran psychiatric population. *Journal of Personality Assessment, 47*, 396–404.

Clark, D. A., Steer, R. A., Beck, A. T., & Ross, L. (1995). Psychometric characteristics of revised sociotropy and autonomy scales in college students. *Behavior Research and Therapy, 33*, 325–334.

Clarke, G. N., Lewinsohn, P. M., & Alexander, C. (1985, Spring). *A psychoeducational approach to the treatment of depressed adolescents*. Paper presented at the Western Psychological Association, San Jose, CA.

Cone, J. D. (1998a). Assessment practice standards. In S. C. Hayes, V. M. Follette, R. M. Dawes, & K. E. Grady (Eds.), *Scientific standards of practice: Issues and recommendations* (pp. 201–225). Reno, NV: Context Press.

Cone, J. D. (1998b). Psychometric considerations: Concepts, contents, & methods. In A. S. Bellack & M. Hersen (Eds.), *Behavioral assessment: A practical handbook* (pp. 22–46). Boston: Allyn and Bacon.

Cooper, P. J., Campbell, E. A., Day, A., Kennerly, H., & Bond, A. (1988). Nonpsychotic psychiatric disorder after childbirth: A prospective study of prevalence, incidence, and nature. *British Journal of Psychiatry, 152*, 799–806.

Courey, L., Feuerstein, M., & Bush, C. (1982). Self-control and chronic headache. *Journal of Psychosomatic Research, 26*, 519–526.

Coyne, J. C. (1976). Toward an interactional description of depression. *Psychiatry, 39*, 28–40.

Cronkite, R. C., & Moos, R. H. (1995). Life context, coping processes, and depression. In E. E. Beckham & W. R. Leber (Eds.), *Handbook of depression* (2nd ed., pp. 569–587). New York: Guilford Press.

Crowne, D. P., & Marlowe, D. (1964). *The approval motive: Studies in evaluative dependency*. New York: Wiley.

Cull, J. G., & Gill, W. S. (1982). *Suicide Probability Scale*. Los Angeles, CA: Western Psychological Services.

Dawes, R. M. (1986). Representative thinking in clinical judgment. *Clinical Psychology Review, 6*, 425–441.

Derogatis, L. R. (1994). *Symptom Checklist-90-R administration, scoring, and procedures manual* (3rd ed.). Minneapolis, MN: National Computer Systems.

Derogatis, L. R., Lipman, R. S., Rickels, K., Uhlenhuth, E. H., & Covi, L. (1974). The Hopkins Symptom Checklist: A self-report symptom inventory. *Behavioral Science, 19*, 1–15.

DeRubeis, R. J., & Crits-Christoph, P. (1998). Empirically supported individual and group psychological treatments for adult mental disorders. *Journal of Consulting and Clinical Psychology, 66*, 37–52.

Dobson, D. J., & Dobson, K. (1981). Problem-solving strategies in depressed and nondepressed college students. *Cognitive Therapy and Research, 5*, 367–371.

Dobson, K. (1989). A meta-analysis of the efficacy of cognitive therapy for depression. *Journal of Consulting and Clinical Psychology, 57*, 414–419.

Dohrenwend, B. S., & Dohrenwend, B. P. (Eds.). (1974). *Stressful life events: their nature and effects.* New York: Wiley-Interscience.

Dozis, D. J. A., Dobson, K. S., & Ahnberg, J. L. (1998). A psychometric evaluation of the Beck Depression Inventory-II. *Psychological Assessment, 10*, 83–89.

Dykema, J., Bergbower, K., Doctora, J. D., & Peterson, C. (1996). An Attributional Style Questionnaire for general use. *Journal of Psychoeducational Assessment, 14*, 100–108.

Dykema, J., Bergbower, K., & Peterson, C. (1995). Pessimistic explanatory style, stress, and illness. *Journal of Social and Clinical Psychology, 14*, 357–371.

D'Zurilla, T. J., & Goldfried, M. R. (1971). Problem solving and behavior modification. *Journal of Abnormal Psychology, 78*, 104–126.

D'Zurilla, T. J., & Nezu, A. M. (1990). Development and preliminary evaluation of the Social Problem Solving Inventory (SPSI). *Psychological Assessment, 2*, 156–163.

Elwood, R. W. (1993). The clinical utility of the MMPI-2 in diagnosing unipolar depression among alcoholics. *Journal of Personality Assessment, 60*, 511–521.

Endicott, J., & Spitzer, R. L. (1978). A diagnostic interview: The Schedule for Affective Disorders and Schizophrenia. *Archives of General Psychiatry, 35*, 837–844.

Endler, N. S. (1988). Hassles, health and happiness. In M. P. Janisse (Ed.), *Individual differences, stress and health psychology* (pp. 24–56). New York: Springer.

Endler, N. S., & Parker, J. D. A. (1994). Assessment of multidimensional coping: Task, emotion, and avoidance strategies. *Psychological Assessment, 6*, 50–60.

Evans, I. (1985). Building systems models as a strategy for target behavior selection in clinical assessment. *Behavioral Assessment, 7*, 21–32.

Feighner, J. P., Robins, E., Guze, S. B., Woodruff, R. A., Winokur, G., & Munoz, R. (1972). Diagnostic criteria for use in psychiatric research. *Archives of General Psychiatry, 26*, 57–63.

Ferster, C. B. (1973). A functional analysis of depression. *American Psychologist, 28*, 857–870.

Foley, S. H., Rounsaville, B. J., Weissman, M. M., Sholomskas, D., & Chevron, E. (1989). Individual versus conjoint interpersonal psychotherapy for depressed outpatients with marital disputes. *International Journal of Family Psychiatry, 10*, 29–42.

Folkman, S. (1979). *An analysis of coping in an adequately functioning middle-aged population.* Unpublished doctoral dissertation, University of California, Berkeley.

Folkman, S., & Lazarus, R. S. (1980). An analysis of coping in a middle-aged community sample. *Journal of Health and Social Behavior, 21*, 219–239.

Frankel, M. J., & Merbaum, M. (1982). Effects of therapist contact and a self-control manual on nailbiting reduction. *Behavior Therapy, 13*, 125–129.

Frankl, V. E. (1959). *From death-camp to existentialism.* Boston: Beacon.

Fuchs, C. Z., & Rehm, L. P. (1977). A self-control behavior therapy program for depression. *Journal of Consulting and Clinical Psychology, 45*, 206–215.

Fullerton, D. T., Wenzel, F. J., Lohrenz, F. N., & Fahs, H. (1968). Circadian rhythm of adrenal cortical activity in depression: II. A comparison of types in depression. *Archives of General Psychiatry, 19*, 682–688.

Gladstone, T. R. G., & Kaslow, N. J. (1995). Depression and attributional style in children and adolescents: A meta-analytic review. *Journal of Abnormal Child Psychology, 23*, 597–606.

Gotlib, I. H., & Asarnow, R. F. (1979). Interpersonal and impersonal problem-solving skills in mildly and clinically depressed university students. *Journal of Consulting and Clinical Psychology, 47*, 86–95.

Gotlib, I. H., & Hammen, C. L. (1992). *Psychological aspects of depression: Toward a cognitive-interpersonal integration.* Chichester, England UK: John Wiley & Sons.

Gotlib, I. H., & Robinson, L. A. (1982). Responses to depressed individuals: Discrepancies between self-report and observer-rated behavior. *Journal of Abnormal Psychology, 91*, 231–240.

Gotlib, I. H., Whiffen, V. E., Mount, J. H., Milne, K., & Cordy, N. I. (1989). Prevalence rates and demographic characteristics associated with depression in pregnancy and the postpartum. *Journal of Consulting and Clinical Psychology, 57*, 269–274.

Gotlib, I. H., & Whiffen, V. E. (1989). Stress, coping, and marital satisfaction in couples with a depressed wife. *Canadian Journal of Behavioral Science, 21*, 401–418.

Graham, J. R. (1993). *MMPI-2: Assessing personality and psychopathology* (2nd ed.). Oxford: Oxford University Press.

Griffin, N., Chassin, L., & Young, R. (1981). Measurement of global self-concept versus multiple role-specific self-concepts in adolescents. *Adolescence, 16*, 549–556.

Gunderson, J. G., Phillips, K. A., Triebwasser, J., & Hirschfeld., R. M. A. (1994). The Diagnostic Interview for Depressive Personality. *American Journal of Psychiatry, 151*, 1300–1304.

Gurland, B. J., Yorkston, N. J., Stone, A. R., Frank, J. D., & Fleiss, J. L. (1972). The Structured and Scaled Interview to Assess Maladjustment. I. Description, rationale, and development. *Archives of General Psychiatry, 27*, 259–264.

Hamilton, M. (1960). A rating scale for depression. *Journal of Neurology, Neurosurgery and Psychiatry, 23*, 56–62.

Hamilton, M. (1967). Development of a rating scale for primary depressive illness. *British Journal of Social and Clinical Psychology, 6*, 278–296.

Hammen, C. L., & Krantz, S. (1976). Effect of success and failure on depressive cognitions. *Journal of Abnormal Psychology, 85*, 577–586.

Hammen, C., & Goodman-Brown, T. (1990). Self-schemas and vulnerability to specific life stress in children at risk for depression. *Cognitive Therapy and Research, 14*, 215–227.

Harrell, T. H., & Ryon, N. B. (1983). Cognitive-behavioral assessment of depression: Clinical validation of the Automatic Thoughts Questionnaire. *Journal of Consulting and Clinical Psychology, 51*, 721–725.

Haskell, D. H., Pugatch, D., & McNair, D. M. (1969). Time-limited psychotherapy for whom? *Archives of General Psychiatry, 21*, 546–552.

Hathaway, S. R., & McKinley, J. C. (1942). A multiphasic personality schedule (Minnesota): III. The measurement of symptomatic depression. *Journal of Psychology, 14*, 73–84.

Hayes, J. A. (1997). What does the Brief Symptom Inventory measure in college and university counseling center clients? *Journal of Counseling Psychology, 44*, 360–367.

Hedlund, J. L., & Vieweg, B. W. (1979). The Hamilton rating scale for depression: A comprehensive review. *Journal of Operational Psychiatry, 10*, 149–165.

Hedlund, J. L., & Vieweg, B. W. (1980). The Brief Psychiatric Rating Scale (BPRS): A comprehensive review. *Journal of Operational Psychiatry, 11*, 48–65.

Heppner, P. P., & Anderson, W. P. (1985). The relationship between problem-solving, self-appraisal and psychological adjustment. *Cognitive Therapy and Research, 9*, 415–427.

Hersen, M., Bellack, A. S., Himmelhoch, J. M., & Thase, M. E. (1984). Effects of social skills training, amitriptyline, and psychotherapy in unipolar depressed women. *Behavior Therapy, 15*, 21–40.

Hill, C. A. (1987). Affiliation motivation: People who need people … but in different ways. *Journal of Personality and Social Psychology, 52*, 1008–1018.

Hoberman, H. M., Lewinsohn, P. S., & Tilson, M. (1988). Group treatment of depression: Individual predictors of outcome. *Journal of Consulting and Clinical Psychology, 56*, 393–398.

Holden, N. L. (1983). Depression and the Newcastle Scale: Their relationship to the dexamethasone suppression test. *British Journal of Psychiatry, 142*, 505–507.

Hollon, S. D., & Kendall, P. C. (1980). Cognitive self-statements in depression: Development of an automatic thoughts questionnaire. *Cognitive Therapy and Research, 4*, 383–395.

Hollon, S. D., Kendall, P. C., & Lumry, A. (1986). Specificity of depressotypic cognitions in clinical depression. *Journal of Abnormal Psychology, 95*, 52–59.

Hollon, S. D., & Kriss, M. R. (1984). Cognitive factors in clinical research and practice. *Clinical Psychology Review, 4*, 35–76.

Hollon, S. D., Shelton, R. C., & Loosen, P. T. (1991). Cognitive therapy and pharmacotherapy for depression. *Journal of Consulting and Clinical Psychology, 59*, 88–99.

Hoover, C. F., & Fitzgerald, R. G. (1981). Marital conflict of manic-depressive patients. *Archives of General Psychiatry, 38*, 65–67.

Huprich, S. K., & Nelson-Gray, R. O. (1998). *Depressive personality disorder: Empirical validity and object loss.* Unpublished manuscript.

Hussian, R. A., & Lawrence, P. S. (1981). Social reinforcement of activity and problem-solving training in the treatment of depressed institutionalized elderly patients. *Cognitive Therapy and Research, 5*, 57–69.

Ingram, R. E., Kendall, P. C., Siegle, G., Guarino, J., & McLaughlin, S. C. (1995). Psychometric properties of the Positive Automatic Thoughts Questionnaire. *Psychological Assessment, 7*, 495–507.

Ivanoff, A., Jang, S. J., Smyth, N. J., & Linehan, M. M. (1994). Fewer reasons for staying alive when you are thinking of killing yourself: The Brief Reasons for Living Inventory. *Journal of Psychopathology and Behavioral Assessment, 16,* 1–13.

Jacobson, N. S., Dobson, K., Fruzetti, A. E., Schmaling, K. B., & Salusky, S. (1991). Marital therapy as a treatment for depression. *Journal of Consulting and Clinical Psychology, 59,* 547–557.

Jolly, J. B., & Weisner, D. C. (1996). Psychometric properties of the Automatic Thoughts Questionnaire-Positive with inpatient adolescents. *Cognitive Therapy and Research, 20,* 481–498.

Jones, R. G. (1969). A factored measure of Ellis' irrational belief system, with personality and maladjustment correlates. *Dissertation Abstracts International, 69,* 6443.

Joshi-Peters, K. L. (1991). *Frequency of self-reinforcement: A children's form.* Unpublished doctoral dissertation, University of Hawaii at Manoa.

Kahnemann, D., & Tversky, A. (1973). On the psychology of prediction. *Psychological Review, 80,* 237–251.

Kanfer, F. H. (1971). The maintenance of behavior by self-generated stimuli and reinforcement. In A. Jacobs & B. Sachs (Eds.), *The psychology of private events: Perspectives on covert response systems* (pp. 219–243). New York: Academic Press.

Kay, S. R., Fiszbein, A., & Opler, L. A. (1987). The Positive and Negative Syndrome Scale (PANSS) for schizo-phrenia. *Schizophrenia Bulletin, 13,* 261–276.

Kazdin, A. E., French, N. H., Unis, A. S., Esveldt-Dawson, K., & Sherick, R. B. (1983). Hopelessness, depression, and suicidal intent among psychiatrically disturbed inpatient children. *Journal of Consulting and Clinical Psychology, 51,* 504–510.

Kazdin, A. E., Matson, J., & Senatore, V. (1983). Assessment of depression in mentally retarded adults. *American Journal of Psychiatry, 140,* 1040–1043.

Keller, M. B., & Shapiro, R. W. (1982). "Double depression": Superimposition of acute depressive episodes on chronic depressive disorders. *American Journal of Psychiatry, 139,* 438–442.

Kerner, S. A., & Jacobs, K. W. (1983). Correlation between scores on the Beck Depression Inventory and the Zung Self-Rating Depression Scale. *Psychological Reports, 53,* 969–970.

Klerman, G. L., Weissman, M. M., Rounsaville, B. J., & Chevron, E. (1984). *Interpersonal psychotherapy of depression.* New York: Basic Books.

Koenig, H. G., George, L. K., Robins, C. J., Stangl, D., & Tweed, D. L. (1994). The development of a Dysfunctional Attitudes Scale for Medically Ill Elders (DASMIE). *Clinical Gerontologist, 15*(2), 3–22.

Krohne, H. W., Egloff, B., Kohlmann, C. W., & Tausch, A. (1996). Untersuchungen mit einer deutschen Version der "Positive and Negative Affect Schedule (PANAS)" [Investigations with a German version of the Positive and Negative Affect Schedule (PANAS)]. *Diagnostica, 42,* 139–156.

Kurokawa, N. K., & Weed, N. S. (1998). Interrater agreement on the Coping Inventory for Stressful Situations (CISS). *Assessment, 5,* 95–100.

Lee, Y. T., & Seligman, M. E. P. (1997). Are Americans more optimistic than Chinese? *Personality and Social Psychology Bulletin, 23,* 32–40.

Levitan, R. D., Rector, N. A., & Bagby, R. M. (1998). Negative attributional style in seasonal and nonseasonal depression. *American Journal of Psychiatry, 155,* 428–430.

Lewinsohn, P. M. (1974). A behavioral approach to depression. In R. J. Friedman & M. M. Katz (Eds.), *The psychology of depression: Contemporary theory and research* (pp. 157–185). New York: Wiley.

Lewinsohn, P. M., Antonuccio, D. O., Breckenridge, J., & Teri, L. (1987). *The Coping with Depression Course: A psychoeducational intervention for unipolar depression.* Eugene, OR: Castaglia.

Lewinsohn, P. M., Biglan, A., & Zeiss, A. M. (1976). Behavioral treatment of depression. In P. O. Davidson (Ed.), *The behavioral management of anxiety, depression and pain* (pp. 91–146). New York: Brunner/Mazel.

Lewinsohn, P. M., & Graf, M. (1973). Pleasant activities and depression. *Journal of Consulting and Clinical Psychology, 41,* 261–268.

Lewinsohn, P. M., & Libet, J. (1972). Pleasant events, activity schedules, and depressions. *Journal of Abnormal Psychology, 79,* 291–295.

Lewinsohn, P. M., & Talkington, J. (1979). Studies on the measurement of unpleasant events and relations with depression. *Applied Psychological Measurement, 3,* 83–101.

Lewinsohn, P. M., Youngren, M., & Grosscup, S. J. (1979). Reinforcement and depression. In R. A. Depue (Ed.), *The psychobiology of the depressive disorders: Implications for the effects of stress* (pp. 291–315). New York: Academic Press.

Libet, J., & Lewinsohn, P. M. (1973). The concept of social skill with special reference to the behavior of depressed persons. *Journal of Consulting and Clinical Psychology, 40,* 304–312.

Linehan, M. M., & Nielsen, S. L. (1981). *Suicidal Behaviors Questionnaire.* Unpublished inventory, University of Washington, Seattle.

Lovibond, P. F. (1982, May). *The nature and measurement of anxiety, stress, and depression.* Paper presented to the meeting of the Australian Psychological Society, Perth.

Lubin, B. (1981). *Depression Adjective Checklists: Manual* (2nd ed). San Diego, CA: Educational and Industrial Testing Service.

Lubin, B., Larsen, R. M., & Matarazzo, J. D. (1984). Patterns of psychological test usage in the United States: 1935–1982. *American Psychologist, 39,* 451–454.

Lukoff, D., Liberman, R. P., & Nuechterlein, K. H. (1986). Symptom monitoring in the rehabilitation of schizophrenic patients. *Schizophrenia Bulletin, 12,* 578–602.

MacPhillamy, D. J., & Lewinsohn, P. M. (1982). The Pleasant Events Schedule: Studies on reliability, validity, and scale intercorrelation. *Journal of Consulting and Clinical Psychology, 50,* 363–380.

Manderscheid, R. W., Rae, D. S., Narrow, W. E., Locke, B. Z., & Regier, D. A. (1993). Congruence of service utilization estimates from the Epidemiologic Catchment Area Project and other sources. *Archives of General Psychiatry, 50,* 108–114.

Markowitz,, J. C., & Weissman, M. M. (1995). Interpersonal psychotherapy. In E. E. Beckham & W. R. Leber (Eds.), *Handbook of depression* (2nd ed., pp. 376–390). New York: Guilford Press.

McLean, P. (1979). Therapeutic decision-making in the behavioral treatment of depression. In P. O. Davidson (Ed.), *The behavioral management of anxiety, depression and pain* (pp. 54–89). New York: Brunner/Mazel.

McLean, P. D., & Hakstian, A. R. (1979). Clinical depression: Comparative efficacy of outpatient treatments. *Journal of Consulting and Clinical Psychology, 47,* 818–836.

Merten, T., & Siebert, K. (1997). A comparison of computerized and conventional administration of the EPQ-R and CRS: Further data on the Merten and Ruch (1996) study. *Personality and Individual Differences, 22,* 283–286.

Michelson, L. K., Bellanti, C. J., Testa, S. M., & Marchione, N. (1997). The relationship of attributional style to agoraphobia severity, depression, and treatment outcome. *Behaviour Research and Therapy, 35,* 1061–1073.

Minkoff, K., Bergman, E., Beck, A. T., & Beck, R. (1973). Hopelessness, depression, and attempted suicide. *American Journal of Psychiatry, 130,* 455–459.

Moorey, S., Greer, S., Watson, M., Gorman, C., Rowden, L., Tunmore, R., Roberton, B., & Bliss, J. (1991). The factor structure and factor stability of the Hospital Anxiety and Depression Scale in patients with cancer. *British Journal of Psychiatry, 158,* 255–259.

Morrow-Bradley, C., & Elliott, R. (1986). Utilization of psychotherapy research by practicing psychotherapists. *American Psychologist, 41,* 188–197.

Muñoz, R. F. (1977). A cognitive approach to the assessment and treatment of depression. *Dissertation Abstracts International, 38,* 2873B (University Microfilms, No. 77-26, 505, 154).

Myers, J. K., Weissman, M. M., Tischler, G. L., Holzer, C. E., Leaf, P. J., Orvaschel, H., Anthony, J. C., Boyd, J. H., Burke, J. D., Kramer, M., & Stolzman, R. (1984). Six-month prevalence of psychiatric disorders in three countries. *Archives of General Psychiatry, 41,* 959–967.

Mynors-Wallis, L. M., Gath, D. H., Lloyd-Thomas, A. R., & Thomlinson, D. (1995). Randomised controlled trial comparing problem solving treatment with amitriptyline and placebo for major depression in primary care. *British Medical Journal, 310,* 441–445.

Nelson, L. D., Stern, S. L., & Cicchetti, D. V. (1992). The Dysfunctional Attitude Scale: How well can it measure depressive thinking? *Journal of Psychopathology and Behavioral Assessment, 14,* 217–223.

Nezu, A. M. (1986a). Cognitive appraisal of problem-solving effectiveness: Relation to depression and depressive symptoms. *Journal of Clinical Psychology, 42,* 42–48.

Nezu, A. M. (1986b). Efficacy of a social problem solving therapy approach for unipolar depression. *Journal of Consulting and Clinical Psychology, 54,* 196–202.

Nezu, A. M. (1987). A problem-solving formulation of depression: A literature review and proposal of a pluralistic model. *Clinical Psychology Review, 7,* 121–144.

Nezu, A. M. (1996). What are we doing to our patients and should we care if anyone else knows? *Clinical Psychology: Science and Practice, 3,* 160–163.

Nezu, A. M., & D'Zurilla, T. J. (1989). Social problem solving and negative affective states. In P. C. Kendall & D. Watson (Eds.), *Anxiety and depression: Distinctive and overlapping features* (pp. 285–315). New York: Academic Press.

Nezu, A. M., & Nezu, C. M. (Eds.). (1989a). *Clinical decision making in behavior therapy: A problem-solving perspective.* Champaign, IL: Research Press.

Nezu, A. M., & Nezu, C. M. (1989b). Unipolar depression. In A. M. Nezu & C. M. Nezu (Eds.), *Clinical decision making in behavior therapy: A problem-solving perspective* (pp. 117–156). Champaign, IL: Research Press.

Nezu, A. M., & Nezu, C. M. (1993). Identifying and selecting target problems for clinical interventions: A problem-solving model. *Psychological Assessment, 5,* 254–263.

Nezu, A. M., Nezu, C. M., Friedman, S. H., Faddis, S., & Houts, P. S. (1998). *Helping cancer patients cope: A problem-solving approach.* Washington, DC: American Psychological Association.

Nezu, A. M., Nezu, C. M., Friedman, S. H., & Haynes, S. N. (1997). Case formulation in behavior therapy: Problem solving and functional analytic strategies. In T. D. Ells (Ed.), *Handbook of psychotherapy case formulation* (pp. 368–401). New York: Guilford Press.

Nezu, A. M., Nezu, C. M., & Perri, M. G. (1989). *Problem-solving therapy for depression: Theory, research, and clinical guidelines.* New York: Wiley.

Nezu, A. M., Nezu, C. M., & Perri, M. G. (1990). Psychotherapy for adults within a problem-solving framework: Focus on depression. *Journal of Cognitive Psychotherapy, 4,* 247–256.

Nezu, A. M., Nezu, C. M., Saraydarian, L., Kalmar, K., & Ronan, G.F. (1986). Social problem solving as a moderating variable between negative life stress and depression. *Cognitive Therapy and Research, 10,* 489–498.

Nezu, A. M., Nezu, C. M., Trunzo, J. J., & McClure, K. S. (1998). Treatment maintenance for unipolar depression: Relevant issues, literature review and recommendations for research and clinical practice. *Clinical Psychology: Science and Practice, 5,* 496–512.

Nezu, A. M., & Perri, M. G. (1989). Problem-solving therapy for unipolar depression: An initial dismantling investigation. *Journal of Consulting and Clinical Psychology, 57,* 408–413.

Nezu, A. M., & Ronan, G. F. (1985). Life stress, current problems, problem solving, and depressive symptoms: An integrative model. *Journal of Consulting and Clinical Psychology, 53,* 693–697.

Nezu, A. M., & Ronan, G. F. (1988). Problem solving as a moderator of stress-related depressive symptoms: A prospective analysis. *Journal of Counseling Psychology, 35,* 134–138.

Nezu, C. M., & Nezu, A. M. (1995). Clinical decision making in everyday practice: The science in the art. *Cognitive and Behavioral Practice, 2,* 5–25.

Nezu, C. M., Nezu, A. M., & Gill-Weiss, M. J. (1992). *Psychopathology of persons with mental retardation: Clinical guidelines for assessment and treatment.* Champaign, IL: Research Press.

Nichols, D. S. (1992). Review of the Minnesota Multiphasic Personality Inventory-2. In *Mental Measurement Yearbook* (pp. 562–565). Lincoln, NB: Buros Institute of Mental Measurement of the University of Nebraska-Lincoln.

O'Hara, M., Zekowski, E., Phillips, L., & Wright, E. (1990). Controlled prospective study of postpartum mood disorders: Comparison of childbearing and nonchildbearing women. *Journal of Abnormal Psychology, 99,* 3–15.

Ohrt, T., & Thorell, L. (1998). Dysfunctional Attitude Scale (DAS). Psychometrics and norms of the Swedish version. *Scandinavian Journal of Behaviour Therapy, 27,* 105–113.

O'Leary, K. D., & Beach, S. R. H. (1990). Marital therapy: A viable treatment for depression. *American Journal of Psychiatry, 147,* 183–186.

Oliver, J. M., & Baumgart, E. P. (1985). The Dysfunctional Attitude Scale: Psychometric properties and relation to depression in an unselected adult population. *Cognitive Therapy and Research, 9,* 161–167.

Osman, A., Gifford, J., Jones, T., Lickiss, L., Osman, J., & Wenzel, R. (1993). Psychometric evaluation of the Reasons for Living Inventory. *Psychological Assessment, 5,* 154–158.

Osman, A., Gregg C. L., Osman, J. R., & Jones, K. (1992). Factor structure and reliability of the Reasons for Living Inventory. *Psychological Reports, 70,* 107–112.

Overall, J. E., & Gorham, D. R. (1962). The Brief Psychiatric Rating Scale. *Psychological Reports, 10,* 799–812.

Overall, J. E., & Klett, C. J. (1972). *Applied multivariate analysis.* New York: McGraw-Hill.

Parkes, C. M. (1972). *Bereavement: Studies of grief in adult life.* New York: International Universities Press.

Paykel, E. S., Weissman, M. M., & Prusoff, B. A. (1978). Social maladjustment and severity of depression. *Comprehensive Psychiatry, 19,* 121–128.

Puig-Antich, J., & Chambers, W. (1978). *The Schedule for Affective Disorders and Schizophrenia for school aged children.* Unpublished interview schedule, New York State Psychiatric Institute, New York.

Raskin, A. (1988). Three-area severity of depression scales. In M. Hersen & A. S. Bellack (Eds.), *Dictionary of Behavioral Assessment Techniques* (pp. 476–477). Oxford, England: Pergamon Press.

Rehm, L. P. (1977). A self-control model of depression. *Behavior Therapy, 8,* 787–804.

Rehm, L. P., Fuchs, C. Z., Roth, D. M., Kornblith, S. J., & Romano, J. M. (1979). A comparison of self-control and assertion skills treatments of depression. *Behavior Therapy, 10,* 429–442.

Rehm, L. P., Kornblith, S. J., O'Hara, M. W., Lamparski, D. M., Romano, J. M., & Volkin, J. I. (1981). An evaluation of major components in a self-control behavior therapy program for depression. *Behavior Modification, 5,* 459–490.

Reivich, K. (1995). The measurement of explanatory style. In G. M. Buchanan & M. E. P. Seligman (Eds.), *Explanatory style* (pp. 21–47). Hillsdale, NJ: Erlbaum.

Reynolds, W. M., & Coats, K. I. (1986). A comparison of cognitive-behavioral therapy and relaxation training for the treatment of depression in adolescents. *Journal of Consulting and Clinical Psychology, 54,* 653–660.

Robins, L. N., Helzer, J. E., Croughan, J., & Ratcliff, K. S. (1981). National Institute of Mental Health Diagnostic Interview Schedule. *Archives of General Psychiatry, 38,* 381–389.

Robinson, L. A., Berman, J. S., & Neimeyer, R. A. (1990). Psychotherapy for the treatment of depression: A comprehensive review of controlled outcome research. *Psychological Bulletin, 108,* 30–49.

Rosen, A., & Proctor, E. K. (1981). Distinctions between treatment outcomes and their implications for treatment evaluation. *Journal of Consulting and Clinical Psychology, 49,* 418–425.

Rosenbaum, M., & Rolnick, A. (1983). Self-control behaviors and coping with seasickness. *Cognitive Therapy and Research, 7,* 93–97.

Roth, D., Bielski, R., Jones, J., Parker, W., & Osborn, G. (1982). A comparison of self-control therapy and combined self-control therapy and antidepressant medication in the treatment of depression. *Behavior Therapy, 13,* 133–144.

Roth, D., & Rehm, L. P. (1980). Relationships between self-monitoring processes, memory and depression. *Psychological Reports, 47,* 3–7.

Rotter, J. B. (1966). Generalized expectancies for internal versus external control of reinforcement. *Psychological Monographs: General and Applied, 80* (1, Whole No. 609).

Rozensky, R. H., Rehm, L. P., Pry, G., & Roth, G. (1977). Depression and self-reinforcement behavior in hospitalized patients. *Journal of Behavior Therapy and Experimental Psychiatry, 8,* 31–34.

Rule, B. G., Harvey, H. Z., & Dobbs, A. R. (1989). Reliability of the Geriatric Depression Scale for Younger Adults. *Clinical Gerontologist, 9,* 37–43.

Rush, A. J., Giles, D. E., Schlesser, M. A., Fulton, C. L., Weissenburger, J., & Burns, C. (1986). The Inventory for Depressive Symptomatology (IDS): Preliminary findings. *Psychiatry Research, 18,* 65–87.

Russell, D., Peplau, L., & Cutrona, C. (1980). The Revised UCLA Loneliness Scale: Concurrent and discriminant validity evidence. *Journal of Personality and Social Psychology, 39,* 472–480.

Russo, J. (1994). Thurstone's scaling model applied to the assessment of self-reported depressive severity. *Psychological Assessment, 6,* 159–171.

Sadowski, C., Moore, L. A., and Kelly, M. L. (1994). Psychometric properties of the Social Problem-Solving Inventory (SPSI) with normal and emotionally-disturbed adolescents. *Journal of Abnormal Child Psychology, 22,* 487–500.

Safran, J., Segal, Z., Hill, C., & Whiffin, V. (1990). Refining strategies for research on self-representations in emotional disorders. *Cognitive Therapy and Research, 14,* 143–160.

Sahin, N., Sahin, N. H., & Heppner, P. P. (1993). Psychometric properties of the Problem Solving Inventory in a group of Turkish university students. *Cognitive Therapy and Research, 17,* 379–396.

Sanders, C. M., Mauger, P. A., & Strong, P. N. (1979). *A manual for the Grief Experience Inventory.* Unpublished manuscript.

Schotte, D. E., & Clum, G. A. (1982). Suicide ideation in a college population: A test of a model. *Journal of Consulting and Clinical Psychology, 50,* 690–696.

Schotte, D. E., & Clum, G. A. (1987). Problem-solving skills in suicidal psychiatric patients. *Journal of Consulting and Clinical Psychology, 55,* 49–54.

Schulman, P., Seligman, M. E. P., & Amsterdam, D. (1987). The Attributional Style Questionnaire is not transparent. *Behaviour Research and Therapy, 25,* 391–395.

Schwab, J., Bialon, M. R., & Holzer, C. E. (1967). A comparison of two rating scales for depression. *Journal of Clinical Psychology, 23,* 94–96.

Schwartz, R. M., & Garamoni, G. L. (1989). Cognitive balance and psychopathology: Evaluation of an information processing model of positive and negative states of mind. *Clinical Psychology Review, 9,* 271–294.

Seligman, M. E. P., Peterson, C., Kaslow, N. J., Tannenbaum, R. L., Alloy, L. B., & Abramson, L. Y. (1984). Explanatory style and depressive symptoms among school children. *Journal of Abnormal Psychology, 93,* 235–238.

Simons, A. D., Lustman, P. J., Wetzel, R. D., & Murphy, G. E. (1985). Predicting response to cognitive therapy of depression: The role of learned resourcefulness. *Cognitive Therapy and Research, 9,* 79–89.

Skinner, B. F. (1953). *The science of human behavior.* New York: Free Press.

Smouse, P. E., Feinberg, M., Carroll, B. J., Myoung, H. P., & Rawson, S. G. (1981). The Carroll Rating Scale for Depression: II. Factor analyses of the feature profile. *British Journal of Psychiatry, 138,* 201–204.

Spielberger, C. D. (1983). *State-Trait Anxiety Inventory.* Redwood City, CA: Mind Garden.

Spielberger, C. D., Gorsuch, R. L., & Lushene, R. E. (1970). *Manual for the State-Trait Anxiety Inventory.* Palo Alto, CA: Consulting Psychologists Press.

Spitzer, R. L., Endicott, J., & Robins, E. (1978). *Research diagnostic criteria for a selected group of functional disorders.* New York: Biometric Research Unit, New York Psychiatric Institute.

Spitzer, R. L., Williams, J. B. W., Kroenke, K., Linzer, M., deGruy III, F. V., Hahn, S. R., Brody, D., & Johnson, J. G.

(1994). Utility of a new procedure for diagnosing mental disorders in primary care: The PRIME-MD Study. *Journal of the American Medical Association, 272,* 1749–1756.

Stark, K. D., Reynolds, W. M., & Kaslow, N. J. (1987). A comparison of the relative efficacy of self-control therapy and behavioral problem-solving therapy for depression in children. *Journal of Abnormal Child Psychology, 15,* 91–113.

Steinmetz, J. L., Lewinsohn, P. M., & Antonuccio, D. O. (1983). Prediction of individual outcome in a group intervention for depression. *Journal of Consulting and Clinical Psychology, 51,* 331–337.

Strauman, T. J., & Wetzler, S. (1992). The factor structure of the SCL-90-R and MCMI scale scores: Within-measure and inter-battery analysis. *Multivariate Behavioral Research, 27,* 1–20.

Sullivan, H. S. (1953). *The interpersonal theory of psychiatry.* New York: Norton.

Sutter, J. (1990). *L'anticipation psychologie et psychopathologie.* Paris: Presses Universitaires de France.

Sutter, J., & Berta, A. M. (1991). *L'anticipation et ses applications cliniques.* Paris: Presses Universitaires de France.

Swan, G. E., & MacDonald, M. L. (1978). Behavior therapy in practice: A national survey of behavior therapists. *Behavior Therapy, 9,* 799–807.

Swindle, R. W. Jr., Heller, K., & Lakey, B. (1988). A conceptual reorientation to the study of personality and stressful life events. In L. H. Cohen (Ed.), *Life events and psychological functioning: Theoretical and methodological issues* (pp. 237–268). Beverly Hills, CA: Sage.

Tanaka-Matsumi, J., Seiden, D. Y., & Lam, K. N. (1996). The Culturally-Informed Functional Assessment (CIFA) interview: A strategy for cross-cultural behavioral practice. *Cognitive and Behavioral Practice, 3,* 215–234.

Taylor, S. E., Lichtman, R. R., & Wood, J. V. (1984). Attributions, beliefs about control and adjustment to breast cancer. *Journal of Personality and Social Psychology, 46,* 489–502.

Teri, L., & Lewinsohn, P. (1982). Modification of the Pleasant and Unpleasant Events Schedules for use with the elderly. *Journal of Consulting and Clinical Psychology, 50,* 444–445.

Teri, L., Logsdon, R. G., Uomoto, J., & McCurry, S. M. (1997). Treatment of depression in dementia patients: A controlled clinical trial. *The Journals of Gerontology: Psychological Sciences, 52,* 150–166.

Thompson, M., Kaslow, N. J., Weiss, B., & Nolen-Hoeksema, S. (1998). Children's Attributional Style Questionnaire-Revised: Psychometric examination. *Psychological Assessment, 10,* 166–170.

Tondo, L., Burras, C., Scamonatti, L., Weissenberger, J., & Rush, J. (1988). Comparison between clinician-related and self-reported depressive symptoms in Italian psychiatric patients. *Neuropsychobiology, 19,* 1–5.

Topol, P., & Reznikoff, M. (1982). Perceived peer and family relationships, hopelessness and locus of control as factors in adolescent suicide attempts. *Suicide and Life-Threatening Behavior, 12,* 141–150.

Tucker, M. A., Ogle, S. J., Davison, J. G., & Eilenberg, M. D. (1986). Development of a brief screening test for depression in the elderly. *Journal of Clinical and Experimental Gerontology, 8,* 173–190.

Tyron, W. W. (1996). Nocturnal activity and sleep assessment. *Clinical Psychology Review, 16,* 197–213.

Tyron, W. W., & Pinto, L. P. (1994). Comparing activity level measurements and ratings. *Behavior Modification, 18,* 251–261.

Vlissides, D. N., & Jenner, F. A. (1982). The response of endogenously and reactively depressed patients to electroconvulsive therapy. *British Journal of Psychiatry, 141,* 239–242.

Wagner, M. K., Holden, E. W., & Jannarone, R. J. (1988). Factor structure of the Heiby Self-Reinforcement Questionnaire. *Journal of Clinical Psychology, 44,* 198–202.

Watson, D., & Friend, R. (1969). Measurement of social-evaluative anxiety. *Journal of Consulting and Clinical Psychology, 33,* 448–457.

Watson, D., & Tellegen, A. (1985). Toward a consensual structure of mood. *Psychological Bulletin, 98,* 219–235.

Weiss, B., & Garber, J. (1995). *The Vanderbilt Depression Inventory: A self-report inventory of depressive symptoms for developmental comparisons.* Unpublished manuscript, Vanderbilt University, Nashville, TN.

Weissman, M. M. (1987). Advances in psychiatric epidemiology: Rates and risks for major depression. *American Journal of Public Health, 77,* 445–451.

Weissman, M. M., & Paykel, E. S. (1974). *The depressed woman: A study of social relationships.* Chicago: University of Chicago Press.

Weissman, M. M., Prusoff, B., & Newberry, P. B. (1975). *Comparison of CES-D, Zung, Beck self-report depression scales* (Tech. Report No. ADM 42-47-83). Rockville, MD: Center for Epidemiology Studies, National Institute of Mental Health.

Weissman, M. M., Sholomskas, D., Pottenger, M., Prusoff, B. A., & Locke, B. Z. (1977). Assessing depressive symptoms in five psychiatric populations: A validation study. *American Journal of Epidemiology, 106,* 203–214.

Wells, K. B., Burnam, M. A., Leake, B., & Robins, L. N. (1988). Agreement between face-to-face and telephone-administered versions of the depression section of the NIMH Diagnostic Interview Schedule. *Journal of Psychiatric Research, 22,* 207–220.

Westefeld, J. S., Badura, A., Kiel, J. T., & Scheel, K. (1996). The College Student Reasons for Living Inventory: Additional psychometric data. *Journal of College Student Development, 37,* 348–350.

Whitley, B. E. (1991). A short form of the Expanded Attributional Style Questionnaire. *Journal of Personality Assessment, 56,* 365–369.

Wierzbicki, M., & Bartlett, T. S. (1987). The efficacy of group and individual cognitive therapy for mild depression. *Cognitive Therapy and Research, 11,* 337–342.

Wilkinson, R. B. (1997). Interactions between self and external reinforcement in predicting depressive symptoms. *Behaviour Research and Therapy, 35,* 281–289.

Williams, J. B., Gibbon, M., First, M. B., Spitzer, R. L., Davies, M., Borus, J., Howes, M. J., Kane, J., Pope, H. G., Rounsaville, B., & Wittchen, H. U. (1992). The Structured Clinical Interview for DSM-III-R (SCID): II. Multisite test-retest reliability. *Archives of General Psychiatry, 49,* 630–636.

Wing, J. K., Birley, J., Cooper, J., Graham, P., & Issacs, A. (1967). Reliability of a procedure for measuring and classifying "present psychiatric state." *British Journal of Psychiatry, 113,* 499–515.

World Health Organization. (1992). *The ICD-10 classification of mental and behavioural disorders: Clinical description and diagnostic guidelines.* Geneva: Author.

Wylie, R. (1989). *Measures of self-concept.* Lincoln, NE: University of Nebraska Press.

Youngren, M. A., & Lewinsohn, P. M. (1980). The functional relation between depression and problematic interpersonal behavior. *Journal of Abnormal Behavior, 89,* 333–341.

Zemore, R. (1983). Development of a self-report measure of depression proneness. *Psychological Reports, 52,* 211–216.

Zemore, R., & Dell, L. D. (1983). Interpersonal problem-solving skills and depression-proneness. *Personality and Social Psychology Bulletin, 9,* 231–235.

Zemore, R., & Rinholm, J. (1989). Vulnerability to depression as a function of parental rejection and control. *Canadian Journal of Behavioural Science, 21,* 364–376.

Zemore, R., & Veikle, G. (1989). Cognitive styles and proneness to depressive symptoms in university women. *Personality and Social Psychology Bulletin, 15,* 426–438.

Zimmerman, M., Coryell, W., Pfohl, B., & Stangl, D. (1987). An American validation of the Newcastle Diagnostic Scale: II. Relationship with clinical, demographic, familial and psychosocial features. *British Journal of Psychiatry, 150,* 526–532.

Zimmerman, M., Pfohl, B., Stangl, D., & Coryell, W. (1986). An American validation of the Newcastle Diagnostic Scale: I. Relationship with the dexamethasone suppression test. *British Journal of Psychiatry, 149,* 627–630.

Zuckerman, M., & Lubin, B. (1965). *Multiple Affect Adjective Checklist (MAACL).* San Diego, CA: EdITS/Educational and Industrial Testing Service.

Author Index

Abrams, R. C., 133, 134
Abramson, L. Y., 61, 169, 170, 180
Addington, D., 12, 124, 125, 126
Addington, J., 12, 124, 125, 126
Adey, M., 137, 139
Ahnberg, J. L., 30
Aiken, L. S., v
Alexander, C., 225, 260
Alexopoulos, G. S., 133, 134
Alloy, L. B., 61
Ambrosini, P., 140
American Psychiatric Association
    (APA), 9, 10, 53, 54, 109, 140,
    294, 311, 316, 328
Amsterdam, D., 171
Anan, R. M., 209
Andersen, J., 87, 88, 89
Anderson, C. B., 238
Anderson, K. W., 191
Anderson, R., 250, 251
Anderson, W. P., 14
Anthony, J. C., 149
Antonuccio, D. O., 13, 241
Antony, M. M., 44
APA: see American Psychiatric Association (APA)
Archer, R. P., 75
Arean, P. A., 15
Arkes, H. R., 17
Arruda, J. E., 158
Asarnow, R. F., 14
Asberg, M., 75, 77
Atkinson, M., 126

Badura, A., 235
Bagby, R. M., 171
Baldree, B. F., 229
Barber, J. P., 265, 267
Barlow, D. H., 44
Bartlett, T. S., 49
Basco, M. R., 66, 67

Bathelemy, K. J., 207, 209
Baumgart, E. P., 213
Beach, S. R. H., 15
Bech, P., 87, 88, 89
Beck, A. T., 175, 212, 255
    1961, 12, 29
    1967, 168, 175, 183, 186, 187,
        188, 190, 210, 212, 230
    1975, 175
    1976, 15
    1979, 15, 30, 177–179, 189
    1983, 253, 254
    1987, 253, 267
    1988, 30, 175
    1990, 44
    1991, 177, 213
    1996, 30
    in press, 252, 253, 254
Beck, J. S., 11
Beck, R., 175
Becker, R. E., 13
Beckham, E. E., 3, 189, 280
Bellack, A. S., 13, 98
Bellanti, C. J., 171
Bergbower, K., 172
Bergman, E., 175
Berman, J. S., 16
Berndt, D. J., 84, 86, 145
Berta, A. M., 168
Bertolotti, G., 45, 46
Bialon, M. R., 60
Bieling, P. J., 44, 252, 253, 254
Bielski, R., 14
Biggs, J. T., 121
Biglan, A., 220
Birley, J., 125
Birmaher, B., 140, 141, 142
Blashki, T. G., 37
Bliss, J., 65
Bojholm, S., 87, 88, 89
Bolwig, T. G., 87, 88, 89

Bond, A., 149
Borus, J. F., 93, 116
Boyd, J. H., 149
Boyer, J. L., 189, 280
Bradburn, N. M., 41
Breckenridge, J., 13, 241
Brent, D., 140, 141, 142
Brewer, D. H., 159
Brody, D., 92, 93
Brophy, C. J., 119
Brown, G., 213, 267
Brown, G. K., 29, 30, 252, 253,
    254
Brown, R. A., 13
Brown, T. A., 44
Burke, J. D., 149
Burnam, M. A., 78, 80
Burns, C., 67
Burras, C., 68
Bush, C., 242
Butcher, J. N., 73
Butler, C., 209

Campbell, E. A., 149
Campbell, S. B., 111, 147, 149
Carey, M. P., 159
Carney, M. W. P., 87, 88
Carroll, B. J., 37, 38, 67
Cattel, R. B., 242
Chambers, W., 140, 141
Chang, C. H., 75
Chapman, J., 221
Chassin, L., 243
Chevron, E., 15, 16
Chiles, J. A., 233, 234, 235
Choquette, K. A., 119
Chorpita, B. F., 44
Christopher, F., 15
Cicchetti, D. V., 213
Clark, A., 119
Clark, D. A., 255

Clark, L. A., 89
Clarke, G. N., 225
Clemmensen, L., 87, 88, 89
Clum, G. A., 231
Coats, K.I., 154
Cohen-Mansfield, J., 135, 290
Cohn, J. F., 111, 147, 149
Cone, J. D., 18, 23
Cook, H., 238
Cook, J. B., 189, 280
Cooper, J., 125
Cooper, P. J., 149
Cordy, N. I., 149
Coryell, W., 88, 89
Courey, L., 242
Covi, L., 91, 118
Cox, B. J., 44
Coyne, J. C., 203
Cronkite, R. C., 192, 195, 197, 263
Croughan, J. L., 49, 52
Crowne, D. P., 193
Cull, J. G., 234, 258
Cutrona, C., 244

Dahlstrom, W. G., 73
Davies, M., 116, 140
Davison, J. G., 122
Dawes, R. M., 17
Day, A., 149
deGruy III, F. V., 92, 93
DeJonghe, F., 71, 72
Delaune, K., 238
Dell, L. D., 206
Dempsey, P., 47, 49
Derogatis, L. R., 34, 91, 117, 118
DeRubeis, R. J., 265, 267
Devins, N. P., 93
Dobbs, A. R., 139
Dobson, D. J., 14
Dobson, K. S., 14, 15, 16, 30
Doctora, J. D., 172
Dohrenwend, B. P., 41
Dohrenwend, B. S., 41
Dozis, D. J. A., 30
Drew, J. B., 209
Droppleman, L. F., 94
Dykema, J., 172
Dykman, B. M., 216, 219
D'Zurilla, T. J., 14, 241, 248, 249

Eber, H. W., 242
Egloff, B., 92
Eidelson, J. I., 267
Eilenberg, M. D., 122
Elliot, R., v
Elwood, R. W., 75
Emery, G., 15, 30, 189, 254
Endicott, J., 108, 110, 173

Endler, N. S., 192, 193, 194
Enns, M. W., 44
Epstein, N., 254
Erbaugh, J., 12, 29
Esveldt-Dawson, K., 175
Evans, I., 18, 20

Faddis, S., 95, 250
Fahs, H., 49
Feighner, J. P., 9
Feinberg, M., 37, 38, 67
Ferster, C. B., 12
Feuerstein, M., 242
Fielding, J. M., 37
Fine, M. A., 207, 209
First, M. B., 114, 116
Fischer, D. G., 204, 206, 288
Fiszbein, A., 126
Fitzgerald, R. G., 15
Fleiss, J. L., 246
Flynn, C., 140, 141, 142
Foley, S. H., 15
Foliart, R., 143
Folkman, S., 262, 263, 264
Frank, J. D., 246
Frankel, M. J., 242
Frankl, V. E., 233
French, N. H., 175
Friedman, M. J., 119
Friedman, S. H., 20, 95, 250
Friend, R., 230
Frost, F., 143
Fruzzetti, A. E., 15
Fuchs, C. Z., 14
Fullerton, D. T., 49
Fulton, C. L., 67

Garamoni, G. L., 172, 230
Garber, J., 181
Garbin, M. G., 30
Garratt, L. S., 204, 206, 288
Garside, R. F., 87
Gath, D. H., 15
George, L. K., 214
Gibbon, M., 114, 116
Gifford, J., 234, 235
Giles, D. E., 67
Gill, W. S., 234, 258
Gill-Weiss, M. J., 21, 150, 151
Gjerris, A., 87, 88, 89
Gladstone, T. R. G., 171
Goldfried, M. R., 249
Goodman-Brown, T., 243
Goodstein, J. L., 233, 234, 235
Gorham, D. R., 32, 34
Gorman, C., 65
Gorsuch, R. L., 39, 91, 230
Gotlib, I. H., 3, 13, 14, 15, 149, 210

Graf, M., 226
Graham, J. R., 73, 75
Graham, P., 125
Greden, J. F., 37, 38, 67
Greer, S., 65
Gregg, C. L., 234
Griffin, N., 243
Grosscup, S. J., 224, 261
Guarino, J., 228, 229
Gullion, C. M., 66, 67
Gunderson, J. G., 208
Gurland, B. J., 246
Guze, S. B., 9

Hahn, S. R., 92, 93
Hakstian, A. R., 13
Hamilton, M., 58, 59, 60, 66
Hammen, C. L., 3, 182, 184, 187, 210, 243
Hammer, A. L., 194
Harrell, T. H., 173
Harrison, R. P., 254
Harvey, H. Z., 139
Haskell, D. H., 95
Hathaway, S. R., 74
Hayes, J. A., 35
Haynes, S. N., 20
Hays, R. C., 172, 173, 277
Hedlund, J. L., 33, 59, 60, 100, 103
Heersema, P. H., 139
Heiby, E. M., 214, 216
Heimberg, R. G., 13
Heller, K., 210
Helzer, J. E., 49, 52
Heppner, P. P., 14, 230, 233
Hersen, M., 13, 98
Hill, C., 243
Himmelhoch, J., 13
Hirsch, M., 140
Hirschfeld, R. M. A., 208
Hoberman, H. M., 13
Holden, E. W., 215
Holden, N. L., 88
Hollon, S. D., 16, 173, 266
Holzer, C. E., 149
Hoover, C. F., 15
Houts, P. S., 95, 250
Howard, B. L., 172, 173, 277
Howes, M. J., 93, 116
Hozer, C. E., 60
Huang, V., 137
Huprich, S. K., 207, 208, 209
Hussian, R. A., 15
Huyser, J., 71, 72

Ingram, R. E., 228, 229, 230
Issacs, A., 125
Ivanoff, A., 235

Jacobs, K. W., 122
Jacobson, N. S., 15
Jang, S. J., 235
Jannarone, R. J., 215
Jarrett, R. B., 66, 67
Jenner, F. A., 88
Johnson, J. G., 93
Joiner, T. E., 61
Jolly, J. B., 228
Jones, J., 14
Jones, K., 234
Jones, R. G., 242
Jones, T., 234, 235
Jonkers, F., 71, 72
Joseph, T. X., 15
Joshi-Peters, K. L., 216
Joyce, J., 12, 125

Kaemmer, B., 73
Kahnemann, D., 17
Kaiser, C. F., 145
Kalmar, K., 14
Kane, J., 116
Kanfer, F. H., 13
Kaslow, N. J., 156, 171, 172, 179
Kastrup, M., 87, 88, 89
Kaufman, J., 140, 141, 142
Kay, S. R., 126
Kazdin, A. E., 151, 175
Keller, M. B., 10
Kelly, M. L., 250
Keltikangas-Järvinen, L., 106, 108, 320
Kendall, P. C., 172, 173, 228, 229, 277
Kennerly, H., 149
Kerner, S. A., 122
Kiel, J. T., 235
Kiluk, D. J., 119
Klerman, G. L., 16
Kobak, K. A., 55, 104
Koenig, H. G., 214
Kohlmann, C. W., 92
Kornblith, S. J., 14, 238
Korotitsch, W., 44
Kovacs, M., 127, 128, 175, 178
Kramer, M., 149
Krampt, P., 87, 88, 89
Krantz, S., 182, 184, 187
Kriss, M. R., 266
Kroenke, K., 92, 93
Krohne, H. W., 92
Krug, S. E., 69
Kurokawa, N. K., 194

Lakey, B., 209, 210
Lam, K. N., 21
Lamparski, D. M., 238

Landsverk, J., 78
Langford, R., 221
Langhinrichsen-Rohling, J., 221
Larsen, R. M., 74
Laughlin, J. E., 69
Lawrence, P. S., 15
Lazarus, R. S., 262, 263
Leaf, P. J., 149
Leake, B., 78, 80
Leber, W. R., 3, 189, 280
Lee, Y. T., 172
Lefebvre, M. F., 185, 186
Legendre, S. A., 158
Légeron, P., 167, 169
Leirer, V. O., 137
Lev, E., 235, 237, 318
Levitan, R. D., 171
Lewinsohn, P. M., 187, 219, 223, 225, 226
   1972, 224
   1973, 13, 226
   1974, 12, 214, 224, 261
   1976, 220
   1979, 224, 226, 261
   1982, 262
   1983, 13, 260
   1984, 13
   1987, 13, 241
   1995, 221
Lewinsohn, P. S., 13
Liberman, R. P., 32, 34
Libet, J., 13, 224
Lichtman, R. R., 95
Lickiss, L., 234, 235
Linehan, M. M., 233, 234, 235
Linzer, M., 92, 93
Lipman, R. S., 91, 118
Livingston, W. W., 93
Lloyd-Thomas, A. R., 15
Locke, B. Z., 41, 93
Logsdon, R. G., 226, 227
Lohrenz, F. N., 49
Loosen, P. T., 16
Lorr, M., 94
Lovibond, P. F., 42, 43
Lovibond, S. H., 42
Lubin, B., 74, 81, 111, 112, 159
Lukoff, D., 32, 34
Lum, O., 137, 139
Lumry, A., 173
Lushene, R. E., 39, 91, 230
Lustman, P. J., 241

MacDonald, M .L., v
MacPhillamy, D. J., 223, 225, 260
Manderscheid, R. W., 93
Marboutin, J.-P., 167, 169
Marchione, N., 171

Margrett, J., 207, 209
Markowitz, J. C., 16
Marlowe, D., 193
Marx, M. S., 135
Matarazzo, J. D., 74
Maticka-Tyndale, E., 12, 124, 125
Matson, J. L., 150, 151
Mauger, P. A., 236
Maydeu-Olivares, A., 248
McClure, K. S., vii, 3, 12
McCorkle, R., 235, 237
McCurry, S. M., 227
McFarlane, M., 250
McKeon, J. J., 96
McKinley, J. C., 74
McLaughlin, S. C., 228, 229
McLean, P., 13
McNair, D. M., 94, 95
Mendelson, M., 12, 29
Merbaum, M., 242
Mermelstein, R., 260
Merten, T., 39
Metalsky, G. I., 61, 169
Metha, P. D., 238
Michelson, L. K., 171
Michielin, P., 45, 46
Miller, C., 204, 206, 288
Milne, K., 149
Minkoff, K., 175
Mock, J., 12, 29
Mokros, H. B., 129
Montgomery, S. A., 75, 77
Moore, L. A., 250
Moorey, S., 65
Moos, R. H., 192, 195, 196, 197, 263
Moras, K., 199
Moreci, P., 140, 141, 142
Morrow-Bradley, C., v
Mount, J. H., 149
Muñoz, R., 9
Muñoz, R. F., 187
Munro, B. H., 235, 237
Murphy, G. E., 241
Myers, J. K., 149
Mynors-Wallis, L. M., 15

Narrow, W. E., 93
Naughton, M., 250, 251
Neimeyer, R. A., 16
Nelson, L. D., 213
Nelson-Gray, R. O., 208
Newberry, P. B., 41
Newman, C., 199
Nezu, A. M., 18, 249
   1985, 14, 192, 195, 197, 231, 249, 263
   1986, 14, 232

Nezu, A. M. (*cont.*)
    1987, 14, 249
    1989, 3, 12, 14, 15, 17, 19, 23,
        241, 249
    1992, 21, 150, 151
    1993, 15, 17
    1996, 19
    1997, 20
    1998, vii, 3, 12, 95, 250
    in press, 248
Nezu, C. M.
    1986, 14
    1987, 14
    1989, 3, 12, 17, 19, 23, 249
    1992, 21, 150, 151
    1993, 17
    1995, 18
    1997, 20
    1998, vii, 3, 12, 95, 250
Nicholas, D. S., 75
Nielsen, S. L., 233, 234, 235
Nolan-Hoeksema, S., 172, 179
Norvell, N. K., 119
Nuechterlein, K. H., 32, 34

Ogle, S. J., 122
O'Hara, M. W., 149, 238
Ohrt, T., 214
O'Leary, K. D., 15
Oliver, J. M., 213
Opler, L. A., 126
Orvaschel, H., 149
Osborn, G., 14
Osman, A., 234, 235
Osman, J. R., 234, 235
Overall, J. E., 32, 34
Overholser, J. C., 243
Overholser, S. J., 143

Paez, P., 140
Parker, J. D. A., 192, 194
Parker, W., 14
Parkes, C. M., 236
Paykel, E. S., 220, 245, 247
Peplau, L., 244
Perri, M. G., 14, 15, 232, 249
Perris, C., 77
Petersen, C. H., 230
Peterson, C., 169, 172
Pfohl, B., 88, 89
Phillips, K. A., 208
Phillips, L., 149
Pinto, L. P., 166
Pope, H. G., 116
Pottenger, M., 41
Poznanski, E. O., 129
Proctor, E. K., 19
Prusoff, B. A., 41, 245, 247

Pry, G., 14
Pugatch, D., 95
Puig-Antich, J., 140, 141

Radloff, L. S., 39, 41
Rae, D. S., 93
Rafaelsen, O. J., 87, 88, 89
Rao, U., 140, 141, 142
Rapp, S. R., 250, 251
Raskin, A., 96
Ratcliff, K. S., 49, 52
Rawson, S. G., 37, 38, 67
Reatig, N., 96
Rector, N. A., 171
Rehm, L. P., 13, 14, 214, 238, 241
Reiger D. A., 93
Reivich, K., 171
Reno, R. R., v
Reynolds, W. M., 55, 104–105,
        152, 154, 156, 255, 256
Reznikoff, M., 176
Rickels, K., 91, 118
Rimon, R., 106, 320
Riskind II, J., 267
Riviére, B., 167, 169
Roberton, B., 65
Robins, C. J., 214
Robins, E., 9, 108, 110, 173
Robins, L. N., 49, 52, 80
Robinson, L. A., 13, 16
Rochat, C., 167, 169
Rohde, P., 221
Rolnick, A., 242
Romano, J. M., 14, 238
Ronan, G. F., 14, 192, 195, 197,
        231, 249, 263
Rose, T. L., 137, 139
Rosen, A., 19
Rosenbaum, M., 240, 242
Rosenberg, R., 93
Ross, L., 255
Roth, D., 13, 14
Roth, M., 87
Rotter, J. B., 242
Rounsaville, B. J., 15, 16, 116
Rowden, L., 65
Rozensky, R. H., 14
Rule, B. G., 139
Rush, A. J., 15, 30, 66, 67, 68, 189,
        307
Russell, D., 244
Russo, J., 49
Ryan, N., 140, 141, 142
Ryon, N. B., 173

Saccuzzo, D., 229
Sadowski, C., 250
Safran, J., 243

Sahin, N., 233
Sahin, N. H., 233
Salusky, S., 15
Sanavio, E., 45, 46
Sanders, C. M., 236
Saraydarian, L., 14
Scamonatti, L., 68
Schalken, H. F. A., 71, 72
Schalling, D., 77
Scheel, K., 235
Schein, R. L., 15
Schissel, B. A., 12
Schlesser, M. A., 67
Schmaling, K. B., 15
Schmidt, S., 250, 251
Schotte, D. E., 231
Schubert, D. S. P., 143
Schulman, P., 171
Schulterbrandt, J. G., 96
Schwab, J., 60
Schwartz, R. M., 172, 230
Schweizer, E., 199
Sechrest, L., v
Seeley, J. R., 221
Segal, Z., 243
Seiden, D. Y., 21
Seligman, M. E. P., 169, 170, 171,
        172, 180
Semmel, A., 169
Senatore, V., 151
Sevall, G., 77
Shamoian, C. A., 133, 134
Shapiro, R. W., 10
Shaw, B. F., 15, 30, 189
Sheffield, B. F., 87, 88
Shelton, R. C., 16
Sherick, R. B., 175
Sholomskas, D., 15, 41
Shumaker, S. A., 250, 251
Siebert, K., 39
Siegle, G., 228, 229
Simons, A. D., 241
Sirl, K., 209
Skidmore, J. R., 191
Skinner, B. F., 12
Smouse, P. E., 37, 38, 67
Smyth, N. J., 235
Snaith, R. P., 63, 64, 65
Society of Biological Psychiatry,
        282
Spielberger, C. D., 39, 91, 230, 250
Spitzer, R. L., 92, 93, 108, 110,
        114, 116, 173
Stangl, D., 88, 89, 214
Stark, K. D., 156
Steer, R. A., 29, 30, 213, 255
    1987, 267
    1988, 175

Steer, R. A. (*cont.*)
  1990, 44
  1991, 177, 213
Steinmetz, J. L., 13
Stern, R. A., 157, 158
Stern, S. L., 213
Stolzman, R., 149
Stone, A. R., 246
Stoppard, J. M., 202, 203, 286
Strauman, T. J., 119
Strong, P. N., 236
Sullivan, H. S., 16
Sutter, J., 168
Swan, G. E., v
Swindle, R. W. Jr., 210
Swinson, R. P., 44

Tabrizi, M. A., 140
Talkington, J., 226, 261
Tan, J. C. H., 202, 203, 204, 286
Tanaka-Matsumi, J., 21
Tatsuoka, M. M., 242
Tausch, A., 92
Taylor, S. E., 95
Teasdale, J. D., 170, 180
Tellegen, A., 73, 89, 90
Teri, L., 13, 225, 226, 227, 241, 262
Testa, S. M., 171
Thomlinson, D., 15
Thompson, M., 172, 179
Thorell, L., 214
Tilson, M., 13
Tischler, G. L., 149
Tondo, L., 68
Tonks, C. M., 245, 247
Topol, P., 176
Triebwasser, J., 208
Trivedi, M. H., 66, 67

Trunzo, J. J., vii, 3, 12
Tucker, M. A., 122
Tunmore, R., 65
Tversky, A., 17
Tweed, D. L., 214
Tyron, W. W., 165, 166, 167

Uhlenhuth, E. H., 91, 118
Unis, A. S., 175
Uomoto, J., 227

Veikle, G., 206
Vidotto, G., 45, 46
Vieweg, B. W., 33, 59, 60, 100, 103
Vlissides, D. N., 88
Volkin, J. I., 238
von Baeyer, C., 169

Wagner, A. L., 238
Wagner, M. K., 215
Ward, C. H., 12, 29
Warren, W. L., 99, 101
Waterhouse, J., 296
Watkins, J. T., 189, 280
Watson, D., 89, 90, 230
Watson, M., 65
Weed, N. S., 194
Weisner, D. C., 228
Weiss, B., 172, 179, 181
Weissenburger, J., 67, 68
Weissman, A. N., 175, 178, 212, 213
Weissman, M. M., 15, 16, 41, 220, 245, 247
Wells, K. B., 78, 80
Wenzel, F. J., 49
Wenzel, R., 234, 235
West, W. G., v
Westefeld, J. S., 235

Wetzel, R. D., 241
Wetzler, S., 119
Whiffen, V. E., 15, 149
Whiffin, V., 243
Whitley, B. E., 171
Wierzbicki, M., 49
Wilkinson, R. B., 216
Williams, J. B. W., 92, 93, 114, 116
Williams, R., 165, 166, 167
Willimson, D., 140, 141, 142
Wing, J. K., 125
Winokur, G., 9
Wisnicki, K. S., 228, 229, 230
Wittchen, H. U., 116
Wood, J. V., 95
Woodruff, R. A., 9
World Health Organization (WHO), 9
Wright, E., 149
Wylie, L. T., 121
Wylie, R., 243

Yesavage, J. A., 137, 139
Yorkston, N. J., 246
Young, R., 243
Young, R. C., 133, 134
Youngren, M. A., 219, 224, 261

Zeiss, A. M., 219, 220
Zekowski, E., 149
Zemore, R., 204, 206, 288
Ziegler, V. E., 121
Zigmond, A. S., 63, 64, 65
Zimmerman, M., 52, 88, 89
Zotti, A. M., 45, 46
Zuckerman, M., 81
Zung, W. W. K., 120